Comprehensive Community Health Nursing

Comprehensive Community Health Nursing

Cecy Correia
Nursing Tutor
Uday General School of Nursing
Cardinal Gracias Memorial Hospital
Sandor, Bangli, Vasai (W)
Thane, Maharashtra, India

Foreword
SA Pinto

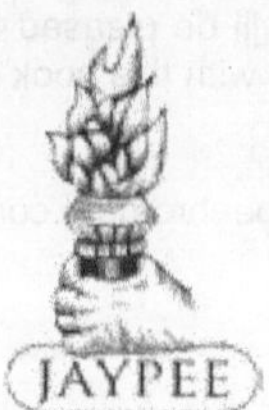

JAYPEE BROTHERS MEDICAL PUBLISHERS (P) LTD

New Delhi • London

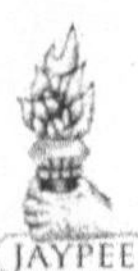

JAYPEE **Jaypee Brothers Medical Publishers (P) Ltd.**

Headquarters

EMCA House
23/23-B, Ansari Road, Daryaganj
New Delhi 110 002, India
Landline: +91-11-23272143,
+91-11-23272703+91-11-23282021,
+91-11-23245672
E-mail: jaypee@jaypeebrothers.com

Overseas Off ce
JP Medical Ltd.
83, Victoria Street, London
SW1H 0HW (UK)
Phone: +44-20 3170 8910
E-mail: info@jpmedpub.com

Corporate Office
Jaypee Brothers Medical Publishers (P) Ltd.
4838/24, Ansari Road, Daryaganj
New Delhi 110 002, India
Phone: +91-11-43574357
Fax: +91-11-43574314
E-mail: jaypee@jaypeebrothers.com

EU GPSR Authorised Representative
Logos Europe, 9 rue Nicolas Poussin
17000, La Rochelle, France
Phone: +33 (0) 6 67 93 73 78
E-mail: Contact@logoseurope.eu

Website: www.jaypeebrothers.com
Website: www.jaypeedigital.com

Inquiries for bulk sales may be solicited at: jaypee@jaypeebrothers.com

Comprehensive Community Health Nursing

First Edition: 2011

Reprint: **2025**

ISBN 978-93-5025-162-1

Printed in India

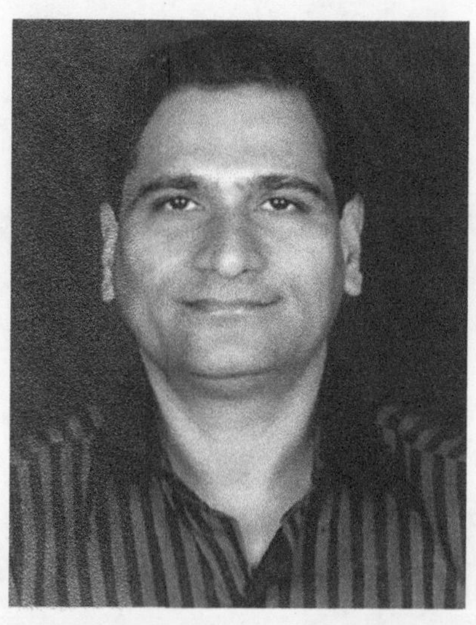

This book is gratefully and fondly dedicated to
my husband Mr Alois Macwan.
He made it possible for me to write this book
through his constant support and inspirations;
and the push I got from him;
otherwise, I would not have been able to write
without him accompanying me all through.
There is an invisible guiding hand behind this work.
That is God. I bow my head in prostration before him
for his guidance and invisible presence.

Foreword

I am indeed delighted to introduce a book titled *Comprehensive Community Health Nursing* by Cecy Correia, a renowned author and lecturer in community nursing. At the very onset itself let me congratulate Cecy Correia for having prepared such a wonderful book, which can be recognized by INC and MNC syllabus.

Cecy Correia has created a niche herself in the field of nursing education with her latest book *Comprehensive Community Health Nursing*. I am sure the response to this book will be no less and index will recommend it as a best book for school of nursing.

As a person associated with nursing education for the past few decades, I have come to realize more and more the vital information of community in the changing scenario of modern nursing profession.

Nurses today have to deal with a good number of communities knowing patients and health care professionals whether working within one's community or abroad. I have no doubt whatsoever that Cecy Correia is just the ideal tool to achieve these objectives.

This book is also great aid to medico-social workers, health and development project holders, voluntary health workers, and both postgraduates and undergraduates.

I hope this book will continue to serve not only the people of India, but also in allied subjects in the country.

My appreciation is extended to Jaypee Brothers Medical Publishers for the great care bestowed in publishing of this book. It will definitely make unique contribution to the world of medical literature available. All this is possible because you are mediator for this book.

SA Pinto
Principal
Uday General School of Nursing
Cardinal Gracias Memorial Hospital
Sandor, Bangli, Vasai (W)
Thane, Maharashtra, India

Preface

'Learned from the Ground' as NGO's point of view, I have worked and lived in the private organization for almost two decades working with grass root level rural poor where I was able to gather lots of experiences, which is treasureable and therefore like to share it through this book. For the students whom I am teaching the subjects on community health nursing: Part I and II, my experience was strengthened and it has benefited them in many ways and they insisted if I could put it into words, which will give them added knowledge on the subject.

As I was teaching and preparing my subject matter, I felt why not put it in to words, the unique way, which I have worked in community through a private organization with collaboration with Government agencies. I realized that I too have worked in rural grass root level for many years and the pattern of work I did and followed also could be put in to words that can help people who implement different integrated schemes and projects on developmental work. It can be good self-help for social workers, and get added knowledge for community health nurse. After all, NGOs, social workers, nurses, and Government agencies: all collaborate to work towards the betterment of people and their wholeness and wellness.

Community health includes first aid and small ailment treatment, home nursing, nutrition, environment, maternal and child health, communicable diseases control, school health, health information services, mobile health services, domiciliary health services, rural occupational health, elements of acupressure and herbal medicine, initiating developmental projects, community organization, innovative methods in health education, communication skills and home economics—which I have tried to integrate into this book. So this book intended to help and will contribute to a great extent to help nurses, voluntary health workers, village health guides, dais, paramedical workers, community health nurses, nursing school students and for library use; and all those who are interested in common man's development who lives in remote village.

It also deals with many useful topics on changing face of the youth, youth towards tomorrow, youth self discovery, old age, facing death courageously, palliative care, common infectious diseases, complimentary medicines, nutrition, supplementary food, balwadis, all-round development and education, women's health, skills and people's day-to-day living and much more; as you turn every chapter, there is something for all.

It is based on experience of living and working in close contacts with different groups of people who are elevated and lifted up on different levels. I have struggled with them in their pain and sickness; and felt one with them, accompanied and walked with them a few miles and felt close with solidarity living close to nature and tried to live their insecurity, and learnt to live for a day. Helped them in health education, mobile clinic, village visits, participated in their cultural activities, celebration, and worships, adopted their foods and got enriched in return. When these come back to my memory as a flash back, it gives me contentment for spending that prime climax of youth, that part of precious life with precious people who are simple yet can teach you the art of living. Without them, I could not be what I am today. So I owe all my credit to these simple rural village people and bow before them in humility and dedicate this book to them who still continue to struggle with difference even today and carry them still close to my heart. Therefore, I humbly salute them.

The importance of taking care of one's body is a top priority. Today, preventable diseases are taking a heavy toll of human life worldwide. Every system of human body is affected by scores of diseases. When we succeed in containing one disease, another raises its head. We have made wonderful advances in medical science—new vaccines, key hole surgery, laser beam in surgery, PET scan, gene therapy, etc., but we can ask ourselves: Are we more healthier than our ancestors who did not have knowledge of these new scientific technologies? In ancient times, people were healthy. Many studies of people who lived to a ripe old age showed that a balanced diet of healthy food, contented minds, unpolluted environment and a focus in life enabled them to enjoy good health till they died naturally at ripe old age.

Noncommunicable diseases are taking away thousands of lives. Majority of deaths are ascribed to coronary diseases, cerebrovascular diseases, diabetes and cancer. Infectious diseases caused by a causative agent can be fought by public health measures like safe water supply, environmental sanitation and immunization. Behavioral factors that are responsible for cerebrovascular diseases and cancer can be changed. They include smoking, excessive salt and sugar consumption, obesity, lack of exercises and stress.

Health is our most precious gift. Be wise to guard your health while you have it. As so many, by the way they live, that they are not diligent to preserve their bodies and eventually reap the unhappy result. 'An ounce of prevention is worth a pound of cure'. Nursing a person at home; treatment you can give like medicated steam inhalation, hot water bottle, and hot pack; handling an injured person, preventing wound infection; and handling common emergencies at home. As it is said in the *Vedas:* Man can live individually, but can survive only collectively.

I express my deep sense of indebtedness and gratitude to all the authors and publishers of articles in different newspapers, health magazines, and books from which references have been drawn while preparing my classes, that I have made use of in writing this book. The inspiration came essentially from people at grass root level with whom I lived and worked almost two decades and the community health nursing students whom I am teaching this subject have requested me to accept this challenging task of writing this book and their constant encouragement; and assistance as a teacher, I have also learnt a lot from them. Do not consider this book to be an ideal one but a humble attempt is made. This will give relevant information to all those who work in slums and in rural villages as well as public health point of view.

Hence, our challenge is to form a progressive community by balancing the interests of the individual and that of the society. When one eye weeps, can the other sleep? At the bottom of everything is the question: What is the meaning of personal and collective responsibilities? Does it mean responding to a situation of caring out a set of work without feelings and concern? What is needed is a human touch, touching the core, sensitivity towards the poor people's woes and helps them to come out from reasons of becoming numb and insensitive. There is no uniform pattern of change, but change is the only thing that is permanent, the rest everything is transitory.

The writing of this book came as an inspiration and was like a gush of fresh air. It gave me a clearer vision, hope and zest for life. Poor only are surviving, now we have to make them 'fully alive and fully human'. Teach them to live life in fullness. Make them realize fear is worthless, it gets reflected in perception of others; continuously ask yourself: Why am I doing this? What is my intention? Is my intention to prove my supremacy? What am I really doing? Am I helping the people at all? Am I really concerned about the people? Have I ever tried to understand the needs of people? Have I made any effort to know what they want? With the change of looking at self and at work should undergo change.

When the child runs away from home? When he does not feel at home in his own home! I would like to say that I have found purpose in life; I have learnt to live life fully. A little intervention will help them to come out of that state of stagnation. A little change in one person's life will reflect in several changes. Isn't it worth giving them a chance to make life worthwhile? In social sector, what is the core of an organization? Is it concerned for the people or the image, efficiency and target achievement? While streamlining the administration, increasing efficiency, are we not taking the risk of losing our direction? There will be a target and our aim and efforts will be to fulfil, the target. When we are preoccupied with the needs like meeting the deadlines, maintaining the name and reputation, keeping up the image, the goal of reaching the people will take a back seat. In the process of working for development, factors like care and concern have become dormant and needs like name, fame, image, recognition and money have come to the forefront. They become so dominant that they start dictating terms. Are we not placing what is convenient above what is necessary? Our aim is to work for the people with care and concern, to treat them equally, to be people oriented, sensitive and humane to address the issues of poverty, socioeconomic injustice, which is human oriented rather than profit oriented. Work should not become monotonous and a conclusion.

We are running for image status, which leads to impression of management, are we being honest with the needy and ourselves when we say we are doing for the benefit of the poor? Can we claim that our intensions are clear? Preoccupation of money, recognition, image which leads to take a break and ponder over where do we stand? What is development all about? Development is the key word around which the nongovernment agencies weave their activities like working for the poor, downtrodden, oppressed, and marginalized.

Where do we end up? In case we have lost our purpose, let us search where we have lost it, individual dream has become the dream of the community. The process of helping a group or a community of people to grow is not an easy task when they are spread over a vast area. Intellectually, mentally and spiritually, women are equivalent to male and she can participate in every activity. "As long as we don't consider girls as natural as our body, our nation will be in dark eclipse" —*Mahatma Gandhi*. It is better to put out spark of fire rather than allowing it to spread and call the fire brigade later. Just as the color of a rainbow varies from one end to the other, the severity of disease varies. Write your own success story. Therefore, develop social consciousness among the masses. Intensify publicity, campaigns, enhancing child survivals, promotion of spacing methods.

Even though some books on community health are available, this book is unique and it will be an immense value to all those who work in social welfare programs and betterment of community.

Welfare cannot be assured without respect for the dignity of each person, all are born free and has equal right and dignity, and no one shall be tortured, degraded and thus social transformation takes place.

The secret of happiness in life is well-being. If you have knowledge of prevention and cure, you will be healthy. In today's world of fast forward ultramodern lifestyle, fast food, modernization, unhealthy competition, tensions and stress at work of heavy responsibilities, unhealthy living conditions, environmental pollution and climatic change have increased diseases like diabetes and heart problem. Therefore, it is vital important in today's world to invest in health and create positive living habits. There are many books available, yet people continue to search better materials to satisfy their health needs. This book will give better understanding in the areas of integrated community development.

Virtue itself spreads the quality of the things. If a doctor is highly qualified and clients get well, his clients themselves make him famous. If the teacher is brilliant, his students will spread the fragrance of his deeds. In addition, all those who read this book will find something for self-help and they will spread the forum, as the flower does not need to keep a board, it will come from deep inside the forum and that is this book will do. Quality of the book is to transform a child into angel and so the hand that rocks the cradle rules the world. Good things come in small packages. A milestone and a stepping-stone. The book is like an onion, you peel it off one page at a time. Do not judge this book by its cover, there is a treasure in the broken vessel, dive deep into it and find the nectar at the core level.

From ancient age until today's modern age, human being has done tremendous progress in all the fields, hi tech, which is unimaginable. Yet if any part of the society is weak, its ripple effect is on whole society. Moreover, it prevents the development of the entire society. Development focuses of totality, as whole. Rural community health also has a lion's share in development process.

At the end of the each chapter, the relevant and appropriate photos are displayed which will enhance the reader to understand with clarity the subject matter better. The readers will get at one glance the clear concept such as women's health care, rural village set up, cancer, health education, tuberculosis, and so on.

The feel of the exact situation/location of the place is easily understood with the pictures, which will have long memory as it gets registers in the mind more easily and readers can understand the concept better. Photographs help the community to come to the classroom. It promotes correlation of information. Photographs are nearer to reality and give valuable association which promote in self-learning.

Every teacher has his/her own unique way of approaching the topic and preparing the subject. Some are born teachers who possess the ability and mastery over the subject, which just flows to capture the complete attention of the group, this is the art and skill of teaching through photographs, which I am sure, will help to enrich the subjects enabling the readers to transform. Poor are the burning bush. We must take off our sandals as we approach the poor because God resides in them.

As the author explains in the script the rural mindset, this book is specially dedicated to the poor, as living God resides in them. May this book be a blessing to all who read it.

Cecy Correia

Contents

PLATE 1

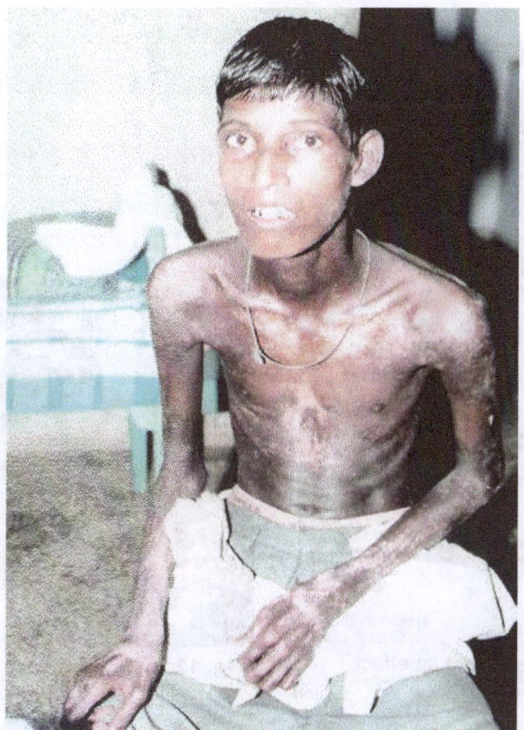

Fig. 7.15: Nurses' role in 'National Health Program'.
Early detection and notification of diseases

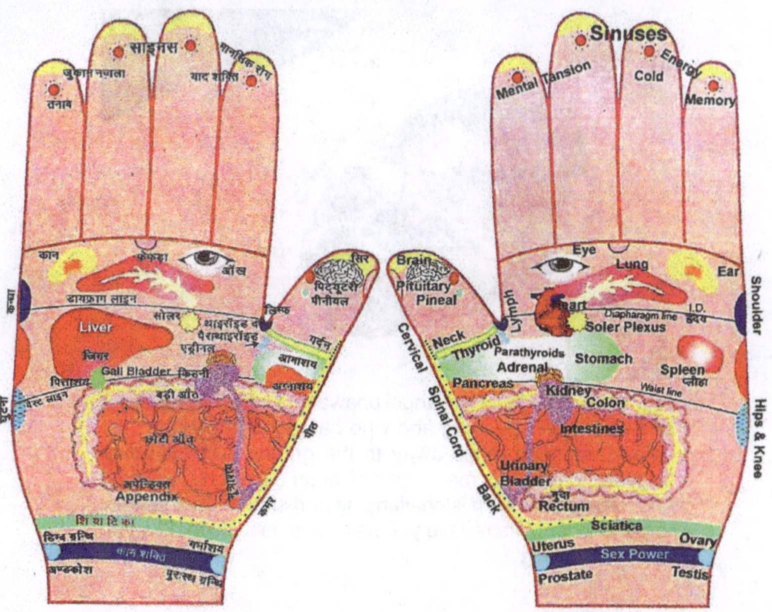

Fig. 9.1: Acupressure. It is a nature cure system originated in ancient India for treatment in which pressure is applied on points to the ailment of body without any medicines

PLATE 2

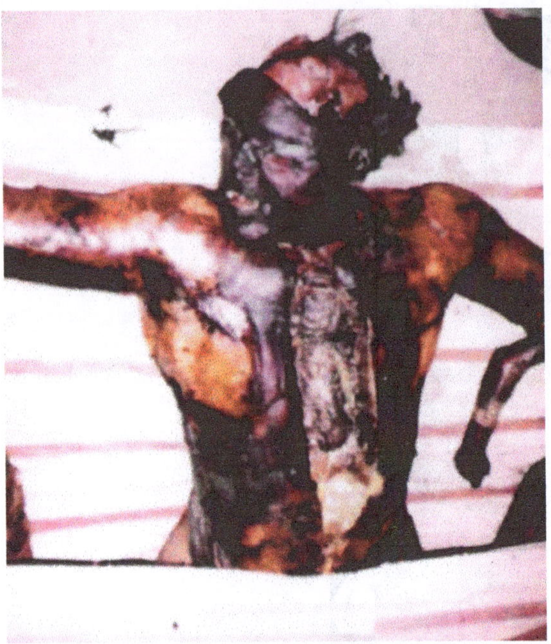

Fig. 12.23: Man-made disaster and its effect on innocent lives

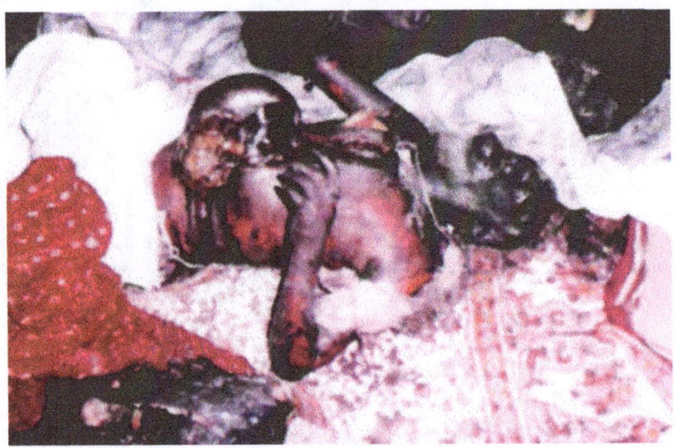

Fig. 12.24: Fundamental respect for human life. Loss of life, pain and suffering that is inconsolable

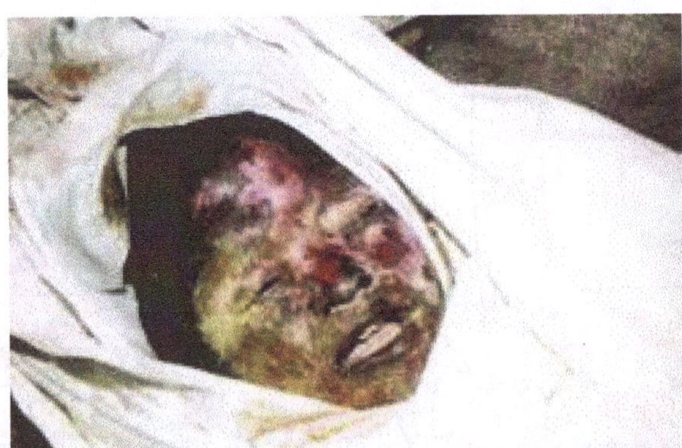

Fig. 12.25: The innocent angel unaware of what is happening and why is it happening and who has done it; precious life before blooming fades away to the ground. The inhuman tragedies caused by man-made disaster cannot be forgotten and forgiven easily. It is challenging and shame on humanity to comprehend, incredible yet the truth of lost life makes you and me thinking

PLATE 3

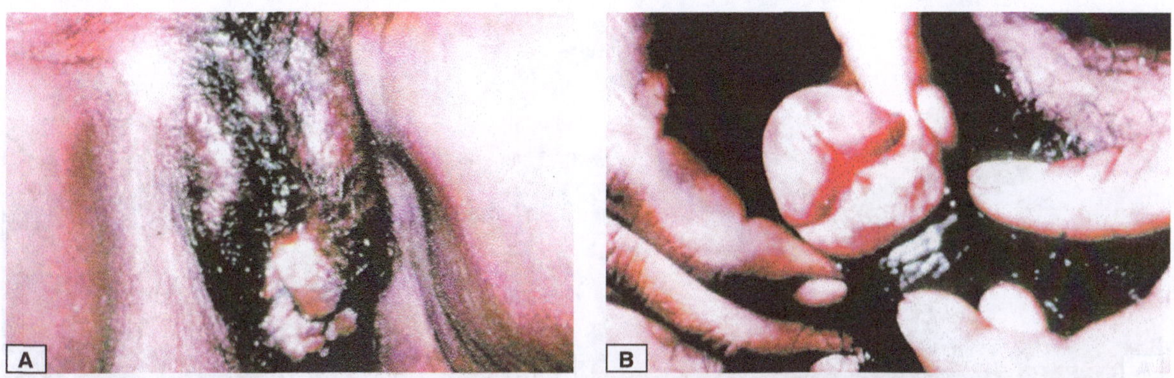

Figs 18.1A and B: Syphilis

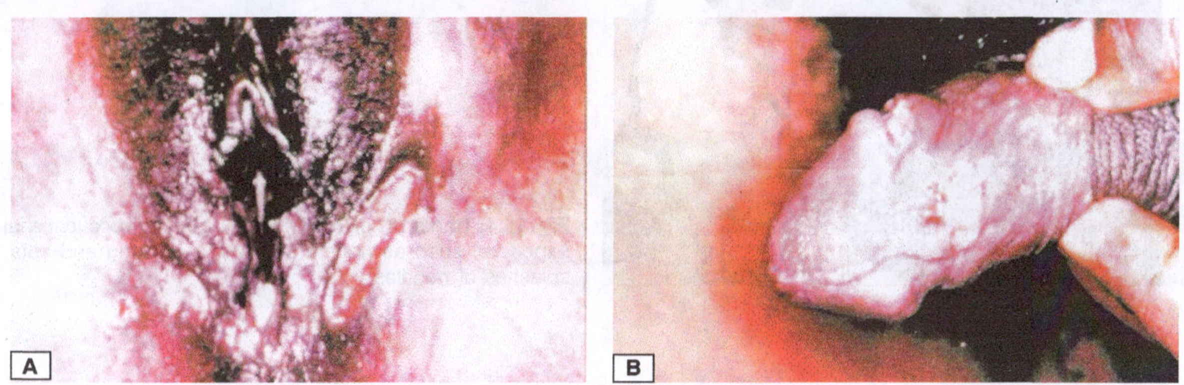

Figs 18.2A and B: Chancroid

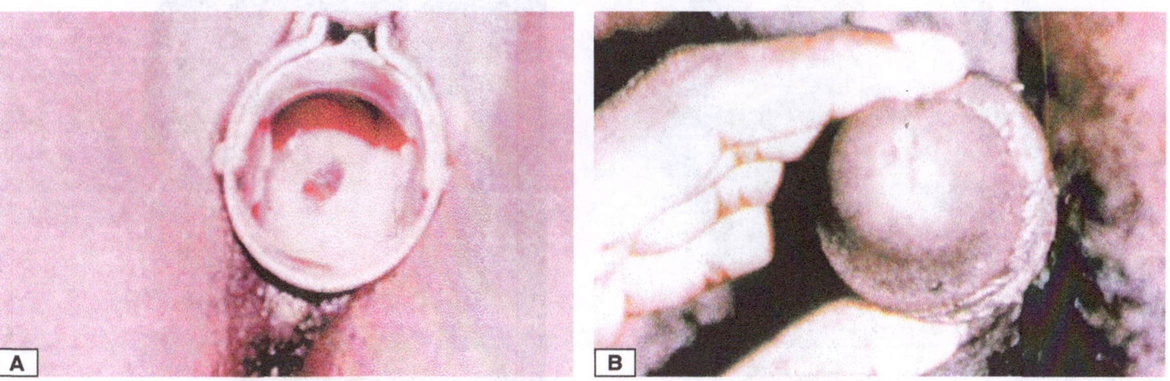

Figs 18.3A and B: Gonorrhea

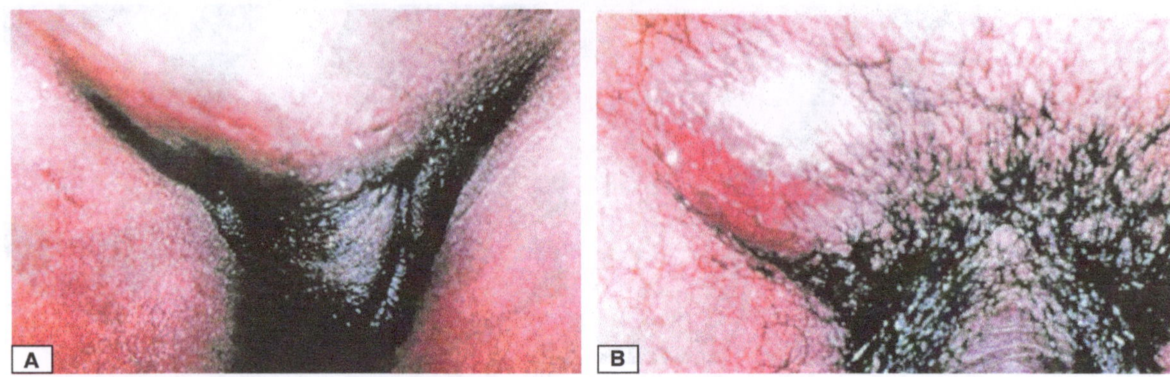

Figs 18.4A and B: Lymphogranuloma venerum

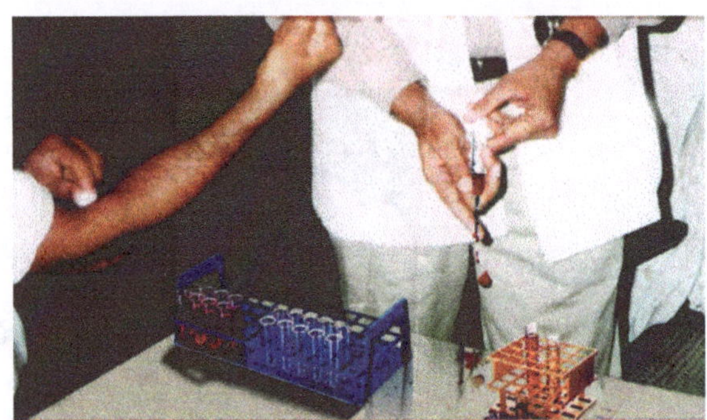

Fig. 19.4: Transmission of HIV infection through occupational exposure, such as needle sticks and pricking and cuts, splashes of needles

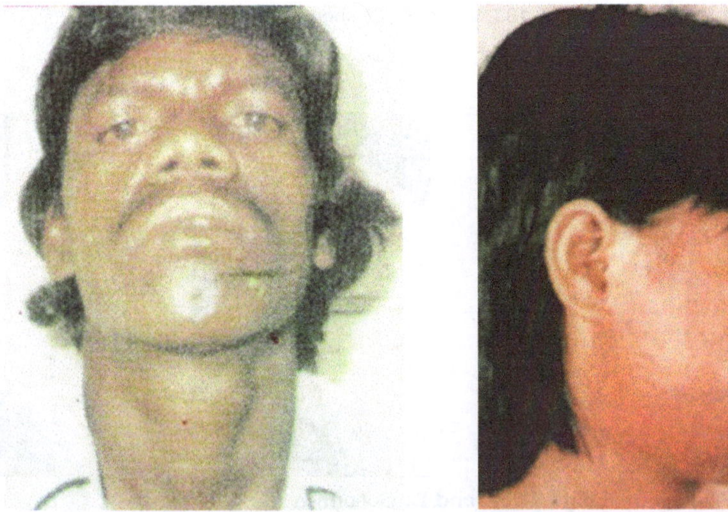

Figs 20.3 and 20.4: Early sings of leprosy–light colored patches on skin, specially the face and ear. Loss of sensation in finger, toes, pain in nerves—do not fear, seek medical aid immediately. Leprosy is caused by bacillus and not by curse or evil spirit or by past sins

PLATE 5

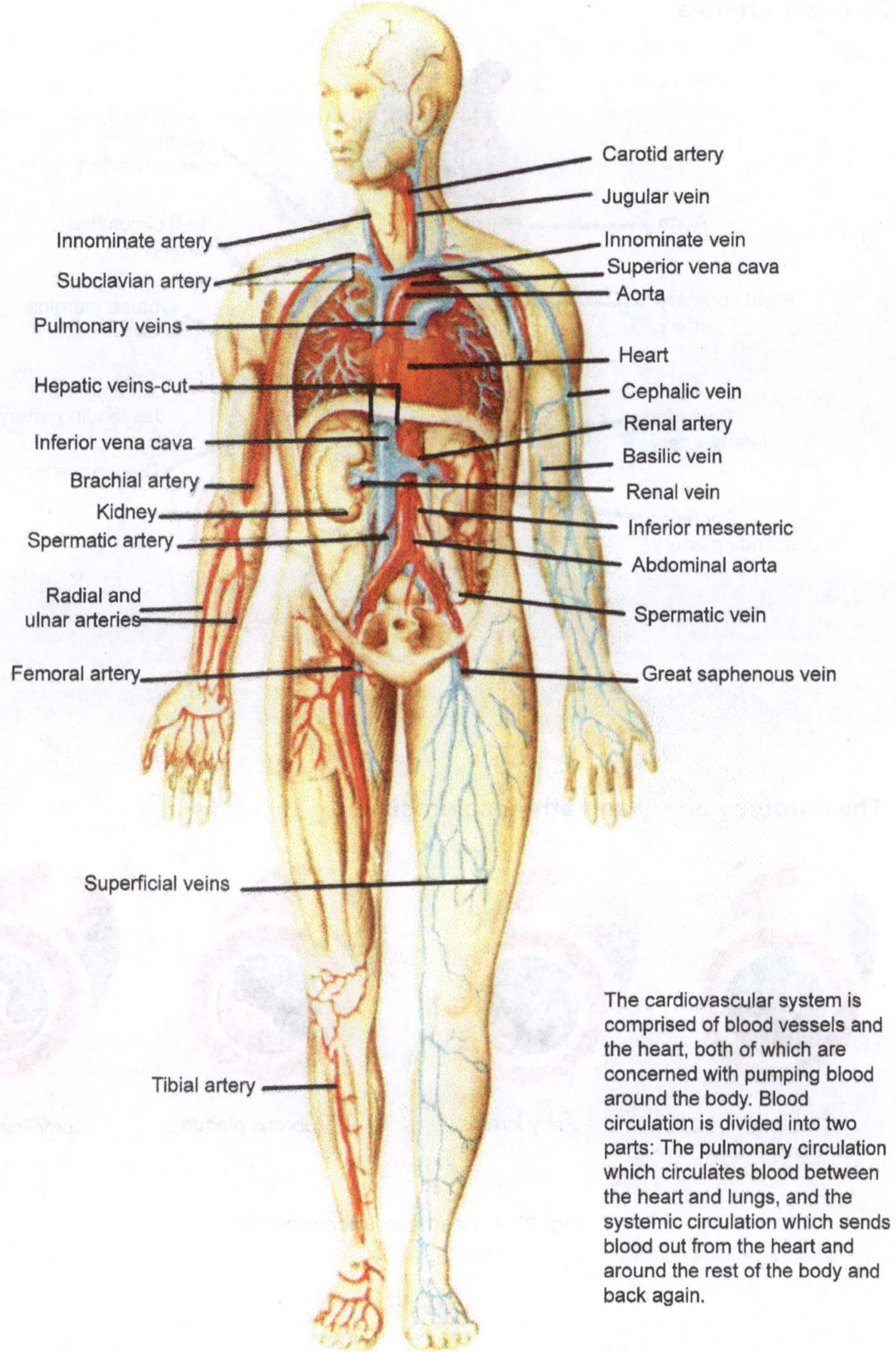

The cardiovascular system is comprised of blood vessels and the heart, both of which are concerned with pumping blood around the body. Blood circulation is divided into two parts: The pulmonary circulation which circulates blood between the heart and lungs, and the systemic circulation which sends blood out from the heart and around the rest of the body and back again.

Fig. 27.1: The cardiovascular system

PLATE 6

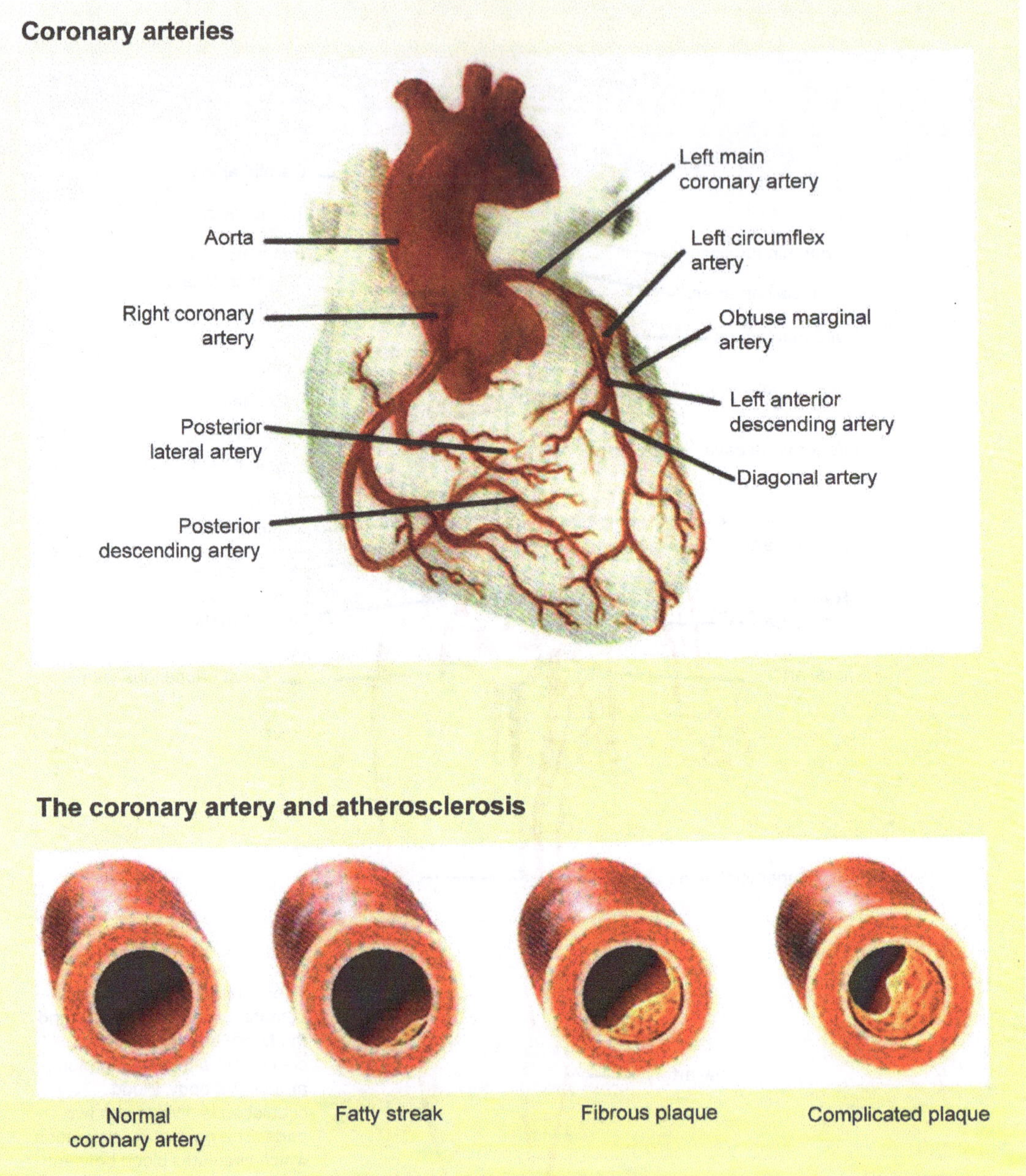

Fig. 27.2: Heart and arteriosclerosis

PLATE 7

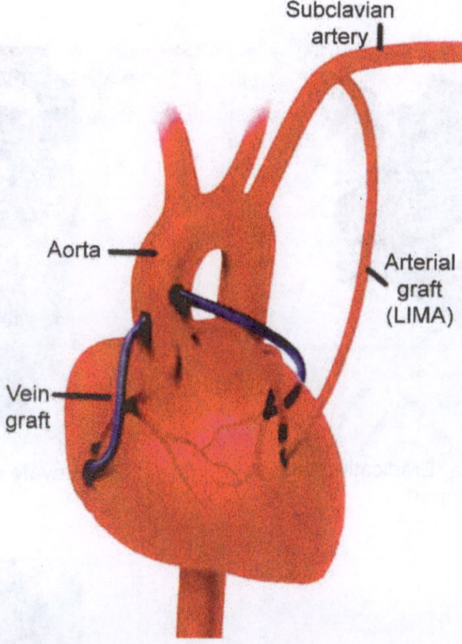

Fig. 27.3: Heart beat: The rhythm of life

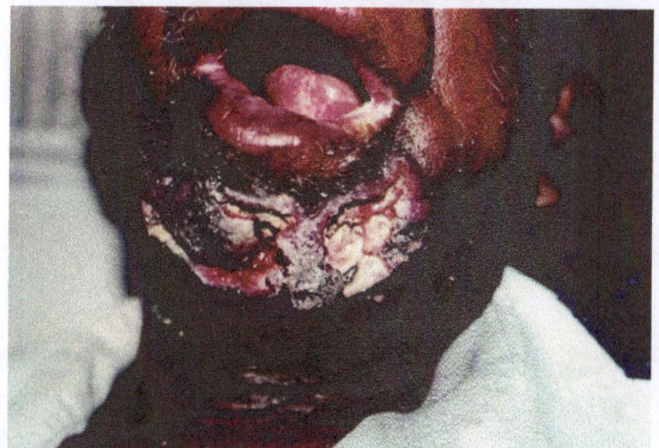

Fig. 30.1: Fundamental right to live with self-respect. Give care and hope

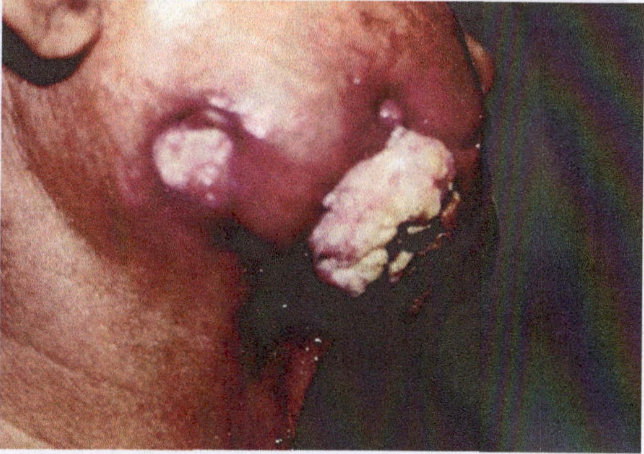

Fig. 30.2: Sharing care and concern for the sick and suffering

PLATE 8

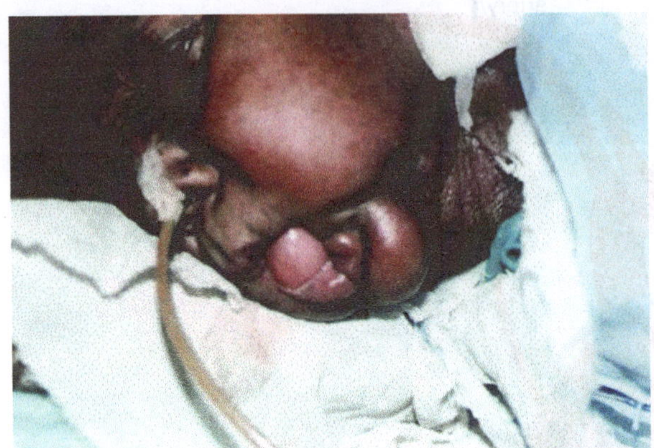

Fig. 30.3: A home from home. Eradicating the crippler. Give support

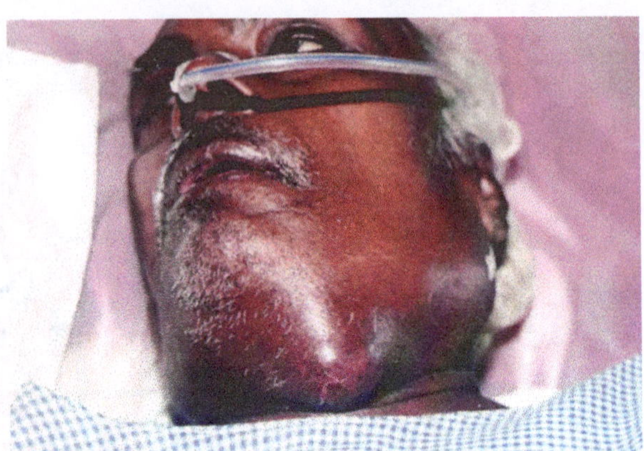

Fig. 30.4: Elevate suffering and pain. Give love and dignity

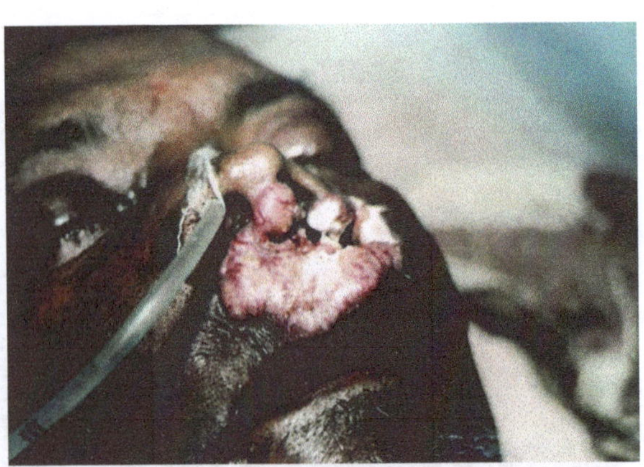

Fig. 30.5: Hold the hands of assurance

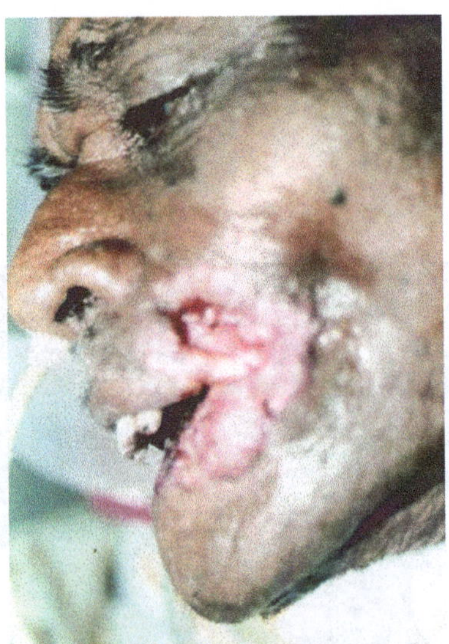

Fig. 30.6: Help to bare pain

1 Rural and Urban Sociocultural Community

Rural community consists of the land and its people. They mainly work as farmers who cultivate and who live in remote area. They live with lack of facilities; among them lack of education and health facilities are important. Villagers evolve their own leadership patterns called **Panch**. Panch originally means '5 member committee'. Five people, who are supposed to be elders and respected people of the village community, formed it. The members of the Panch are normally elders with wisdom and experience who look after and govern the community regarding its harmony. The identity of the community is to maintain by this local Panch and the community will respect this body. It is a healthy step towards the community unity and smooth functioning.

India has been a land of villages; **Panchayat** is a part of village life from time immemorial. It maintains justice, law, and order; distribution of land, tax collection, maintaining peace and harmony, public welfare work, education, and health, all these come under the orbit of Panchayat. Though punches have no pay, yet they have certain important responsibilities. They have grip and hold on community such as protecting water sources for drinking, imposing regulations to keep the village clean and make villagers to construct their own latrines and drainage. It is their task to get illegal construction demolished, to get labor from the villagers for public work construction and repairs of roads, constructions of village roads and provide for streetlights; Panchayat is traditional system today they are elected through the election – politics.

They are looking after the property of the Panchayat, and organizing mela and exhibition. They take initiatives for the development of agriculture and are teaching new techniques of agriculture, making provision for better quality manure and seeds, establishing cooperative societies, cottage industries, improving quality of animals and treat them well. They are making provision for library and reading-room facilities, radio and television, which is for entertainment kept in common place for all to watch.

Involvement of local self-government institution is vital. The role of local self-government institution in the health sector has been appreciated. Their participation as a part of the implementing body can be ensured through the following steps: Health Center of the village can be put under the supervision of Panchayat for ensuring proper and efficient functioning. A standing committee at the village Panchayati Raj Institution level has to be set up for this purpose. The Panchayati Raj Institution can also be involved while transferring the local health center professionals. Whatever mode of education

– health awareness must be dispersed through local bodies, i.e. Panchayat. The voluntary sector works for people's need and welfare are therefore natural partners. The government has the infrastructure and resources; the voluntary sector has the ideas, initiative and inspiration.

Being the children of the land, villagers have capacity to enjoy life. Hardships, failure of crops, the struggle to survive has given them the gift of the **dance** of life where they blend with nature and accept joys and pains as they come. **Music and dance** are the life-breath of the villagers. It is part of an expression of their urge for creative art, which enliven their otherwise human life, feasts, festivals and fairs, and of course weddings, provide them with many opportunities to express themselves in joy with full gusto. The rural communities have **distinctive culture** and mode of living. They have their own rights, customs and ceremonies. They have peaceful co-existence with each others in villages. **Agriculture** is the main occupation of the rural with paddy as their main crop, which is harvested during monsoon once a year. They also grow jowar and pulses. There is a little or no surplus for the coming year.

Usually the spirits and gods who must be appeased and feared determine the people from rural area, who have their understanding of life, death, health and sickness, harvest and drought.

In the villages time concept is different from ours. For them time is not a commodity as for us in today's competitive world. When we take up work we need waiting capacity for hours together with patience, as their time is not controlled by clock. They hardly have any private space; walls and boundaries do not confine space for them. They feel comfortable within the space of the whole village; they have everything under the **same roof even the animals**. They feel familiar with all and they know everyone in the village. They are united in the **village as a community**, take part in birth, death, marriages, and follow their own rituals.

PLIGHT / SOCIOECONOMIC CONDITION

Even though **poverty alleviation** has been on the national policy agenda for more than fifty years poverty is still an existing phenomenon that poses threat for the development of the nation. The trend in rural poverty shows a very close similarity with trends in agricultural wages. Rural poverty is more directly affected by food grains harvest because it is the major source of both employment and of the supply of the basic necessity consumed by the poor. They have to guard their family health.

Rural problems are many and complicated, social evils are deep rooted. The most glaring fact of massive de-humanizing poverty in rural villages even today they are confronted with poverty, deprivation, and violence of human rights by unjust power capitalist. Although our country claims to be a secular democratic republic our people in towns and the numerous villages do not experience for themselves the implication of this ideal. They are torn apart by object of hunger and powerlessness, social discrimination, and exploitation. They are living with poverty and **struggle of daily life,** they do not even get what is justly theirs, and this is the stark reality.

Death continues of the small **farmers** even today. They see the **empty skies** and scanty crops have driven them to take loans from banks or worse, put them at the mercy of ruthless money lenders, exposes the horrible reality of the under privileged farmers life. A sensitive, stark tale of a poor farmer cannot determine the price of his crop himself. He has to face the tyranny of intermediaries who buy at a below price when the supply is high then make huge profit for themselves. Difficulties of an average farmer today have become even tougher even he can barely exist, and he barely has the strength to keep going.

Widespread poverty forces individuals, families and communities into the alienation and a life of dignity is impossible in the midst of poverty. While looking at the gloomy picture of development, what gives hope is by various ways and means ordinary people make themselves happy and try to adjust to the situation as it comes.

Development is not going to come from the President, Prime Minister or Rulers of the World. The alternatives which are emerging at the National and global levels through experiences developed by people at the grass-root level will continue to give meaning and define and redefine the development of the nation. To make them **economically self-supporting** we need to mobilize the savings of the poor themselves as a first step.

Bharat Nirman National Rural Health Mission connects rural India to improved health care facilities; and building blocks of a new freedom by sarva shiksha abhiyan, national rural employment guarantee Act; creating community institutions for better health facilities and link workers serving in villages.

Yet if one looks around from urban to rural set up can obviously be able to note the point that there is a concentration of doctors up to 80% in urban areas where only 20% of population live. In addition, where there are 80% population lives only 20% doctors are provided, such a vast disparity. This is due to mal-distribution, which is attributed to absence of amenities in rural areas, lack of job satisfaction, professional isolation, lack of rural experience and inability to adjust to rural life.

Young doctors head to the west for lucrative salaries and better working conditions. We cannot ignore the rot in our system that is making them leave. The poorly equipped hospitals in rural health care system, the poor pay scales and poor working conditions making a potent push mechanism. We need to understand the cause of brain drain in order to find effective solutions. Villages in India have government funded rural sub-center that provide only the very minimum medical care. A roof over the poor man's head instead of star lit sky and economic empowerment of women to feed their starving children. India's health care scenario will change for better completely, the brain drain notwithstanding. India's doctors go over seas, there are enough to take care of the ill at home; provided the working conditions and infrastructure in the rural areas is upgraded.

Having aware of the fact the health sector plans and implements various national health programs and makes broad policies and gives directions to the work, by looking after the health problems and medical care. Whole of this system is well planned and organized to achieve set target, objectives and goals. It acts like a network, like a web, a chain that is integrated.

In this context the community nurse helps to develop realistic view of existing rural health care service to the community to identify the major health problem of the area. She can acquire knowledge about various rural development schemes required for lifting up villages. To aim comprehensive and all round development of people to give better living, an attempt to bring about a social and economic transformation through the effort of the people themselves. A special training to be imparted in modern techniques of agriculture and leadership at grass root level for employment to agricultural labor in the season; helping in **constructions of cheap** and hygienic **houses**, tube wells, hand pumps, free textbooks and note books, stationary and even free hostels. Through cottage industries an effort is made to alleviate the problem of unemployment, poultry, farming, development of handicrafts, and assistance provided to sell their goods at reasonable prices.

The ecological degradation, poor agriculture and insufficient livelihood have had a deleterious effect on the health. The close contact of the agricultural workers with animals of their products increases the probability of contracting certain zoonotic diseases. Agriculture accidents, insect and **snakebites** are an additional health problem.

How long will they able to survive an isolated existence? Steps are to be taken to bring this community into the national mainstream or else they may be disintegrated tomorrow. Various facilities offered by high tech medicine today are not quite relevant to the needs of the poor. Medical technology is advancing by leaps and bounds from the past few decades. New diagnostic and therapeutic discoveries are being made every year. Yet indicators show that women's physical well being is very low. The reasons are poverty, illiteracy, and male's attitude towards female, reproductive diseases, over burden of work etc. often physical well being has a lot to contribute to one's mental health. Added to this is the very stressful living situation. Reducing the rural poverty of people living below poverty line, construct roads; electrify houses and streets, connecting them to the towns and cities.

During summer months villagers look for part time jobs, men of the family work during the summer on other farms, constructing bunds, **brick factories** and repairing roads for the government with the forest department. The women too work along with the men, in seasons other than monsoon. The available land in its present state cannot give gainful employment to the people.

As they have not enough to eat and are unemployed they migrate, there they live as daily wagers in subhuman conditions. Urban slums are breeding centers of diseases and different kinds of crimes. Urban man is engaged in diverse occupations like industry, trade, factories, shops, building modern roads, railways, and individualism and commercial he has artificial environment. Urban communities are large, population is in lakhs, millions or in crores, in small area large number of people reside overcrowding, concentrated, diversity of language, age, religion, and culture is present.

Villages have to be developed so that the rural people do not migrate in large scale to the cities. **Community consciousness** in rural community is much bigger than in urban community. Rural community here is not mechanical but natural, spontaneous; their interests are common in the villages, whereas in urban slums it differs.

Every aspect of community life affects cultural influences, beliefs, values, rules and structures, food habits, socio-economic factors, lifestyle patterns, educational backgrounds, the coping ability and the capacity to deal with drastic, unexpected eventualities. Either there is too much rain or too little rain, either there is floods or drought, to some other natural disaster. As number of rural people still depend on **favorable weather conditions** for their farming and agricultural work. Community nurse cannot ignore and avoid seeing and noting all these factors when she works in the field.

She will have to take appropriate measures in protecting people and understand the basic needs and the concept of the community where the people are susceptible to ill health. Community nurse is concerned with people who are not only sick physically but well as well taking into consideration the total population with a holistic view. She has to make an effort to maintain, support, control, care, contribute, educate, manage and coordinate and follow-up with regular evaluation of the family, individual and community needs. Her task today is demanding to meet the needs of the society and work for well being of whole community.

Her quality of work affects, as she is responsible for the **group organization**, so her vital service is to give top priority to work within the framework of the unit entrusted to her care. Health of the people is a great concern in today's society. The field of health science is rapidly expanding due to the latest development, new concepts and improved technology in all the spheres of medical world is a challenge to her to keep abrase and be up to date. Nurses are instrument in conveying this knowledge and promote and guide the activities and prevent health hazards of an unhygienic way of living.

There is no single measure of health as health is multi-dimensional and it various, with cultural and family characteristics, Community nurse has to help them develop healthy attitudes and acceptable behavior in altering attitudes and to be sensitive to the community point of view.

Lack of proper housing facilities in urban slum and rural village causes serious health and social problem to the lower middle-income group of people. In rural area still huts are widely found which are dark and inadequate for the family, which do not protect them from extreme weather, climate of hot, cold and monsoon, which is unpredictable, and that hits the poor hardest. Good house is essential for good health, security, shelter, and comfort where one can satisfy one's physical, emotional and health needs; and live with human dignity and respect.

NGOs can be an important institution to provide advocacy for the vulnerable sections of society in identifying problems and working towards improving the quality of life through various activities, projects and programs. To ensure effective participation of NGOs, there has to be a clearly defined support system on the part of the government. It is a general observation that the process of funding is the biggest barrier between government and NGOs partnership; this needs proper evaluation and monitoring for effective networking.

This implies attempts at alteration of lifestyles and a new mindset and a new attitude. So attention has to be paid in nutritional need, educational awakening and social development; water, the liquid of life and food that build your body. One has to find happiness in simple lifestyle; adapting to simpler and healthier lifestyle with minimum damage to the environment.

However, certain accepted parameters of health have not shown the desired improvement; the various health projects and the schemes being implemented under various programs. Health is a subject closer to everybody's heart. Improvement of one's health and health of one's family is a universal aspiration. Right to healthy life is integral part of the right to life. Any threat to health care must be considered as the denial of the Right to Life.

Infectious diseases continue to pose a threat to the lives of large sections of our people. The alarming increasing number of tuberculosis, and new cases reported, so too malaria, gastroenteritis, AIDS, and hepatitis do take heavy toll of deaths; in addition diarrhea and acute respiratory infections. Due to lack of access to quality health care the number of women dying from preventable causes related to pregnancy and childbirth.

Due to poverty and powerlessness illnesses associated with malnutrition, poor living condition and lack of basic requirements; further aggravate the problem and health for many remains a distant dream. Keeping all this in mind we have to focus backward and marginalized communities to enable to attain and maintain health-care with reasonable quality at reasonable cost; making health as our top priority opting for the poor, by reaching to the unreached and becoming the voice of the voiceless; burning till burn out, with tireless effort centered on integrated development of the poor rooted and grounded in rural focus.

Specific health cares services for the women, aged, adolescents, the slum-dwellers, which needs special attention. Only screening of the health conditions of the occupational workers is not sufficient. It must be the responsibility of the employer to take care of the health of these employees with medical aid. It is well evident that there are not enough health care facilities available for the slum-dwellers, so there is a need to have health care provisions for this section of the society.

A holistic approach for improvement of rural and urban slum infrastructure and environment has to be adopted. Rapid urbanization has led to an alarming deterioration in the quality of the city dwellers. Slums suffer multiple problems like infrastructure deficiencies, poor sanitation and hard waste disposal, water shortages, polluted natural water resources, water logging in monsoon, frequent epidemic, inadequate health care, depletion of green areas, poor roads and transportation, dust and air pollution, proliferation of slums growing illiteracy, lack of support for socially and economically disadvantaged communities.

Urban poor living in the slum has many problems. Increasing population, meant mushrooming growth with unhygienic living conditions, living below poverty line, with low monthly income, ill maintained and unusable public toilet; open drainage often contaminate water, many slums not connected by sewage to the city system and the hips of garbage collection in these areas. Moreover, the problem they face when slum huts demolition by bulldozers leaving slum dweller with no choice but to move out their belongings.

Help people in empowerment process, people's process, is neither project-oriented nor money-oriented. Community workers need dedication and commitment **teamwork** and generous hands to elevate the sufferings of the poor specially slum dwellers, remote villagers and Adivasis.

It is important to motivate the communities, in mobilizing resources from the slum dwellers with community interaction an alternative sketch proposal for discussion with community group. This prepares them to change and involves them in garbage collection of their areas. Thoughtful planning can improve knowledge and the sensitivity towards the surrounding environment.

When I worked with them in Mumbai certain slums, wondered often how can they live like this in sub-human condition, there are still many poor slum dwellers who do not know how the sum of money they receive at the beginning of the month is going to last till the end. Due to their irregular jobs and financial insecurity, they are not sure, when the income will cease to come. In emergency of bodily sickness or social need, they have no resources to draw from? There they feel the shame of the unpaid bill, there is an anguish of the counting on money to see how far it can reach. Silence of the wife, the unsatisfied children, the minimum expenses, the worn-out clothes, the worn out cot, mended spectacles, teeth that have never seen a dentist, the insufficient meals, and the cruel uncertainty, even this may not last because circumstances are difficult, the job is uncertain. In addition, moreover, in such situation to keep the nobility of the character that the difficulty will end with a sense of pain.

When all the money in the house counted, all the drawers searched, all pockets emptied, when all the coins had been piled together and counted and recounted the sum does not come even to half of the amount required. When several mouths to feed and bodies to cloth, a house rent to be paid and school fees to be met and no money for it. Day after day and month after month what that state of insecurity can be when it is prolonged for a lifetime is beyond imagining.

How to live with this situation day by day in a poor house with old furniture, fear of sickness, inability to pay children's fees – such daily night mare is the hardest trail that can be conceived for a person who otherwise has to put up a front smile as though all were well within, God knows what heart suffers while a face smiles. Love has hands to help others. It has feet to hasten to the poor and needy. It has eyes to see misery and want. It has ears to hear the signs and sorrows of others. When, when will I look beyond me to see that there is a treasure in broken simple lives? Learn to look beyond my needs and not judging them by mere appearances. They too have talents, capacities, but due to poverty they are incapacitated and crippled and handicapped like an injured bird unable to fly or a man with both the hands cut utter helplessness he feels is the same experience when one lives in the slum or rural poor areas.

Migrant workers we see them like big group of animals, huddled together at the railway station. We see them as sardines packed together in the unreserved compartments of trains. We see them silently sitting in the market place waiting to be hired. We see them standing at bus station like lost travelers. We see them gathered together at the big and small slums. We see them staying in their thatched huts in open space in the fields and side of the highway or in thatched roof made of empty cement bags near factories or multi-story buildings. There only wealth is their body and the ability to do manual work to eke out a living and work very hard to earn a living. No fix hours or days of work. They work often in the open in the **heat of summer** and the bitter cold of winter. They have no protection of proper clothing or shelters against the heat, rain or cold. They are defenseless and physically and mentally penalized by unjust and corrupt owners. They too are the children of the great nation mother India just as you and me. Only living and working with them one experiences the born morrow reality at the gut level and the hands of yours go raised above to the creator what have I done special to get such a good life whereas my own brothers and sisters are still so unfortunate because they did not get the change and opportunity as me and are born in poor family.

A ray of hope to come from helping hand; to raise their income **train them skills** like tailoring, electric gadget repairing, two-wheeler repairing which will lead them to their empowerment and increase their self-confidence and self-esteem, to discover their uniqueness by improve the earning ability and where they can move upward to join the main streamline.

One of the greatest investments that we can make for them is to invest in health, for there is no other investment like health insurance, success and happiness insurance.

Health then, holds a mirror to human civilization. What we see today is not very ennobling or dazzling. Yet we owe it to our future generations not to be dwarfed, debilitated by our inability to act today.

The health system in India has considerably improved during the past five decades with the spread and accessibility of modern medicine and considerable improvement in the health status. But compared to other developing countries the health status in India shown a lower level of improvement.

Malnutrition one of the major illness that is affecting our people and it is the social evil. Most of the malnutrition is due to hunger and poverty. Though this strictly is not a disease condition it is a health hazard that needs all round measures.

Health care today entirely expensive, far beyond the resources of the poor, investigations gone highly sophisticated, where our poor and marginalized suffer silently, poverty and malnutrition related diseases, scarcity of clean drinking water, no proper sanitation.

For this concerts, radical and people-oriented planning is needed. It is necessary to understand the ways and means of making proper plan at proper time for a healthy living. Plan making is one of the essential life-skills that help us to deal constructively and helps to solve problems. An action without proper plan is bound to create problems. So identify problem, analyzing, naming the choice and alternative involved in your plan, gathering information and listing the advantages and disadvantages of each choice, which will provide direction and help; Vision and awareness and perception of reality. Time to time evaluation will tell us where we are, time-to-time monitoring of activities will prevent conflicts, confusion and sidetracking. The quality of plan will depend on goal focus, resources available, timing, feasibility, and adequacy. So that planning can become successful.

Create a new humanity of hope and love. "Bread for me is a material question; bread for my neighbor is a spiritual question." Words without deeds are empty and deeds without words are ambiguous. Being poor and illiterate does not incapacitate a person to make choices.

Illiteracy is one of the main reasons that have led to their degradation and exploitation. The villagers by nature are introvert, non-expressive, shy and quiet when it comes to verbal communication. They seldom revolt or raise their voice against any injustice done to them. **Education** helps them to get out of this situation. Awareness through education becomes a tool in their hands to counter exploitation. They become aware of their social status and demand human dignity, rights, freedom and justice. They are easily prone to various diseases and lose their lives to very minor illnesses due to non-availability of medical facilities and lack of knowledge.

Our role is total Liberation and fulfillment of the whole human person-in-community. To include the whole cosmos and to embrace whole human lot who suffer in the universe. The whole creation itself might be freed from its slavery to corruption and brought into the same glorious freedom as the children of God. Human life is stunted, relationships are strained, growth blocked and dignity violate; where freedom is curtailed, decisions are merely imposed, and selfishness, poverty of affection, unbelief and refusal to forgive, have the upper hand. Solidarity with afflicted in attitude and practice, from a sub-human through educational, social and medical apostolate. We are **challenged by these realities.**

The creation of an enabling environment in which rural can identify their needs and properties and with **professional support**, organize them to improve the quality of their lives. To **empower** rural and urban slums communities and groups, particularly the underprivileged and the women. Help them to take control over their lives and manage their environment, to create a better and more equitable society.

The betterment of rural communities is by providing direct support to local communities to promote activities and develop models for sustainable natural resource use and development of human resources. Establishing and strengthening village institutions within the communities is the key focus underlying all programs. Rural development is influenced by many social, economic, as well as environmental factors. Relief and rehabilitation work to be taken up.

The importance of Healing Ministry, offer us a health from all dimensions of human person; to approach people and heal them in all aspects. To transfer this spiritual energy that is within which ultimately brings healing. Thus with this healing touch we can free people from all negative forces. And for this, one has to believe and be convinced of the importance and challenges of Medical Care. The progress we have made in the field of Health challenges the 3rd Millennium is forcing us to face.

Today there has been a greater awareness then ever before to the concept of health, that health is an asset not only for the individual but also for the whole community and that it is desirable to maintain and promote it. This responsibility rests both on the self and the community. Health continues to be a neglected despite lip services. Other needs like wealth, power, prestige, knowledge, security is more important. If money, wealth were all-important then all the rich wealthy people would be happiest. It is taken for granted and its value is not fully understood.

It is an inner disposition, attitudes and positive outlook towards life, it is in contentment in all you have and do. During few years, there has been a **reawakening** that it is an essential and important to improve the quality of life. Health is **multidimensional process** involving the well-being of the whole person – soundness of body, mind and spirit, which will help the community to live a good spiritual, social and economic productive life. The secret of happiness in life is well being holistic living. It is **self-responsibility**. It is to be at peace with self, community, God and cosmos. Community health is also **state's responsibility**.

Community health results are not immediately observed. It takes months and sometimes years to see accomplishment. Make sure that your time is used wisely and people are able to use your services well.

It needs a fresh thinking to evaluate the progress achieved. Every person has right to healthy and wholesome living. All problems cannot be tackled at the same time, so first thing do first. Have right attitudes in using and maintaining harmonious relationships. **Every family is different** no one pattern will fit for all situation at all time. People resist change just as you and me do. Some families face illness realistically and hopefully able to discuss problem and differences with objectivity and reasonable emotional control, the way they manage family budget and the kind of discipline that prevails.

Accept the patterns of behaviors and maintain up-to-date scientific knowledge. Develop an action program, set up a goal, and make a professional judgment. We have always less budget comparing to the size of health problem we meet, we have to concentrate on the most urgent health needs and manage with the available resources, which are realistic; **placing people's health in people's hands.**

Our finance minister P Chidambaram announced a people friendly budget in the parliament **'aam addmi'** budget 2008–2009. The budget has brought good news for women and children. Schemes for women and children, the budget attempts to provide a counter cyclical support for growth through greater allocation to agriculture. Tax relief to individuals and small service taxpayers is a positive step. Focus on education, health care and urban infrastructure is rightly placed. Over all it is good budget full loan waiver for 4 crores small, marginal farmers. Short-term crop loan with 7% interest, irrigate and water resources, finance crop to be set up. Rain-fed area develop program to be started. A great budget for socialists and are happy with schemes for education. The focus on a knowledge-based society is high. The proposal lying of additional infrastructure better broadband connectivity between institutions is very good. A lot of emphasis is laid on expenditure to bring social justice. What difference it makes to the **average person** is vital.

So let us hope for the best for the years to come to see rural and urban poor live happy with self-esteem and with human dignity as the proud children of the mother India.

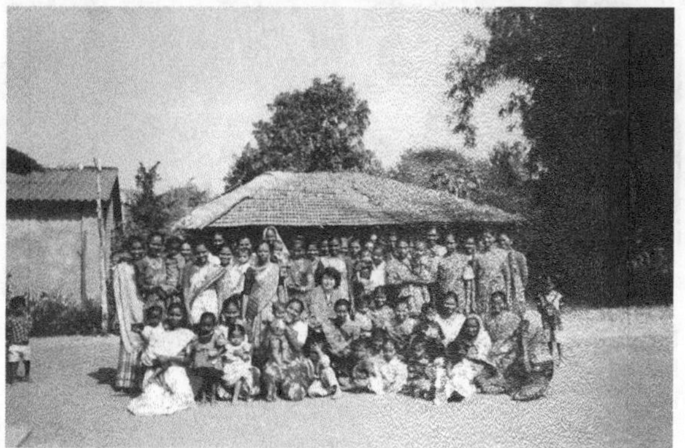

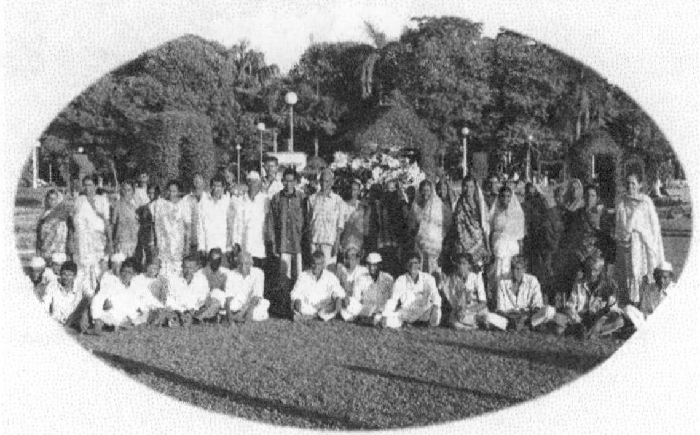

Figs 1.1 and 1.2: Community health is formed by a group of families living in a specific geographic location, having similar needs, goals and common ends

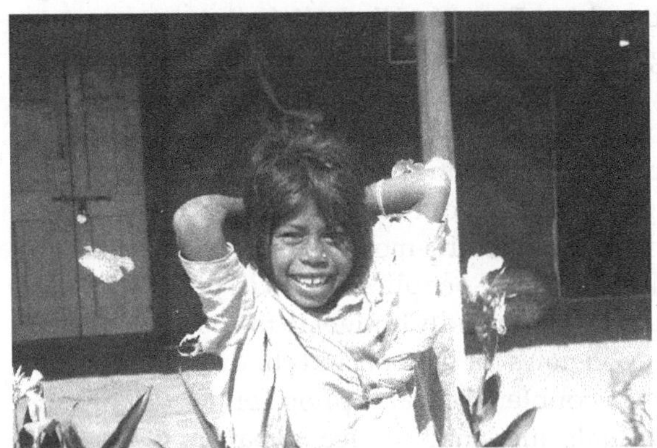

Fig. 1.3: Save and empower the girl child

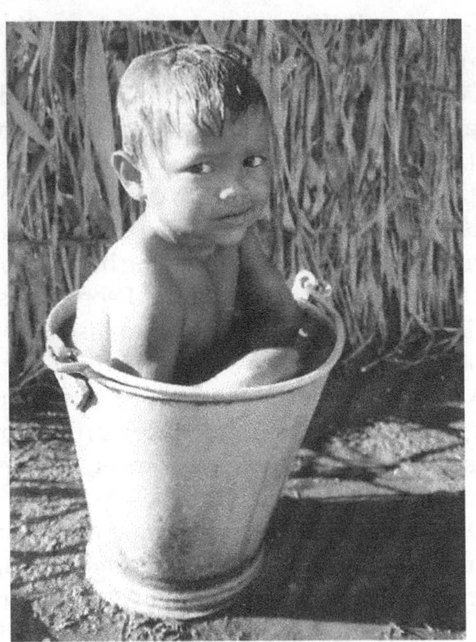

Fig.1.4: Rural child development

Public health is science and art—promoting health, preventing disease, and protecting it through organized community efforts

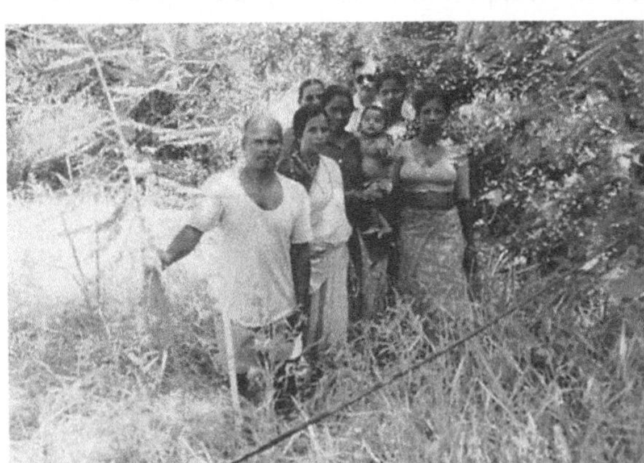

Fig. 1.5: To reach health to the unreached remote areas

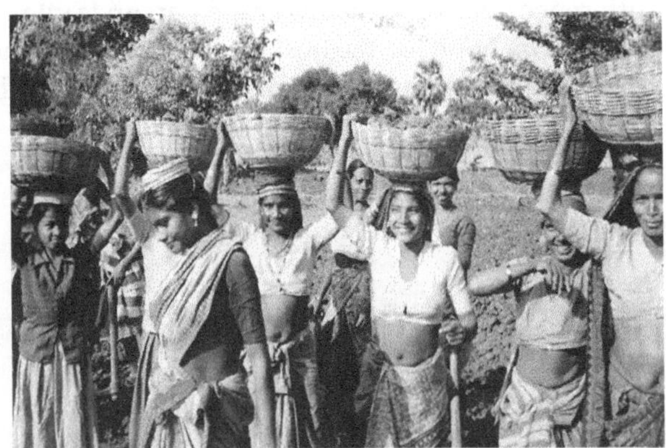

Fig. 1.6: Community organization for social awakening. Moreover, economic conditions, daily work activity to improve families' health. Rural health mission

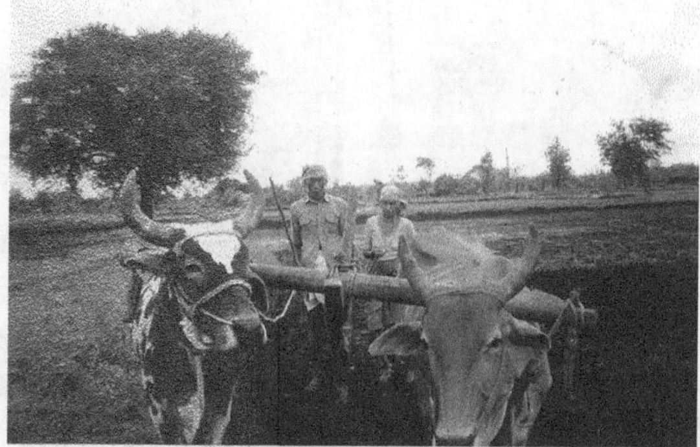

Fig. 1.7: Agriculture and farming is a backbone of the rural village community that provides food and employment. Improving a level of health that will permit people to lead a socially and economically productive life

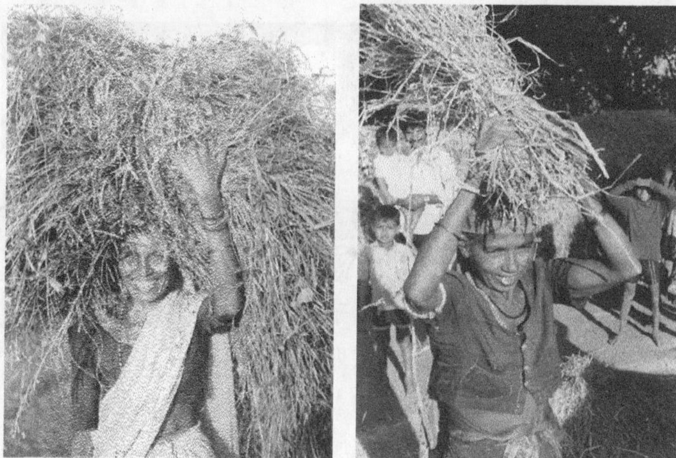

Figs 1.8 and 1.9: Status of women. Poverty and the hard labor of the rural poor. Common sight of the rural people who work from hand to mouth. Assist in coping ability. Health is self-responsibility, it is to improve the quality of life

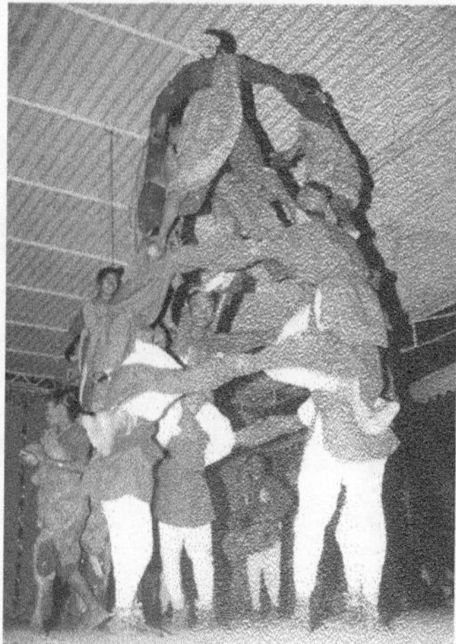

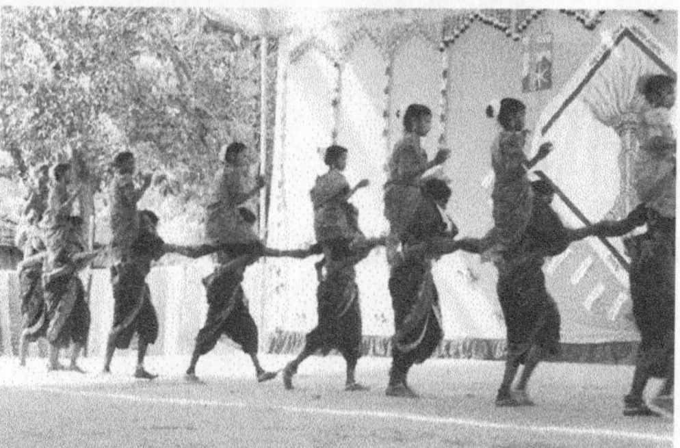

Figs 1.10 and 1.11: Dynamics of the culture. Sociocultural views affect health system. Each tribe has their own cultural background, which is reflected in their way of dressing, foods, houses and way of living

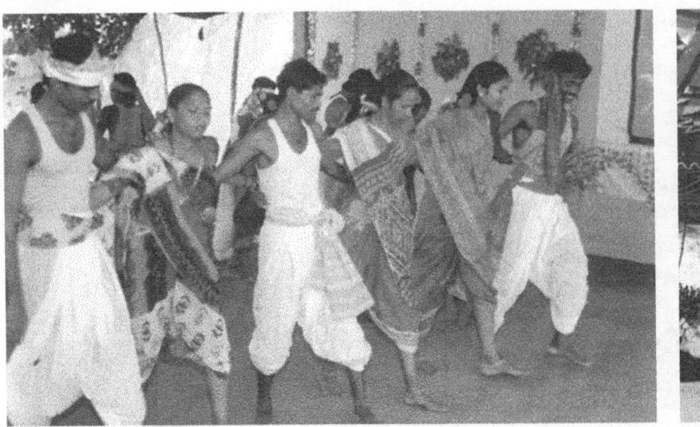

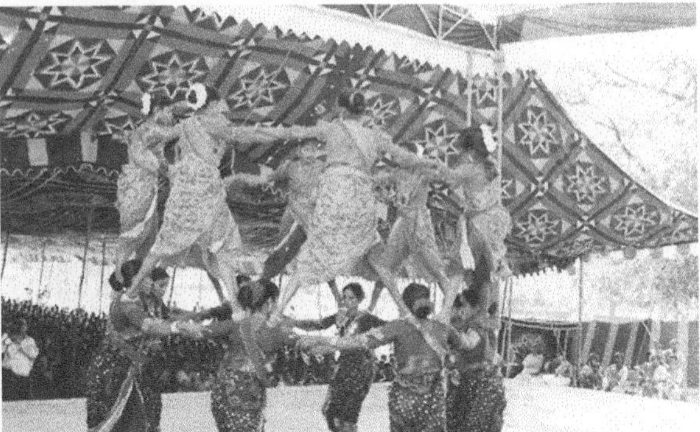

Figs 1.12 and 1.13: Community health nurse needs to identify and incorporate cultural factors to provide effective health care. She is a sheet anchor and a change agent who links community to the center

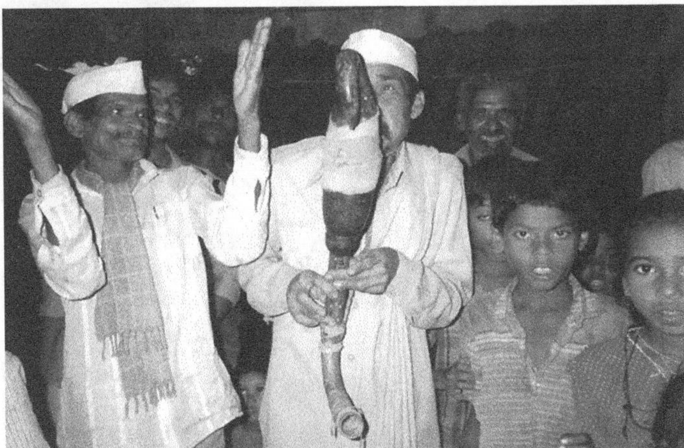

Fig. 1.14: A typical rural cultural instrument. Celebrating feasts and festivals and enjoy simplicity of life where whole community gathers and takes part in typical dance

2 Family: The Center of Community

The family as a social institution has existed from the beginning of time in every corner of the world. It is the oldest institution in the society. It is the smallest group, which satisfies persons' basic needs like food, shelter and clothing. It is most stable, enduring and social universal and cultural form. An economic provision is common and the members of the group share it. There is an economic and social security to each member, because the eldest person sees the welfare of every member of the family. The health of one member of family affects the welfare of the rest of the family. During sickness or unemployment, the other member shares the duties and protects him.

Home is where the heart is. Our entire life revolves around our home. Home is the place of our dreams. It is alive with countless warm memories. To be happy at home is the ultimate result of all ambition. Today nuclear family gaining prominence in today's times family ties are loosened. Pressures of city life add to mental isolation of individual who do not have any one to talk to. In moments of adversity your family can support you.

Health nurse must understand family ways, tradition and customs of the people when some eventualities take place to one person the entire family comes to his rescue. Nature can teach invaluable lessons. **Mother is the center of the home**. A human home is far more complex. Every home is a little heaven on earth. It is based on unity. In the family physical, psychological, cultural and spiritual needs are met. Family functions as a buffer against any odds. Love is a basic and foundational feeling for one another. Self- sacrificing, caring and sharing. There is a natural setting, freedom and space for growth. They experience strong emotional bonds, understanding, loyalty and accountability with commitment. As they relate by birth and bounded by blood relationship. Joint families are still found in rural places though due to modernization and urbanization joint family is slowly disappearing.

Every person is born into a family. The child has the right to be part of the family and reach adulthood receiving care and protection from other members, especially parents. It is there that he/she receives new experiences, and newer relationships. His/her first experience of love, affection, kinship, and support of the other members is not from anywhere else. This child's attitudes and values are very much the same as those prevailing in the family. He/she also grows into a healthy person who possesses physical, mental, social and spiritual well-being as long as he/she lives in a healthy family environment. It is a well-established fact that anyone who comes from a less than healthy family suffers from several forms of maladjustment. The family is the foundation of health. Wherever the foundation is weak and on loose ground, the family breaks the building collapses.

The child should be received as wanted and eagerly awaited, not as an unexpected guest. Ensure childbearing as one of peace and harmony. There should be careful efforts to reduce the stress related to daily life and avoid interpersonal conflicts. Special care should be taken to maintain adequate nutrition and for providing sufficient rest and relaxation to the mother-to-be. Avoidance of alcohol, tobacco, drugs etc. is a must. Parents should be willing to share the parenting responsibilities. Parents should be ready to spend quality time with the children.

The child must be planned. If the child is not wanted their happiness and rejections will be transmitted to the child through their attitude and behavior towards the child. Child needs love and security, parents to set examples of caring, sharing, discipline, understanding, counseling, dialogue here they feel secure and confidant. Here they will develop respect, good qualities like truth, honesty, integrity, and tolerance. With love and protection of parents the child grows. Together with firmness and gentle punishment to be given when a child does some wrong thing repeatedly. Children are very inquisitive and ask all sorts and embarrassing questions they should be honestly told and replied.

Both partners should convince themselves that they should function as an organic unit, bonded in love and concern for each other. The husband and wife will develop due respect for each other and understand each other's strengths and weaknesses.

Why some home fail? Avoid quarrels, mending a broken home, is an important aspect of good discipline is a price of happy home. Little things mean a lot, avoid confusions. Counseling, sharing so that children build self-confidence, develops respect, have value for truth, honesty, punctuality, integrity, tolerance. Learn to pray and trust God. If family is negative, restricted, do this, do that, don't do this, then members feel isolated.

What is the importance of family in your life? Your goals and objectives of family care? Poverty leads to sickness and sickness to poverty. People suffer from various illness and they cannot get adequate medications due to poverty. They are not able to cope up with the family demands because family income is low which leads to family insecurity, inadequate nutrition and low standards of living. Health gets impaired, and they become susceptible to any infections. This causes malnutrition, negligence.

Every person is born into the family. Child from **birth to adulthood** gets care and protection in family. It is the family he receives new experience of love, affection and support. The child's attitudes and values are the same as those prevailing in the family. Careful efforts to be made to reduce stress related to daily life of avoiding interpersonal conflicts one of peace and harmony.

Spent quality time with the children, talk to them, play with them, take them out for a walk the bounding takes place as a result of time spent together is a lasting experience. Develop due respect for each other and understand the strength and weakness of one another. The harmonious relationships sends the message of security, warmth, feeling of belonging, children will grow emotionally healthy and physically strong. The family that prays together, spends time together, eats and celebrates together lives together. This family is vibrant and lives happily. That is a family. As family is a universal concept and they are same in rural areas and in urban places.

To improve the quality of life family welfare has to help in education, nutrition, health, employment, shelter, and safe environment. **In the homes of the people the secret of national health lies.** They are backbone of community health and its planning. The development of health is a holistic process related to the over all growth. It depends on many supportive services, which are to be made available and assessable to the family and community. Nurse's role is coordination and provision of essential services to build a self-reliant family. Community Health Nurse (CHN) aims at the elimination of poverty, ignorance and ill health to raise the quality of life. She has to strive towards securing satisfactory basic needs of people, by over coming barriers and obstacles of progress.

Remember this. Happy parents create happy homes. Happy homes produce happy children. Happy children make a happy family and a happy family a happy community and happy communities make a happier nation/world. Real homes are built on love that endures. The true center of every home is the mother. No one else can ever take her place. If you look into the community, you will find that all the interests and activities of a happy **family center on a mother.** If she is kind and cultured, her home will reflect her fine ideals. The success of the family, the community, the nation and the world depends on the young women of today and the kind of homes they establish. Happiness does depend upon the amount of money one possesses, but rather a wholesome personality and outlook on life. Little joys, kindness and happy surprises really make family life worthwhile.

When children are given opportunities, they discover their own potential and dreams, they are glimpse a promising future and they have hope, despite deprivation, 'across to education' has created a hope in their life and opened new vistas for them. Self-confidence, self-respect, self-reliance, and wisdom – these four elements comprise the **process of learning**, which is based on life experiences.

When a community nurse works in the field urban slum/rural villages she has to do survey of the family which is also important, which will help her find out family origin, their native place, years of living in the area, years expected to be in the area. This background supporting information will help her in her work that she is going to carry out into those areas. She can find out also their income pattern annual, daily, monthly. Their pattern of expenditure on food, education, health, electricity, water etc. What is the family social status—do they have a ration card? Do they have any savings? Do they actively take part in social activities?

Does the family own the house of their own or take on rental basis where they live? Are their health services available-government/private? Are they educated, what education they have completed or weather any body in the family has discontinued schooling? What is the reason for this, is it due to poverty and economic condition or lack of awareness. Are any of the family members suffering from any disease? Diseases such as tuberculosis, asthma; are there any water-borne diseases such as typhoid, cholera, and diarrhea. Jaundice; is there an insect-borne diseases such as malaria, filaria, dengue.

Are the women healthy or do they have reproductive diseases, menstrual problem, discharge, and pain. What other health problems exist such as psychological problems, skin problems, diabetes, blood pressure, and heart disease, cancer. What kind of customs and culture do they follow? Are there people with addiction, smoking, alcoholism, drug abuse, and tobacco/gutkha?

'Family' forms the connecting link between life and death for a victim. The tension and rupture of this vital link often is the root cause among addicts to give up on recovery. With our society becoming more educated and aware everyday, the rights of a woman to raise her voice, to react to her victimized state are being strongly encouraged to redefine her family life.

The alcoholic parent becomes increasingly dysfunctional and has difficulty maintaining a responsible role as parent, marital partner, homemaker and breadwinner. Psychological stress produces physical ailments in family members that may go unattended as the focus of attention remains on the effects of the drinking behavior. The family is, and will always remain, the corner stone of social stability. At its best, it is also the firmest foundation for recovery from addiction.

Describe the demographic concept of the family. Assess nutritional status of the family members. Understand environmental condition of the family. Evaluate immunization status of the family. Identify major health problems and render nursing care accordingly. Motivate use of birth control measures to eligible couples. Plan and prepare family budget. Skill and develop nursing care plan and give comprehensive nursing care to the family.

In family health nurse contacts the head of the family, write their address, and occupation, their income, and religion they follow. Community nurse will have to record the date of first contact with the family and the total numbers that make the family. Type of family that need to be mentioned as nuclear, joints, broken, family economic status, number of earning members, total income of family, and how do they plan their budget expenditure of food, physical condition, clothing, education, how much or in what form do they keep house saving specially for future or for unexpected happenings.

She has to assess and see the house built, is it slum/pucca/well built up, and how many rooms in the house, is the ventilation adequate/inadequate; the source of light, water supply, sources of fuel, excreta disposal, do they have latrine/open defection/community latrine/household latrine, how do they refuse disposal. Is mother pregnancy at present, number of pregnancy, duration of pregnancy weeks, injection tetanus vaccination taken, anemia observed, any other information about maternal health, immunization status of the children, Family planning followed, any eligible couple observed any one using contraceptives, or willing for permanent sterilization.

Present approach of a health care system is doctor-centered, drug-based and cost-effective. Healthy lifestyles are the key to staying fit. Human being is too complex to be narrow concepts and that the body, mind, and spirit form an integral complex which defines man; emotions can influence the functioning of several organs in the body. The working of the heart, blood vessels, lungs, stomach and intestines is obviously affected by emotional states. Persistent negative emotions like anger and depression can affect the functioning of the internal organs to lead to many psychosomatic diseases.

Mental health of a family is like a barometer of the social life of a population. Many new issues have come up in the family with implications for mental health. The most notable are alcohol, violence in society, the growing population of elderly persons, urbanization, disaster, migrants and refugees, street children, and stress at work place.

What is stress in family? What causes it? And what happens when family under stress? More importantly, how to prevent it? It could be poor work environment, excess noise, too much or too little work, long working hours, boring or monotonous work, machine-paced work, unreasonable production targets, shift work, social isolation at work, discrimination, sexual harassment, conflict with management, interpersonal conflict and tension, could be some of the common sources of the stress in the family.

Courage makes family stand for convictions and act according to principles. Life brings along with it a number of challenges and these challenges call for the ability to face them squarely and not to run away. Courage is the strength or ability to face, setbacks and adversities. Courage is inherently dynamic. It motivates family to fight for principles and values. It prompts family to face any situation and stand boldly and face even death.

Courage coupled with love makes family even sacrifice lives. It bestows superhuman powers leading family to heights of heroism. True courage is linked with deep faith. It is the only force that induces even to meet disaster with calmness and confidence. Courage makes one face new challenges and shoulder responsibilities. It calls for accepting the hard realities of life and also one's own limitations. It is courage that turns failures into stepping-stones to success. Courage makes family stand for their own convictions and act according to principles. It makes them stand for truth even in the face of losing popularity. It is here the real test of family greatness lies.

The role of positive emotions, especially feelings of love and forgiveness increase peace of mind and anger and hatred reduce peace of mind, every action as well as reaction is significant. So is family way of feeling and dealing. Deciding on what lifestyles to adopt and what to give up. Wealth can perhaps be inherited and transferred, but health is to be earned through proper habits of daily life. The present-day medical system, which is disease-oriented, needs to be corrected and made family health-oriented.

Any family has stress related conditions such as headache, anxiety, depression, work tension, family conflict, and addiction. Is there any child who needs special attention in the family? Do they need rehabilitation if person is suffering from polio, paralysis, blindness, deafness, speech problem, mental retardation, learning disorder? Is there any need to take such people to the center through the contacts with social organization that can come forward to help them and can be refer them to specialist treatment?

Where does family take treatment when they are sick? Is there any death during the past 3 years? Do they have any pregnant woman in their family? Is all Immunization of children below 5 years done? Health, hygiene and nutrition—What is the source of water? How do they store water? How do they purify water? What type of latrine does their family use? How long did mother breastfeed her child / did they practice bottle-feeding?

What kind of snacks does family give their children? Is there any problem of insects like mosquitoes / cockroaches in family area? Does anyone come to spray pesticides? Reproductive illness awareness—What is the cause for HIV / AIDS? Are they practicing any method of family planning? Intake of food / type of foods do they have healthy habits. Any family member is involved in income generation activity.

Concept of marriage—Any problem in the family- marital conflict, dispute with neighbor, conflict with relatives, financial crisis, extramarital affair, wife beating, alcoholism, property dispute. All this is very important to find out before implementing any program in the rural village. Community nurses approach and attitude towards the family is vital. All these things are very important to know if one wants to help them and work for them in upliftment and progress of the downtrodden.

A child's world centers on the home, school and the local community. Homes should be healthy places where children can thrive, protected from disease. Many environment threats to children's health are aggravated by persistent poverty, conflicts, natural and man-made disasters, and social inequity. Children have a unique vulnerability. Children with chronic disease and long-term disability will not grow up to be healthy and productive people. Children are particularly vulnerable to environmental hazards because they are constantly growing, and consume more food, air and water than adults do in proportion to their weight. Their immune, reproductive, digestive and central nervous systems are still developing and they spend their time closer to the ground where most dust and chemicals accumulate.

Many children are born at home, and spend a major part of their young lives there. But from conception, their health may be adversely affected by hazards in the home such as lack of sufficient water, indoor air pollution, inadequate hygiene, contaminated food, and many others.

Safety precautions to be taken in your home to store water in covered containers safe, clean and cool places, promote the use of improved stoves and cleaner household fuel, wash your child's and your own hands with water and soap before preparing food and eating, and after defecation, keep your child away from smoke during peak cooking times and do not smoke near children, store household cleaning products, pesticides, fuels and medicines away from children's reach, use insecticide-treated bed-nets to prevent malaria, open fires in the home can generate toxic fumes and cause burns to children, indoor humidity, moulds, dust and pets can trigger asthma and allergies, unsafe electrical wiring, poor construction and building maintenance can cause injuries, water from lead pipes and lead-containing paint and dust in the home may affect a child's health and intelligence.

In your community make public places smoke free, organize waste management to promote a healthy community, clean up streams, advocate for safer roads and organized traffic, eliminate the use of leaded gasoline, take care of children in swimming areas, or when playing in ponds and creeks, maintain slides and swings to avoid injuries, plant trees to provide protection from the sun, excessive and unsafe use of pesticides represents a risk to children, stagnant water favors malaria and other infectious diseases, children playing in unsafe, polluted waters may get diseases.

As poor families live a hand-to-mouth existence; health care is out-of-pocket, poverty, inequality and ignorance are the greatest diseases of our society. In fact, the key barriers to good health are not lack of technology but inequity in health system and radical poverty of the masses. Where are we today? Health of a family is greatest possession, for it lays a solid foundation for healthy nation.

Statistics to be updated in formation on modern trends, new concepts and improved technology to be updated as health of the people is becoming a great concern in today's society. Health care and its delivery systems are changing rapidly in order to meet the needs; Socio-cultural, political factors that play a significant role in health and illness, newer medical technology, newer drugs, innovative methods in diagnostic procedure, computerization to facilitate quick diagnosis and scientific research. Health is a community concern.

Sometimes community nurse has to change the way of her thinking and adjust to the patterns of family's lives to be integrated into it. In Indian, culture, this has deep-rooted family values. We have tremendous loyalty to the family. For instance, parents make enormous sacrifices for their children. They support them until they can stand on their own feet. On the other side, children consider it is their duty to take care of aged parents. In fact, all the other siblings respect the eldest brother or sister. As for marriage, it is held to be a sacred union – husband and wife are bonded, most often, for life. In rural areas joint families are still found, the entire family woks towards the welfare of the family. There is so much love and affection in our family life. This is the essence of Indian values and one of our key strengths. Our families act as a critical support mechanism for us, supporting them through the tough times.

Our attitude towards family life has to reflect in our attitude towards community behavior. And we do not have to be apathetic towards the common good. So that we can contribute care more for the society than we do. To enhance the quality of life we have to sacrifice more for the society. To create more respect for the public good like parks, clean streets, public toilets, all these are instances of care for the public good. In India, we keep our houses clean and water our gardens everyday, same way when we go to a park, individual's responsible behavior towards the community as a whole. Example of putting the interest of oneself, at best that of one's family, above that of the society.

Public vigor in solving community matters should not held us back from making progress, which is otherwise within our reach. When we see serious problems around us we have to try to solve them. We have to show in our deeds that as if the problems do exist and affects it and me is not somebody else's but of the community in which I live. Public issues belonged to each one of us and it is our responsibility in solving them. Aristotle's words: "We are what we repeatedly do." So we have to repeat to do public and community good and set an example for others to follow. So that we get the joy of giving our care wholeheartedly to the family and the society to build our rural society thus build our nation.

The family is subjected to a lot of suffering and hardships after a cancer, stroke strikes a family member and its effects are borne by the family for a long time. Hence, it is important to include the families in planning acute and long-term care of all patients, especially the severely disabled families that need regular discussion on patients' condition and prognosis. Diet is now considered a major factor in the prevention and treatment of cancer. Tobacco-related cancers account for about half of all cancers among men and one-fourth among women. Tobacco smoking is a leading cause of ill health.

The family plays a vital role in caring for the sick person. A wholistic approach to sick persons should be viewed from a physiological, psychological and spiritual perspective. Illness is not merely a physical and a biological phenomenon, but an event that occurs in a social context. Essentially, all patients and their families have various kinds of emotional reactions to illness. The responses may vary greatly depending on the variety of factors such as personality, age, family, social conditions, employment, way of becoming ill, nature of illness, its treatment and possible outcome.

Family shares common kitchen and common purse. Community health nurse (CHN) has to interact to tackle the situation. Certain disease runs via genes in family. Meet people in their family setting and help in their health problems.

Family, being universal primary social unit, is the first social contact for every human being. It is regarded, as the most significant part of one's adjustment to illness is better than when they are stressful. The significant attributed to the family's role in relation to illness family problems may precipitate illness in a vulnerable individual or it may be the consequence of certain illness. Its importance in the field of health and illness is paramount.

Alcoholism is another major problem, which has wreaked havoc in the lives of many family members. Alcoholism, which has been termed as a 'family illness', is known to affect at least 2-3 members in each family. It wreaks destruction upon all that is dear to the spouse like family life, economic resources, well being of the children and status in the society. Children who need a great deal of love and attention for development of a healthy personality may have difficulties in this area, leading to psychological and behavioral problems. Most families function as a buffering agent during recurrent crisis and hence they need special care to help their patients. Well-informed families could reduce stress in the sick persons and remain a good support during convalescence.

People are denied what they really need to know. We are today equipped with the latest information, advanced medical technology and the latest intervention modalities that can enhance health care services. Medical video conferencing and global consultation have become possible thanks to medical media development. The patients and population at large are much better informed about prognosis of diseases and treatment patterns and above all the risks involved in complex medical procedures and their outcome.

Electronic data processing is comparatively cheaper and can provide limitless information. It can reach any part of the globe almost in the twinkling of an eye. The Internet has impacted almost every aspect of human life. But it seems a paradox that despite the information revolution and the easy access to information, super specialized people know less. It is not easy for ordinary people to exploit the benefit of the IT revolution. And the power relation between the rich and the poor, the ruled and the ruling still remain very much the same and this happens especially because people are denied what they really need to know. The privileged few get the vital information that really matters. Let us also keep in mind that it is the family the center of the community and its welfare is the welfare of the nation.

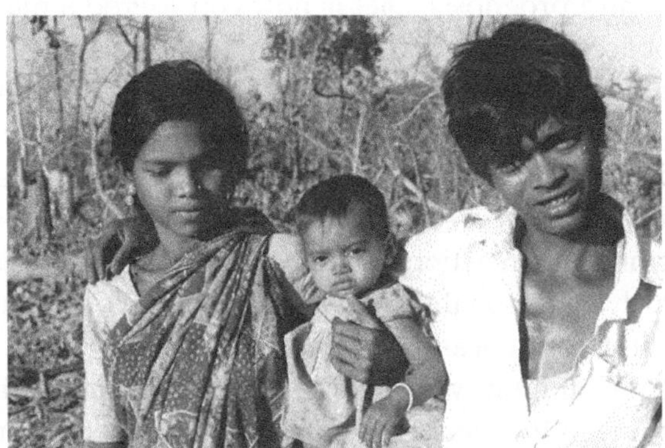

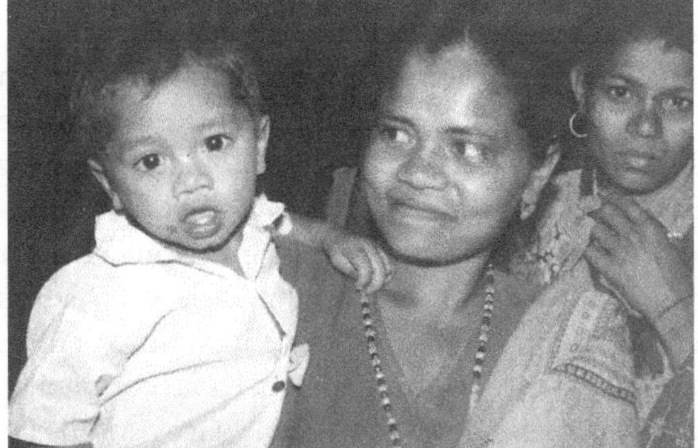

Figs 2.1 and 2.2: Family the center of community health work. Family is the oldest social institution in the society. Every family has its own ways, traditions and customs. Family, the most stable and universal cultural form. Family functions as a buffer

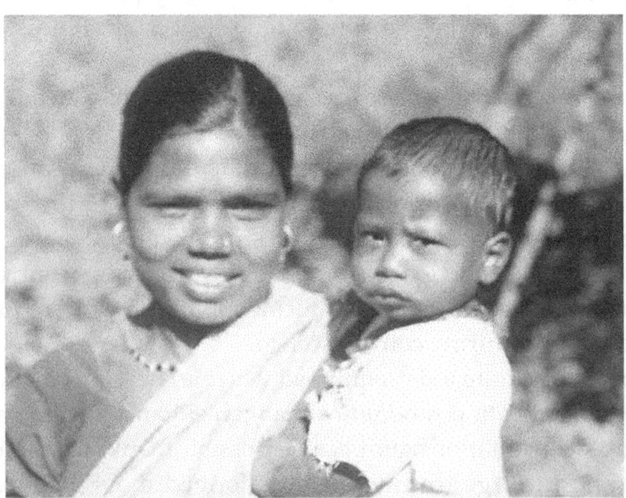

Fig. 2.3: Mother is the center of home and love is the basic and foundational feeling where child receives care and protection

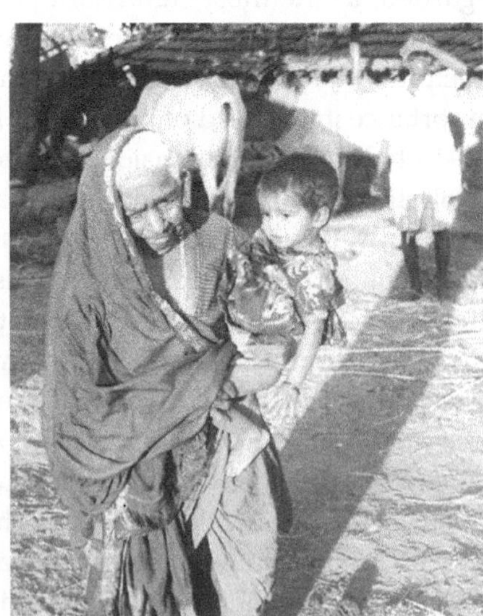

Fig. 2.4: Every person born into the family, it is journey from childhood to old age

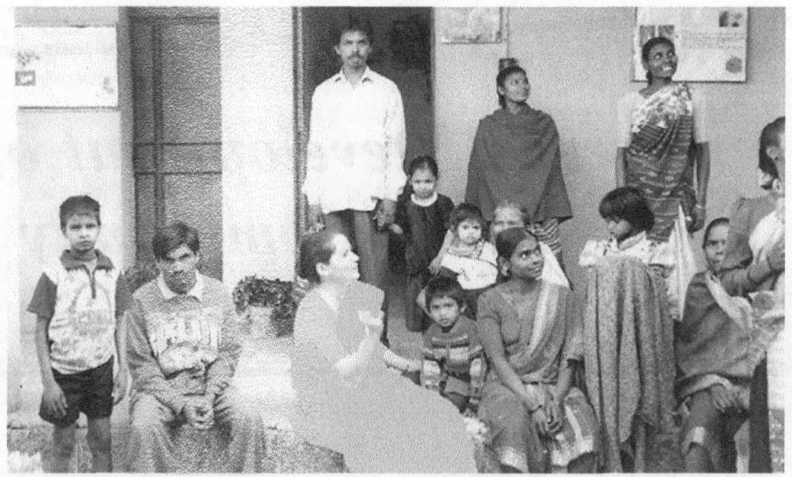

Fig. 2.5: Roles and responsibility of the community field functionary

3 Integral Development of the Rural Community

Integral development is a movement around, the rural community itself, which focuses on health indicators, the cycle of malnutrition, poverty-related health issues, socioeconomic dimension, levels of health care system, community participation. To provide sanitation facilities, to promote health education program, to provide water supply, adequate nutrition, and above all give them self- respect and human dignity to live uprightly in society. In order to liberate the poor from the horrid clutches of exploitative forces, and to affirm itself educationally, socially, culturally, politically and thus availing themselves to join in the mainstream-line of India, yet keeping alive their **culture and identity.**

The program to be envisaged not only to build houses but also to build communities as a strong unit; the process of enabling the community towards self-reliance and empowerment will have to be the focus. "Community development defined as a process designed to create conditions of economic and social progress for the whole community with its active participation and the fullest possible reliance upon the community's initiative".

Today large sections of our people continue to be exploited and oppressed and many of our societies are torn apart by hatred and intolerance; passing through a period of rapid change, which affects social structures, political institutions and the economy. Traditional values are under threat from new forms of development and technologies as well as political authorities and economic organization that manage these changes.

In particular, the marketization and globalization of economies with digital sky jet world are changing the balance between the private and the public, the state and the international community, and worsening the situation of the poor and the disadvantaged. These changes threaten many valued aspects of life, the result of the dehumanizing effect of technology, the material orientation of the market, and destruction of the community. People have decreasing control over their lives and environment. There is a massive exploitation of workers, with wages that are frequently inadequate for even bare subsistence and low safety standards that put the lives of workers in constant danger. There are people who earn and become multimillionaires and the poor who help them in this process working day and night to build are paid very little and never come up and remain in subhuman condition life long, this is the disparity of certain development programs.

Development has to bring people who are below poverty line to certain stander where they can enjoy certain statues in life. World is moving forward very fast and still if we look we can see rural villages are still without light, clean water, improper roads or inadequate health and educational facilities.

Under the modernization chemicals are being used increasingly in agriculture either as fertilizers, insecticides or pesticides. Agriculture workers are exposed to toxic hazards from these chemicals. The agricultural worker may be exposed to extremes of climatic conditions such as temperature, humidity, solar radiation, which may impose additional stresses upon them. Inadequate ventilation and working in uncomfortable positions for long periods of time. Exposure to dusts of grains, rice husks, coconut fibers, tea tobacco, cotton, hay and wood are common where these products are grown which gives rise for diseases.

Home based work, which includes pounding masalas, rolling beedis and agarbatis. Here, not only the workers themselves, but also their family members are also exposed to the toxic fumes of tobacco and masalas powders. Women workers spend long hours in a sitting posture which results in pain in the lower abdomen, irregular periods, leucorrhea, anemia and frequent miscarriages. This causes rheumatic problems, bodyache and back pain.

Even this modern era with scientific advancements still maternal death is of great concern. Community nurse should be aware of existing beliefs and practice to provide meaningful care to the mother and take up this as a challenging that no death in area of your work should take place. She has challenging opportunities in terms of observing these practices and habits of people in the care of expectant mother, reassurance to be given to mother. Life saving obstetric aid to motivate all **expectant mothers** to utilize the available health services, healthy mother healthy nation.

The nation will be shaped and moulded into a healthier and stronger one, if its children are strong and healthy. In rural community lot of help and guidance is necessary on these matters. The seed of good habits needs to be sowed at very early stage. The nurse has tremendous opportunity and great responsibility in promoting the healthy of community. Community is key factor in rural area. Nurse has to convey the correct ideas, needs to use various aids to convey message, it requires skill to convey the right ideas. She must offer right explanation, guidance to clear fear, doubts or anxieties about the program, should keep abreast with current development as she plays significant role in national welfare services. Make use of community resources to help the individual, family to deal with social and emotional problem. Promote self-reliance of a community.

People living in poorly designed low-cost shelter houses develop air-borne infections and vector-borne diseases. Women and children who spend prolonged periods in poorly ventilated houses get exposed to smoke emanating from bio-mass fuels. They contract the following diseases such as chronic obstructive lung disease, heart disease, acute respiratory infections and so on.

In the cultivation of wheat and paddy they spend more than 12 hours in a squatting posture. This creates pressure on the uterus and result in premature delivery. Backache and pain in the leg are common due to the sitting posture while weeding. **Women carrying head-loads of bricks** and mortar, and crushing bricks in a construction site is common scene. While head loading causes fatigue, muscular pain, gastro-enteritis and intestinal problems, they are also susceptible to accidents due to collapsing and scaffolding, inadequate illumination, blasting, handling of heavy metals etc.

Women hawkers and vendors have a long working day, beginning at early dawn and stretched until the late evening. Outdoor work and carrying of heavy weights give rise to stiffness of hands and hips. Urinary tract infections are also common due to the lack of toilet facilities. Ocular deficiency is common with workers engaged in the handloom sector, especially in embroidery, lace making and zari work. Spondylitis, due to the bent posture while stitching, and tuberculosis because of congested living and working conditions.

Marine products constitute a major export commodity and the fish processing industry in India is booming in the past few decades. Standing and working in ice-cold water for long hours while cleaning, sorting, shelling, grading and packing of shrimps and fish is the task of women in fish processing. Added to the exhaustive work, often they are deprived of any safety equipment like gloves, masks, which make working condition all the more precarious. Chest congestion, skin infections due to the bacteria in fish, numbness as an outcome of working in the cold and damp processing units and bruises while peeling prawns is common.

Development is full of contradictions. There is massive and deepening poverty in the midst of growing affluence of some sections of the people. Levels of health, nutrition and education of large numbers of our people are appalling, denying the dignity of human life. On the name of Welfare our natural resources are being depleted most irresponsibly and the environment is so degraded that the quality of life has worsened immeasurably, even for the better off among us; priority is to be given to the care of the poor and the disadvantaged.

There is increasing awareness among the peoples of the importance of rights and freedoms. They realize the connection between their poverty and political powerlessness and the denial to them of these rights and freedoms. They believe that political and economic systems have to operate within a framework of human rights and freedoms to ensure economic justice, political participation and accountability, and social peace. We believe that rights are universal, every person being entitled to them by virtue of being a human being. Cultural traditions affect the way in which a society organizes relationships within itself.

Technology must liberate, not enslave human beings. Natural resources must be used in a manner consistent with our obligation to future generations. We must never forget that we are merely temporary custodians of resources of nature. Nor should we forget that these resources are given to all humankind, and consequently we have a joint responsibility for their responsible, fair, and equitable use. Corruption, **violation of human rights,** blind faith in globalization and liberalization are destroying the very fabric of democracy in our country and lowering the quality of people's lives. Time has come to educate our people. India's prosperity and stability are based on agro-economy. Progress is good, we have to march and compete with the world but not on the cost of the poor who are side tracked, overthrown or displaced on the name of progress.

The health and prosperity of a nation, together with many other things, depend on the health of its workforce. If people have to work in unfriendly, unhealthy or unsafe surroundings, their health will be affected which, in turn, will affect the work ability, productivity and economy. Public awareness is vital not only to save workers but also the whole community from the clutches of occupational hazards. And anything could be done only when people get proper knowledge and information. The employees should be given proper knowledge and information about the material they are dealing with and the need for safety measures. They should be taught the need to observe a healthy lifestyle, which also plays a role in ensuring occupational health.

Family members often constitute the workforce. Not infrequently, children accompany their mothers to the workplace. Child work represents a large part of the workforce. Some of the new hazards are stress in the workplace, increasing job insecurity, violence at the workplace, and ergonomic problems etc. Workplace health risks are high in the informal sector and the small industry, which are key areas of action on poverty alleviation. Nurse must have interest in people, her observation, perception and judgment establish contact with community and understand human behavior and learn from people. She has ample opportunities to promote, educate and counsel people to get basic services. Who are entitled to bring about desired change in attitudes and practices.

Effective measures have to be taken to elevate people from the cause of poor health; India with such a vast country with huge magnitude and health need. The population explosion has affected economic development and the quality of the living of underprivileged. The problem of environmental sanitation is truly gigantic and mind blowing. Modern medical care is not accessible to the bulk of the rural people. Voluntary agencies will function as an interface between the local community and the national health system at the peripheral level. What we see is only tip of the iceberg for the progress of the society. The pattern of disease in hospital is quite different from that in the community. Community health team has responsibility for rural health and a step forward. The emphasis is simplicities rather than complexities.

All persons have the right to live in peace so that they can fully develop all their capacities, physical, intellectual, moral and spiritual, without being the target of any kind of violence. We all have right to literacy and knowledge, to food and clean water, shelter and to medical facilities for a healthy existence, entitled to share the benefits of the progress of technology and of the growth of world economy. We believe that in this way we would establish fair and humane conditions for our individual and ensure social justice, to build up the human community. Not only promoting the economic status of the people but to build up a new life. New life where there is justice, peace, equality and brotherhood. Thus, building peoples dignity to man as man.

Human beings flourish as human resources in a society, if opportunities are created. A change of approach is needed to tackle the various health problems. Social and health securities through insurance measures, nutritional security through community gramin banks, water security, through village water banks, self-help groups and gender equality; low cost construction.

People who have lost dignity and confidence in their daily lives because of their social system. Development means to work for poor for their food security, security for life that is shelter and standard of life that is clothing. To achieve this we have to build the capacity of the people by giving them knowledge and skills. Impact of work is to be created to give greater self-confidence in people, which will help them in return.

To bring about all this a community nurse shall uphold the dignity and honour of her profession. She should be an upright person, instructed in the art of healing, pure in character and be diligent in caring for the sick; conducting herself with propriety in her profession and in all the actions of her life. She should merit the confidence of clients entrusted to her care, rendering to each a full measure of service and devotion. She should try continuously to improve medical knowledge and skills and should make available to her clients. Ready to respond to the calls of the sick and the injured, practice methods of healing; learn value based, effective ways of bringing health care to rural people and city's poor; where she has to walk many miles still long way to go.

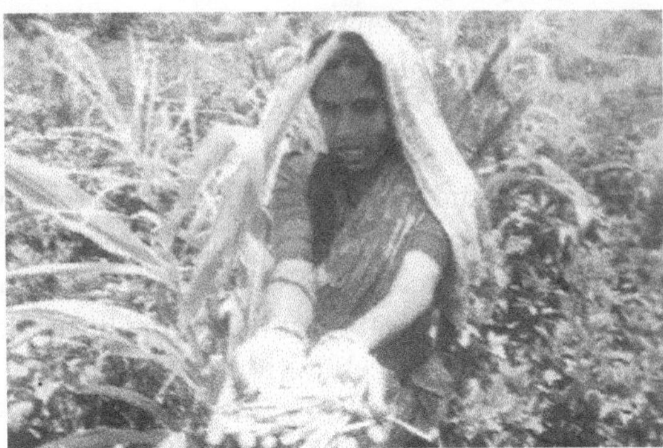

Fig. 3.1: Kitchen garden: Woman benefited by vegetables grown on vada: water from group well

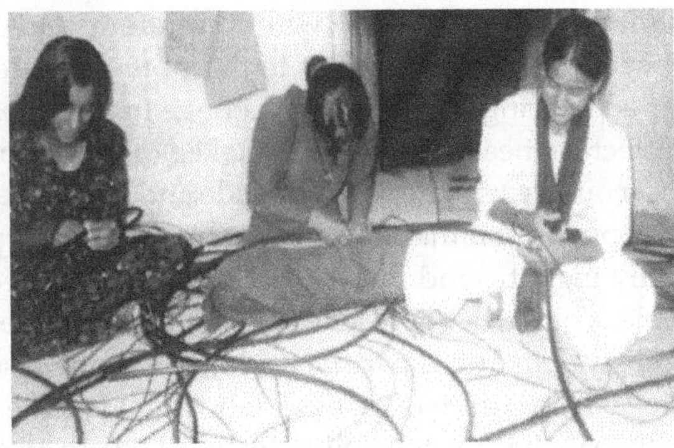

Fig. 3.2: Activities of community development, improvement of arts, crafts, and cottage industries. Mobilizing community involvement in family welfare. Income generating and skill development

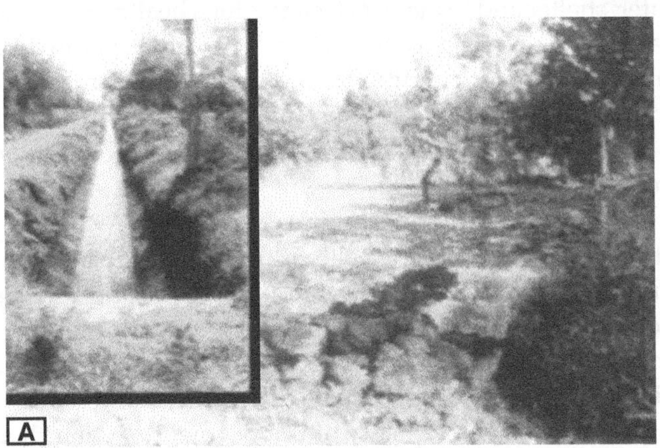

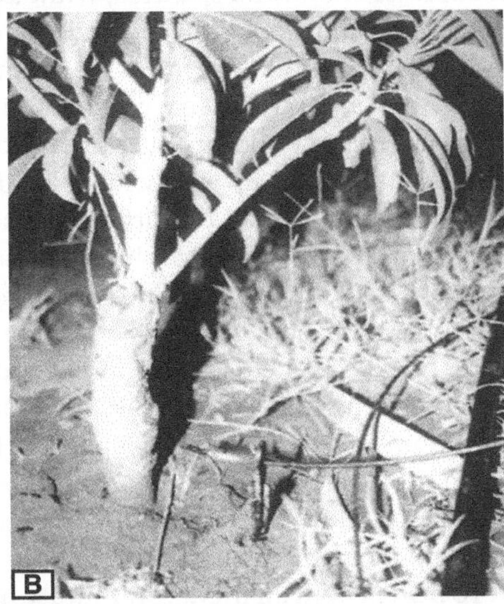

Figs 3.3A and B: Drip irrigation can save the water and get good harvest. Thus, water is used in minimum which helps in areas of scarcity of water yet get maximum benefits

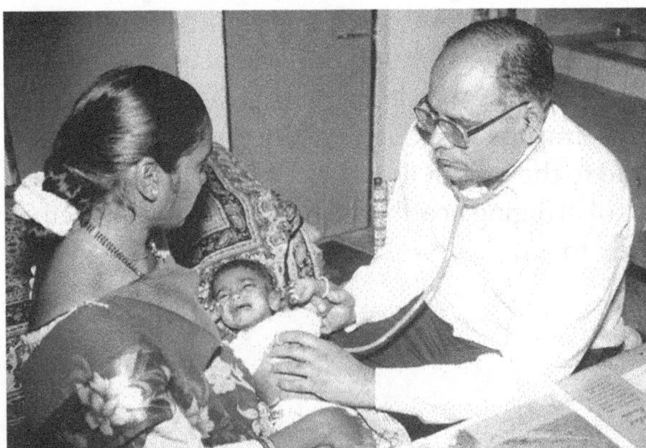

Fig. 3.4: Health care services essential in community. Health care practice. Health is multidimensional

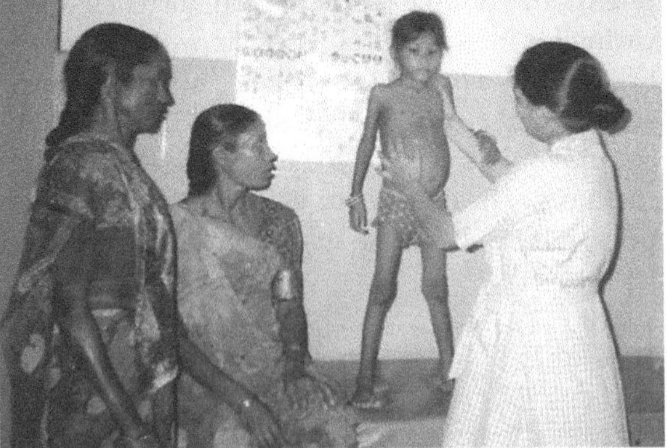

Fig. 3.5: Roles and responsibilities of field functionary: Developing rapport with family and its issues of health. Process involving the well-being of whole person

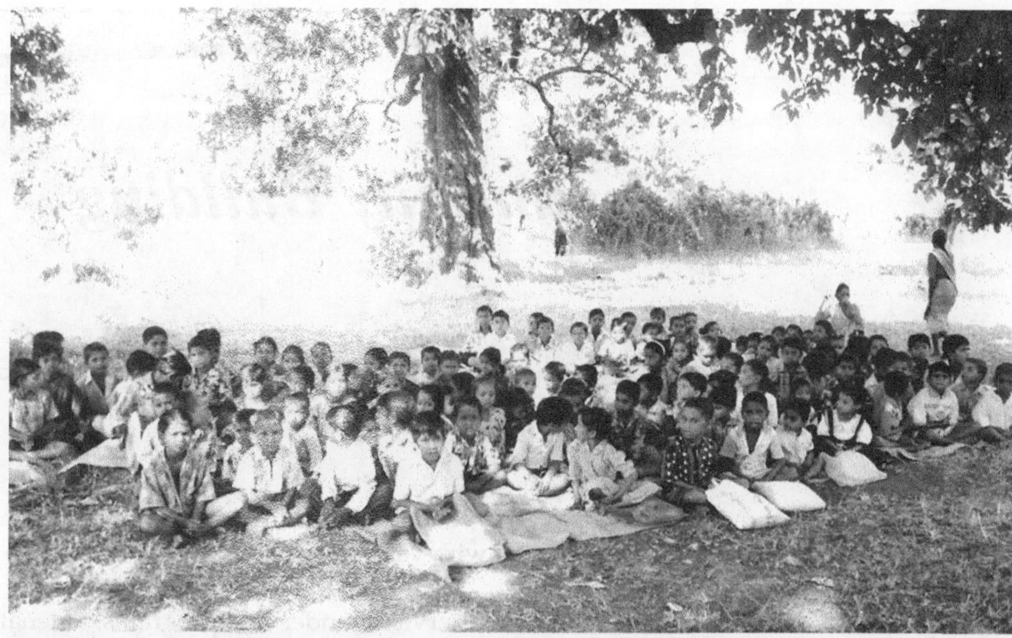

Fig. 3.6: Health and education of children are foundational; education is the only thing that will change the face of the society, building the future of the nations depends on this children. Towards tomorrow together

4 Community Building

To build community we have to teach people ways of achievement to motivate for further building community by taking initiatives at various levels with various activities and awareness to pool in resources and increase own contribution.

Nature of activities can be focused are Curative services, under five programs, antenatal care, tuberculosis, leprosy, health workers, health education, organizing Mahila Mandals. Other works such as land development and land leveling, irrigation and drinking water schemes, seeds and fertilizers for agriculture, forestry in a few places, dairy co-operatives, education formal and non-formal, Free legal aid and other programs. By which they are empowered and community building is enhanced.

To achieve this we have to use modern approach to build the capacity of the people by giving them knowledge and skills through the schools, vocational training, courses, tailoring, embroidery. So they are prepared to see for themselves and to feel that this is my community program for my community welfare. This needs a defined and well-documented program planning, modified in relation to situation and resources and manpower available.

Aim is to improve the pathetic condition of the families by improving their status in the community; help to build in confidence in their lives to restart life in a meaningful way. The feeling of having something of own will be achieved by this planning. Every improvement in health and other development will have an impact on the social and economic sphere.

Improvement in water system restoration to their houses will definitely improve the condition of women. Providing formal and non-formal education; literacy level will go up and regular attendance in the school will increase with less dropouts. They themselves will be responsible for school building maintenance. They will benefit from community center and village administration offices. The community organization program along with livelihood will create overall impact on the lives of the community. The quality of the life will improve, as the livelihood of many families in the village will be rejuvenated. The income level will increase which will lead to quality improvement in social life, economic life and cultural sphere. The villages will live as one community with less caste and communal difference, which will lead to the nation building process.

What is rural community and community health? Why do nursing schools include community health in their syllables? Without health can you think of happiness? No. The secret of happiness in life is fullness, wholeness; when health is a way of life, well being follows, that is optimal living. Health is considered to be superior to wealth. Health itself is wealth. So you have to invest in health, which will give you hundred fold back on maturity day that no other investment is ever able to give you because you will have sound mind sound body in sound soul and you will enjoy peace and harmony with self and with the universe that is surrounded by you. You will live long healthy life.

In today's sky jet age people just run after wealth and lose their health and later in life they lose wealth to get back that lost health, Then it becomes too late and no amount of wealth is able to give your health back that you have lost. They become miserable and are not able to enjoy wealth collected as their lifeline is shortened or they will be suffering from one or more major diseases. Therefore, health is well defined as a state of complete physical, mental and social, spiritual well being and not merely an absence of disease or infirmity. So if you learn how to live healthy balanced life, you can prevent 80% of life-threatening disease, which are prevented by following living healthy lifestyle.

As the nursing profession makes big strides forward into the new millennium the quality of nurse as a leader in all level and in all areas need to rise as a modern styles of leadership, intellectual, skills, sensitive towards current social issues and commitment to the cause of social justice, to work with integrity, creativity, dynamism; where wider horizons are open to enhance professional knowledge. Learning new skills to strive new vision, achieve extraordinary results.

Today health is considered as one of the fundamental rights of man. To protect and promote the health of its citizens is a primary duty. It has been observed that in regions where better public health action took place health level went up. In today's world of fast forward ultra model life, globalization, privatization, and liberalization, fast food modernization, unhealthy competition, tensions of heavy responsibilities, unhealthy living has increased disease like diabetic, heart problem, cancer.

There is a significant relationship between poverty and the poor health status. On an economic point of view in the develop country take great care of public health. They have so many schemes for the welfare of public. Their people are very healthy because government takes care of them. Old, crippled, handicapped, widows, are very well looked after by government.

Whereas developing country like India, health care is determined by poverty; some rural areas where they lack basic needs have neither money nor resources people die of hunger, starvation, Poverty and lack of food first hits the women and children the most. Government is responsible to provide universal education, safe drinking water. Poor people cannot afford to pay the health services so government has to have a health budget higher for the free services of rural public. Where they too deserve the quality services that is holistic and affordable.

Doctors trained at huge public cost are not available to serve the rural areas. Modern health services are generally urban based and elite orientated. Majority of people in this country after independence have no meaningful form of health care. In spite of progress made by modern medicines, millions of people in India are deprived of the most basic form of health care.

The problem of disease, malnutrition; psychological oppression and waste of human potential resources are linked with the socio-economic reality where low wages, bonded labors, exist where health system is only a part. The distribution of health care is unjust and uneven. The many who suffer chiefly from poverty and poverty related diseases in the rural areas and urban slums are the marginalized people. We need to focus on basic factors like health education and nutrition.

There is imbalance in the health of a public, which results in illness or disease due to social environment like social norms, taboos, customs, culture, religion, economic status, standard of living too affect the poor both physically and mentally. People in the community belong to different castes, classes, which has varieties of beliefs traditions. The balancing between these is crucial.

In order to keep good health it is necessary to improve the living conditions of people who live in urban slum and rural community. In order to make people aware of their health, community health nursing is very important and is taught in nursing schools.

As community is an agglomeration of families living together in a fixed locality/specific geographical area for fulfilling the common end that is economical, social, religious and political.

Whenever the member of any group, small or large live together in such a way that they share, not this or that particular interest, but the basic life, we call that group a community. The community may be described as the entire population occupying a certain territory held together by a common system of rules regulating the intercourse of life interrelated. And this is the community need building all round.

The closer the hospital to the community, the more will be the utilization of health services. Whereas people from slums are exposed to a greater risk of falling victims of infection than people living in a sophisticated area.

Community health is people oriented. Our approach, our focus is group, **people's movement**, issues related to people's needs. It was the community and not the individual who came to be considered as the entity for which health services are needed. Therefore, the individual who is a part of a family, which in turn is a part of a community, were required to be healthy as a healthy individual is a part of healthy nation.

The community health is aimed in prevention of diseases through good nutrition and immunization. Community health nursing is science of caring. The first nurse on this earth must have been the mother with her motherly instinct. She nursed her baby, with her maternal cum nurse like feelings to the sick and ailing.

Nursing and medicine go together. Medicine is the science of curing while nursing is the science of caring. Religion too has always helped people to be kind, generous, and helpful towards the young, old, invalids and sufferers. Nursing was considered a part of ones religious duty. The early religious sects devoted their life to nursing the lepers and sick and injured people. This raised the status of nursing as a profession. Women from rich, noble families, elderly women, widows and virgins joined the religious sects to render nursing services to the poor, sick and ailing. They build monasteries and hospitals in Europe like St Benedictine, St Demonic, St Francis of Assisi, the well known monks, who personally visited places in search of the ailing and sick and provided them with nursing care.

Florence Nightingale was the founder of modern nursing. She was born on 12th may 1820 in well -to-do family. She wanted to serve humankind. When Crimean war broke in 1854 between Britain, France and Turkey on one side and Russia on the other, she saw the condition of the sick and injured were deplorable and many were dying want of care. She offered her service with 38 nurses and builds hospitals and started her work, giving priority to cleanliness. Due to her devotional service the mortality rate came down from 42 to 22 percent within one year.

She used to take rounds of the ward holding a lamp even in the midnight so she was nicknamed the lady with the lamp. Her work at war casualty not only helped the military hospital but also raised their quality of work; she helped to raise the status of nursing. On her return to Britain after the war, she founded Queen Alexandra's imperial military services. In 1914, they recruited women for nursing.

After independence it came to know as an Indian military service. Evolution and development of community health nursing in India during the Vedic age, importance was given to health. The ruins of ancient civilization—Harappa showed relics of planned cities and houses built with public baths and underground drainage system, which suggest that they observed proper environmental sanitation. The ayurveda and siddha system of medicine also indicate the importance of health. During period of Buddhist and Jain rulers, importance given to tree plantation, wells to provide clean drinking water for travelers together with human and veterinary hospitals indicates their awareness of the health problems in India. All these facts show that the profession of nursing existed even in ancient India.

In 19th century, public health era gave importance to good sanitation and environment, mother and child health, communicable disease, family planning and Geriatrics. In 20th century, concept of community health was accepted.

In 1952, community development program was launched on 2nd October for development of rural areas. In 1978, the watchword health for all by 200 AD came into light.

India is a vast country with varieties of culture, variation in geographical factors, such as climate, people, and their eating and clothing habits, the dialect of language, religion, custom, traditions, cast and creed. India is second largest country in the world having the largest population with such a vast variation found everywhere she has large problems to deal with in all aspects of life.

Community health has a shift from Hospital, Health Centers, to strong community participation, self-help contribution to self-reliance. Rural community who need most of our attention, holistic health is an answer.

It is the felt need of the people and there is a growing need for Primary Health Care facilities for all sectors of society, especially the most remote and poor. It involves people's participation at all levels of planning, implementation and review. Sixty percent of the diseases can be cured by preventive and promotive measures that any rural health worker or housewife can learn, without the specialized skills of a doctor or the expensive amenities of a hospital.

Health apparently does not claim to have all the answers nor does it promise the solution of a Utopia. What is rather tries to convey is that Health is a concern of the Nation at large where people matter.

UNICEF findings about child-one kid die in India every 15 seconds. In India, 2.1 million children die annually before reaching their 5th birthday. Fifty percent of them not survive even 28 days. Globally the number stands at 9.7 million annually. The statistics are equally shocking among neonates, children newborn to a maximum age of 28 days old. While around 4 million children die within the 1st 28 days of life across the planet every year. India records around one million of the cases. Of the 19 million infants in the developing world who have low birth weight. 8.3 million are in India that is 43% of all the world's infants who are born with a low birth weight are in India. Malnutrition continues to affect newborns and young children and has been found to be the underlying cause of up to 50% of under five deaths. About 55 million or 1/3 world children under five are under weight. India's future lies with these children. Immunization, exclusive breastfeeding, vitamin A supplement can greatly reduce child death.

Total life foundations are being laid and built during these years of their lifetime; where most of his health habits and attitudes are formed. Life and happiness depended on the protection he gets. Total childcare, the child must be cared for with due respect, fed, nursed, helped, educated, sheltered and his talents must be developed. Teach mothers the signs of malnutrition, inspect and find in home visits, give adequate protection against diseases conservation, urge prompt advice ways of medical help, observe child's social habits and behavior, detect early symptoms of deviation and help them to understand normal signs of growth and development. Inspect the child at regular interval.

Maintain resistance through good **nutrition** give dal soup, eggs, scrapped meat, demonstrate how to prepare, cook and introduce new foods in diet. How you approach family and how they receive you. What can be done when need comes into surface. When you perceive family needs what action you plan to solve that need which family can get benefit. Your logical thinking is vital. People must understand the reason for change; there are varied possibilities for health promotion.

Modern public health is designed to prevent disease, prolong life and to promote physical and mental efficiency through organized community efforts. Attempts to control and eradicate prevalence of disease from the community effort made to persevere the customs of people and prevailing social and economical condition of the people. Many agencies working towards a common goal to enrich and rise standard of living of the community, cooperation and coordination with all welfare groups.

We have to keep in mind the basic principles of community development. Activities undertaken should be initiated in response to the felt needs of the people. The community should be encouraged to actively participate in their own program so as to become independent in local self-government by trained local leadership. Encourage participation of women and youth in community and tap the resources of the voluntary non-governmental organizations.

The **self-help projects** of the community must be encouraged by intensive and extensive assistance from the state. Leading rural population from chronic underemployment to full employment, agricultural underproduction to full production by application of scientific knowledge, and cooperation by making rural families credit worthy. The local people have to contribute an equal amount in work, materials and money.

Community development program is the responsibility of the block development officer and the Panchayat Raj, the local self-government since 1958. District collector is link between the govt. and the people. Self-help to uplift our villages on an organized and continuing basis arouses and encourages the people to utilize their resources fully for the development of the area. It has to promise cooperative way of life in the community based on the ideals of manual aid and thrift leading to rural upliftment.

Health is an integral part of the community development because standards of health care closely linked with economic and social structure of the community. The community projects are bright, vital and the dynamic sparks, which radiate rays of energy, hope and enthusiasm. Let community workers strive to add and to the sparks, so that he who toils in the fields on India will enjoy optimal health, to keep the torch of democratic freedom alight in the free India.

Work experience of community building and people's awakening— In remote area my work began with visiting the villages, which were quite far from the center, daily, visiting and knowing the family and family needs and health problems things begun to take shape, malnutrition and tuberculosis, was a prominent health issue. Found that people had lack of health education knowledge, due to poverty they did not have enough food to eat. They could not afford the medicines and even seriously ill could not reach to the center for first aid due to lack of roads and vehicle facility and no money. First work was conducting a free medical camp and then doing the follow-up. Organized immunization camps and people who needed the specialized treatment shifted to civil hospital and even private doctors who were ready to do the treatment at nominal charge. Ordinary simple people lacking basic necessities of life and were living in below poverty line, food they had was not nourishing worked hard even to get that, they were miserable living in utter poverty. The life in the village becomes silent by eight, as they are too tired working in hot sun when it turns dark they go to bed and get up early to walk back to the place of daily wages or fields.

Starting were very difficult to gather them to talk to them and to do follow-up consumed lot of time and energy, some times they would give us the timing of meeting and when you reach there no one to be seen and again go visiting and motivate them to come together.

Slowly and steadily were able to win the confidence when they knew we really were interested in their welfare and all that happens to them and together we could find solution. Initially women use to be in covered faces and lacked confidence, it was hard to convince them, but women who had some leadership qualities were motivated; and taken to the center for training; for health education, to overcome blind beliefs, that illness are caused by virus and not by evil spirits, first aid medicines; on small illness like cold, cough, diarrhea, fever etc. drew the pictures of this sickness and stuck them on the medicinal box so that they can remember with action what sickness the medicines are.

Also with test and color would recognize the drug. On and off three months initial training gave then just few medicines, which were good, and no side effect. Surrounding people started coming to them in time of pain and sickness and we could see with our own eyes our hands reaching out and extending through this ignorant women begun excelling and building confidence and slowly people begun accepting and trusting them and started reveling their problems, all that they could handle they use to handle and the difficult case they would accompany them to the center and the chain of work was formed. They began excelling and became a challenging force.

While training we use to demonstrate to them diet with bringing the potatoes, dal, rice, pulses etc and what each thing contains, so they could remember, few points only drilling over and over again and revising it again they would learn a concept and its importance. There were times one is to feel good and happy there were times of defeat and frustration and I have asked myself am I wasting my time will any good come from here, but as time went by things slowly and steadily were working and bad habits were becoming lessen and superstitious beliefs were reduced, such as lot of snake bit cases were treated with prompt action by reaching them in time to the hospital.

As NGO point of view its use to be difficult at times to manage all aspects of health, people wanted all the medicines free which use to be costly antibiotics, if we tell them to get it they would not complete the course and would not retune back to the clinic, starting I use to feel is it my need or it is the need of the people, why cannot they come in time for medical care, my way of thinking and there was different, they had so many other social problems embedded into their bone marrow and so many customs and cultures took long way to understand. But as some one has said where there is will there is way there are great miracles, and every problem has a solution only one needs strong determination and will power to do it.

Experience that for good work if one wills helping hands come and patients never went without medicines or treatment. Even the most serious and chronic cases once we took up some ones help reached. While working in the rural areas I realized one has to be committed, dedicated, and available always with consistency, ready to take risk and challenges. As time went by I was able to find a place in this peoples heart, even hungry and thirsty but received lot of respect and love from simple and humble people which's memorable and treasureable which I learnt by living and working with this people the art of living happy life. Taught me simple living and high thinking, less laughed and more comfort. Which left the footprints on the hearts of people whom I touched and they touched me remains imprinted until this day. Though there were time you felt supported there was time you did not feel it, at times neglected and other times full of zest and vitality life went through difficulties. Together with health workers training, formed Mahila Mandals, and cooperated into other developmental programs. Due to a enriched experience we were able to conduct mega medical camps, and celebrate elder's day and run mobile clinics, and take rural poor to different cities for exposure.

Mobile clinic experience too was unique, just to reach to the people as a medical person learnt driving and with ambulance use to go 60-65 km away in the jungle areas where people were living, a day was fixed and the people would be waiting in one hut/house. As soon as you reach over huge crowed of patients would be already there, you alone with one helper start examining and giving treatment, from morning 8 O'clock to night 9 you reach home tired and exulted but with deep satisfaction that you were able to elevate and take away some pain and suffering of people who were my unfortunate brethren and children of mother India but poor and living in remote deep jungles. They had very few needs, life was full of simplicity.

Villages where I worked had needs and problems of poverty, malnutrition, immunization, housing problem, sanitation and every other problem together with lack of finance and education. Whenever conducted my gathering or program we had to give them the incentives that provides food and travelling fair and the daily wages. Just for educational purpose, they had no time, so initially incentives to be given. Showing them a film, puppet shows, role-play they use to feel happy, some novelty by which we could give them the message. I have never seen an obese person in the areas, they were below normal weight and at times to get things had to walk miles and miles away.

One has to mingle with people with their way of talking and in a way; they find it comfortable to approach you. They must feel that you are part of them and you become part of their family. You had to go keeping in mind do not know when you will return, for them time moves slowly and we have to move with their space. Here we run jet age but still there are people living far behind the modern times. They have still the curiosity, innocence, and novelty when they see something new. Though today technology is advancing fast and villages are being connected and people have started having TV, radios, mobiles but vast of them still to be covered and lag far behind.

Always getting permission of the elders of the village and giving them the importance and respect they deserve is vital. They would be listening to you with spell bound attention if you speak their language I realized there is an inner thirst to know more about self and about positive thoughts that builds once lives thirst for truth.

They have taught me the herbal medicines which use to grow in the seasons, they know which roots, which leaves useful and how and when to give. So I have tried to use there own knowledge to women who can use this harmless herbs and cure themselves.

The test of living with such a simple people, eating with them talking part in all there rituals and ceremonies is an unique experience, as you loose something you gain some things, you learn to live happy and contented life with few things that needs one to be happy. There you find value in sacrificing part of your life for them, especially when you have to make a carrier and build your life you opted for something deeper facially not valued. When you go the shy but welcoming smile, the food from their scarcity sharing with you and trying to give the best they have, their generosity and spirit of helping each other and the common solidarity they feel when any joyful or a sad situation arise. They have their group spirits and one bond which united them as one family.

During my years of work with the rural set up lots of good experience I had such as in time reaching to the patient have saved life specially during an emergency when a *dais* is trying to conduct delivery and in spite of prolonged difficult labor and risk she fails to see the need of shifting I have reached and rushed the patient to the nearby hospital and thus saved mother and the child. Due to the presence of mind there have been need for artificial respiration , cardiac massage and reviewed patient back to life, and seeing this the faith and trust of the people have increased due to skilled and technique of my profession. Knowledge is power and when it used in right place can help tremendously. There were time a poisonous snake bits have come and I have rushed them to the hospital in time patient gets treatment and life is saved, there are numberless such experience during my service in the community which has helped large villagers. I have tried to train the health workers and Mahila Mandal women's on different issues related to their way of life in a areas set up where they live and work.

Children whom given proper nutrition and have improved from pigeon hold chest and rickets, I realized villagers body have not experience lot of drug or antibiotics consumptions and so with little sickness due to lack of stamina they become serious and also recover with proper short time interval and very well react to the medicines.

No one by birth born great we are product of training and education we have received, villagers no way inferior to any person given them chance they excel was my personal experience. Starting when I came in first contact with them I found some of them do not even know the difference between dirt filth and cleanliness, they hardly cared about personal hygiene such as once on my visit when they gave me tea they wiped with the end of sari with which they have wiped the buttocks of a baby after defecation, they have served food with scabies hand, children after defecation do not use water but stone or leaves or just wipe themselves sitting on mud, always nose leaking, spitting anywhere, the towel they used is used for so many purpose one time you see at the wrapped around west and next moment wiping the face, the water they get looked like a tea, from the river just raw without boiling have it, the mothers who feed the babies if they come near you one will get foul smell as they never change the blouse and all the milk that oozes out dries and the feeding continues, mouths will be smelling either with tobacco, liquor or lack of oral hygiene, all and much more they had been doing because they have never seen he world beyond them, they have no idea what so ever how the plain looks like, what is the ocean with so much water and so vast and limitless, and the tall building etc.

But with constant effort and exposure education things are changing, now they send children to schools, their house is clean, they have better personal hygiene, they look decent, and many of the bad habits that use to affect their health are seen changed and better situation created. We cannot blame people alone for the rural situation and their health condition, everyone is responsible in one way or the other we contribute, we have to give some of our precious services to this outreached downtrodden people who needs to be brought to the mainstream without them no progress is possible. It would be like white washed tombs outside good and inside dead manes born. Preciousness of life is same for all may he be poor or reach all have to live with human dignity as children of god from same place we came and to the same place all will return. If you want to test the sweetness of a meal eat with the poor they do not have much ingredients and simple little oil and masalas but the test they have however you try you will not able to have it, it is a nature who provides for all needs only one has to share time and talents and joint hands for the common cause of community building and building the nation.

There are series of pictures in this book which shows different angels of community health, such as clinic set up, mother and child health, training of health workers, conducting Mahila Mandals meetings, health education and training of *dais*, youth capacity building and training, under five clinic, suppliantly diet, growth monitoring, elders health, tuberculosis treatment, out reach mobile clinics, school health, balwadis and Anganwadi, rituals and programs, life style of people, malnourished all these will give in one flash in nut shell all the ideas about the rural work and its set up where 72% of our India lives there day-to-day life. The real face of India is total urban elite group moving forward with rocket speed and the snail speed the interior remote villages where our brothers and sisters who live. Progress and development has its own prose and corns and its own advantages and disadvantages.

As rural people have lot of peace they work only for the day they never think of the next day what will happen, when they do not want to work they do not, no rush and push, get up early and go to bed early. Life passes by, time is not an important commodity, live for the day, follow the natural law of nature and God fearing simple people with less accumulation and less tension, no loss or gain, whereas in cities the picture is different, lot of tensions and stress to compete, the more higher you climb the more you need and harder you work and less time for yourself and the end become the bundle of diseases. Who is happier the modern man or the rural man. Health is sum total of all this balance healthy way of living nothing too extreme. Villages we have more malnutrition in cities we have obesity related illness, both are bad they become anemic, get more respiratory disease and here we get diabetics, cardiovascular problem. Poor throws away clothes when it tears and the rich throws away when the fashion changes. The more sophisticated you are more the harder effort to cope up. They have less but more comfort, so to achieve total health balance in work, rest, food.

I prostrate before God for having accompanying and enlightening inspiring me to contribute a part of me to the society. A constant guiding light of God and the simple love of the poor that showed me the way to wisdom, knowledge and understanding.

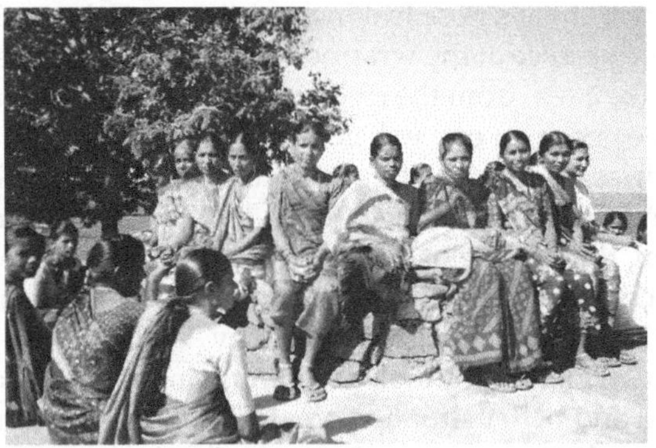

Fig. 4.1: Given an opportunity, people grow. Planning care according to the health needs. No one by birth is born great, it is through process of learning and hard work one can build self and community

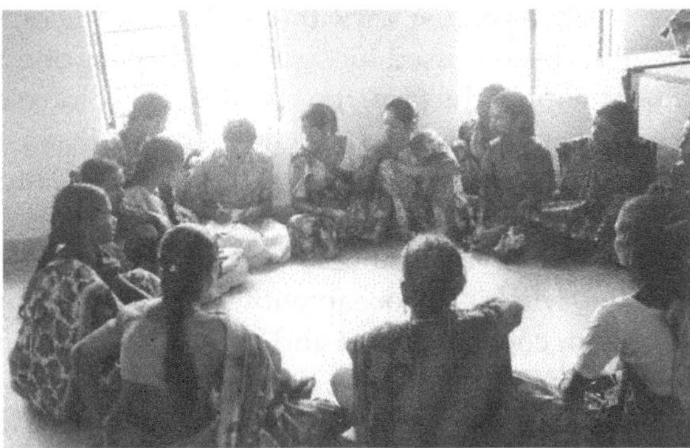

Fig. 4.2: Community decision through dialogue: a process of transforming social and economic life of women with active participation and community initiatives through community efforts, thus awakening, improving their own condition as a group

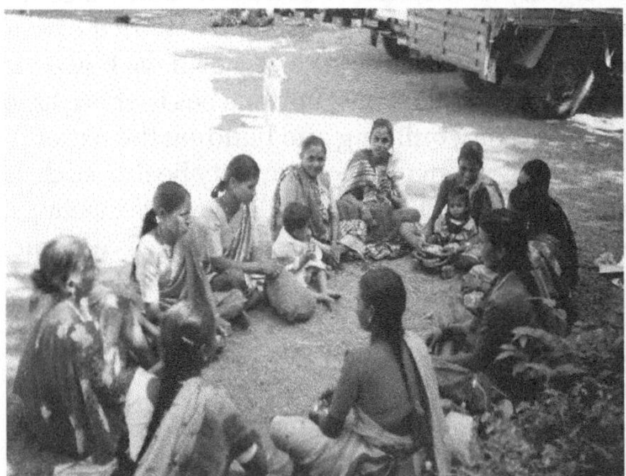

Fig. 4.3: United we stand. Communicating effectively and discussing common issues affecting the lives of rural women's community

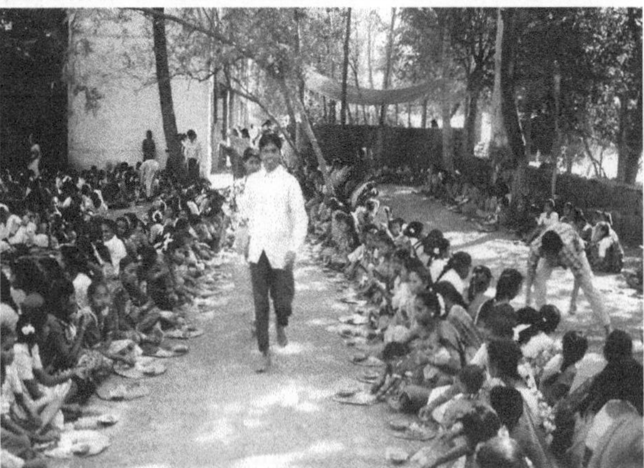

Fig. 4.4: Sharing life and using opportunities for health awareness and bonding together

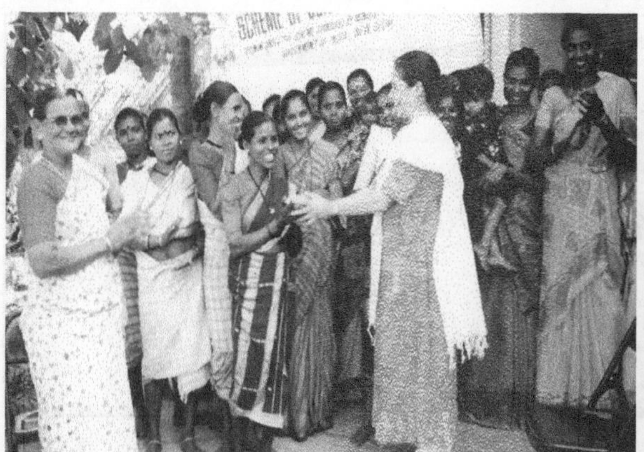

Fig. 4.5: Placing people's health in people's hands. Health in your own hands, we are just facilitators

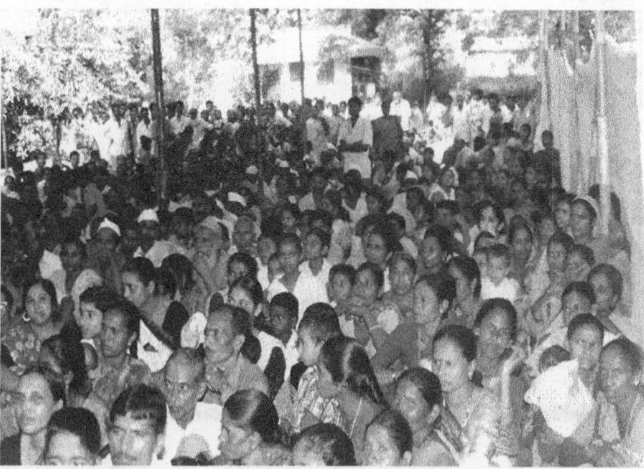

Fig. 4.6: Increasing collective action and bargaining power. Empowering community through education, planning and organization

5 Community Welfare

The word prosperity most frequently refers to increase in material wealth. Not so often, it refers in a wider sense to all round development of individuals and society, with justice and social equity being the corner stone. There is perhaps no society, past or present, in which all sections of people have become prosperous, especially in the latter sense; right of every human being to life, liberty and the pursuit of happiness. Any holistic view of prosperity should therefore consider its social or human costs at least as seriously as its material costs. In today's India, prosperity is the privilege of the few at the cost of the needs and dreams of the majority who are the socially and economically backward classes regardless of their religion.

The narrow concept of prosperity is increase in material wealth, neglecting natural justice and social equity in an ambience of greed for power and material possessions that has made the world what it is today.

Prosperity of society as a whole, which includes justice and equity, enhances the quality of life of the individuals in society.

Whereas prosperity of an individual material wealth and comfort rises, the standard of living of the individual but does little for the quality of life of society.

A process designed to create conditions of economic and social progress for the whole community with its active participation and the fullest possible reliance upon the community's initiative. In community health nursing to study the various health problems the study of national program is necessary, Nurses have a magnificent role to play in implementing Primary Health Care in the community. **School Health Services** are considered very important and integral part of the total community health services.

We know how important it is to focus on the right interventions. Health systems need to reach all and not only the fortunate few.

What are the challenges? Those living in absolute poverty are five times more likely to die before reaching the age of five and two-and-half times more likely to die between the ages of 15 and 19, than those in higher-income groups.

Why is better health an important component of poverty reduction? Ill-health is both a cause and a consequence of poverty. llness can reduce household savings, lower learning ability, reduce productivity and lead to a diminished quality of life – thus creating or perpetuating poverty. Today, effective medicines and control strategies are available to dramatically reduce ill health.

Which health strategies are effective in reducing poverty? Poverty undermines development. Poverty is an attack on human rights and human dignity. Poverty creates political and social instability. Countries cannot afford massive poverty. The goal of having the number of poor people by 2015 is achievable. But it will require broad effort from all of us. By reducing risks through a broader approach to public health, focusing on the health problems of the poor, ensuring that health systems serve the poor effectively; Perception—Change is crucial.

Skilled managers can tap the talents of their employees through various motivational strategies. By adding variety to routine actions, the work itself becomes a group effort that is fun and challenging and produces a sense of achievement for the entire team.

Enhancement of purchasing power, creation of adequate employment opportunities and redistribution of economic growth can together improve the health of the rural people; but to achieve these we need to mobilize and channellize the available resources.

Developmental welfare help the community towards socio-economic sustainability through Bunding, Check dams, excavation of old ponds, grow nursery, plant trees, orchard growing, organic farming, construct low cost latrine, land leveling by constructing farm pond and re-generate the life of wells.

Recognition of artwork, developing **youth capacity** by giving training skill to upgrade, establish network, provide economic viability, build low-cost houses, and construct cattle camps during drought, construct smokeless Chula, distributing saplings, get them land for cultivation, poultry farming. Welfare and **income generating schemes,** scholarships for poor children and provide health services affordable and accessible for all.

People's court to solving local disputes, land disputes, matter of fidelity and ill treatment of women, anti-liquor campaign, and elicit distilling, excessive drinking, organizing village fairs-and festivals, and new agricultural development, teach to distinguish different kinds of seeds, how to use fertilizers, pesticides and how to irrigate, care and maintenance of pumping installations, through basic education meetings to exchange views and experiences, to give feedback.

This helps them to live better quality of life and show them how to improve their own condition, where people learn to rely on their own inner strength in the struggle for better life. It becomes a **people's movement,** and have livelihood with dignity.

Public health services in rural area need proper reviewing in the functioning to be effective and successful. That means to have more funds to invest in modern infrastructure, human resources, drugs and vaccines at affordable costs, adapting to the sociocultural factors and economic resources of the community. Today's sophisticated technology will be unaffordable to the rural poor who have low income, limited education, and inadequate diet.

Reduce the distance and long waiting hours, which discourage people using **public services. Community nurse** has wider role, as she is involved with client as well as client's family at their homes and community, which includes culture, customs and tradition. She is a link between families, doctor and rural community. She is an important pillar and an important member to provide significant and comprehensive health. She has to build a bridge and cement between the healths services to the community and the families.

She has collective responsibilities, which includes all dimensions of holistic health. She has to plan and organize regular in service program. Her role demands that she possesses a thorough knowledge, innovative ideas to provide leadership. Where she can assess and mobilize, provide, maintain, collaborate, and motivate community involvement. So that care is made available, accessible and affordable and appropriate to all.

She is directly related in linkage system of the community based. She has to be well orientated with other groups and agencies working in the community, which are helping to uplift and promote the total health needs and their statues. So that services that are reasonably inexpensive and have the basic essentials required by rural population is provided. So that marked change can be expressed in terms of lives saved, death prevented, cases treated and life expectation prolonged.

Give to every other human being every right that you claim for yourself. It is difficult to reach everybody everywhere at all times so together with government other agencies have to fill this gap coordinating, collaborating, and establishing health care activities. Community nurses have to coordinate her work with different social welfare services. As one never knows when an ailment is going to strike.

Today the community Health Nurse has a tremendous job in the control and eradication programs. Her job will be to visit the cases periodically in the homes, maintain adequate records and see that regular treatment is taken. Certain diseases have great sociological and psychological implications for the clients and their families. Therefore, it is important she has right attitude about the disease prevention. Utilize other resources and help from various agencies to open fresh paths in the lives of clients.

To provide basic nursing, administer medications and treatments prescribed by PHC doctor, observe the illness, prevent any complications, teach the family regarding, prevention of disease and promotion of health, provide comprehensive care to the individual and community by teaching at various levels, participate in research works related to health, conserve life and to promote health. 72.2% population live in rural communities and due to shortage of doctors nurse in this area will be involved both in caring for clients with serious and fatal infectious diseases and in helping to develop public health programs for their control.

Nurses' important function in child health, high birth rate, high IMR, fetal diseases being diarrhea, pneumonia and protein or calorie malnutrition in early childhood. Nurse builds up a relationship by altering the behavior patterns and convincing people to build trust for positive health, infant welfare, and immunization. Family planning involves the nurse in helping parents to avoid too large families, which over extend their financial resources and burden the mother with the care of too many children and constant pregnancies may ultimately affect the mother's health.

Nursing today has all the hallmarks of a profession; it mirrors their diverse roles and new tasks, which are more complex. With use of computer, clinical investigation advanced in scientific knowledge the role and function of a nurse has been extended. Techniques which were formally regarded as the doctors province may now be cried out by the nurse like dialysis the doctors relies on the nurse to report any change in patients condition or any adverse treatment she has observed which may lead him to alter his line of treatment.

To meet common good to develop value system that enhances the trust, confidence and commitment of members of the community. It includes putting the community interests ahead thus our collective progress is predicated on sound values. There are two pillars of the cultural value system – loyalty to family and loyalty to community.

The most important attribute of a progressive society is respect for others who have accomplished more that they themselves have, and learn from them. If we have to progress, we have to change this attitude, listen to people who have performed better than us, learn from them and perform better than them. You are held accountable for what you do.

However, is it an organization or society, there are different people performing different roles. For success, all these people are required to discharge their duties. This includes everyone from the CEO to the person who serves tea – every role is important. We do not seem to respect the other person's time. The Indian Standard Time somehow seems to be always running late. Deadlines are typically not met. How many public projects are completed on time?

Right from a very young age, parents have to teach their children to be independent in thinking, where child can grow up to be strong, confident individuals. We need to overcome this attitude if we have to succeed globally. "People that values its privileges above its principles soon loses both." Our duty is towards the community as a whole, as much as it is towards our families.

We have to remember that fundamental social problems grow out of a lack of commitment to the common good. Most of our behavior comes from greed, lack of self-confidence, and lack of respect for the society. To borrow Gandhi's words: "There is enough in this world for everyone's need, but not enough for everyone's greed". Let us all be responsible citizens who make our country a great place to live.

Develop rapport with family and collect information about family. Provide home care and perform simple procedures at home. Gives appropriate health education; evaluating with follow-up, recording and reporting. Assesses health needs, maintains safe, conducive environment, apply scientific principles, and meet health needs of client, as planned. Evaluate clients' responses to given care, re-examines and modifies care plan. Report accurately, record precisely and promptly.

Assist in the examination of household contacts specially children. Help the family, understand the nature of disease, Observe and demonstrate nursing care. Assist with diagnosis and treatment. Encourage the family to come regularly for the treatment. Teach about care of hands and feet, home isolation is important; see the drugs are taken regularly, emphasis on footwear, ulcers to be dressed regularly. Establish confidence, to convince client of the need for treatment. Take history with confidentially and tactfully.

Community Health Nurse (CHN) can assist in the care of aged by helping the family to provide safe housing good diet, happy surrounding and some kind of recreation. This will help them to overcome infection, mental strain and frustration. Clients who are bedridden due to illness, she frequently visits demonstrates feeding, bath back care, if required placement in old age homes; it is a challenging responsibility and a new dimension of community health nurse. She must learn, understand and practice many new skills such as detection, prevention handling of hazards and first aids.

Community nurse to be aware of infectious diseases that pose threat to people's lives, emergency care in acute conditions requiring immediate treatment, such as heart attack, accidents, poisoning, burns, labor etc.

The all pervasive and extreme poverty has haunted the human conscience throughout the recorded history. Humanity has triumphed over many insurmountable obstacles, conquered several afflictions and survived many conflicts to surge forward with grit and perseverance. But the enigma of poverty never ceased to be a drag on human progress. Poverty reduction is happening, but not at the speed with which it is required.

What promise does the future holds for our poor after 58 years of Independence? Are more windows of opportunities opening for the poor? More public action, private initiatives and voluntary movements are to be involved, giving the poor greater choices and opportunities. To spare no effort to free our fellow men, women and children from the object and dehumanizing conditions of extreme poverty.

Development has often bypassed the poorest people, and has even increased their disadvantages. The poor need direct action to bring them into the development process and create conditions for them to escape from poverty. **Income** is the most common criteria for measuring poverty and the standard method used for identifying it. But poverty cannot be seen merely as lowness of incomes. Poverty is deprivation and lack of opportunities in accessing social services as well as financial resources for the people.

Poverty determines the level of people's ability to meaningfully participate in society's economic, cultural or political activities. Poverty has a dehumanizing effect. It keeps people from realizing their inherent human potential, forces them into unequal relationships that severely limit their freedom.

Poverty is not just a matter of being relatively poorer than others in the society; but of not having some basic opportunities of material well being the failure to have certain minimum capabilities.

It is easier to steal from the poor precisely because they are poor. They neither see nor understand program guidelines, false measurement books of work done, false receipts of payments made. Health status of a community helps assess its poverty level and vulnerability. Any improvement in the health status of the poor will lead to better productivity and greater earning that will help rise from the state of poverty. Disasters like drought, flood, natural calamities etc. aggravate these situations.

Social mobilization leads to empowerment and development of human resources and helps to bring in radical social changes; meeting the basic needs including minimum food, shelter, clothing, health care and education entitlements of all the poor; providing income-generating opportunities; Paying special attention to women in poverty with a view to freeing them from their perpetual entrapment. Mobilizing unemployed youth through various skill development and vacation training programs. Taking special care of socially disadvantaged people through **various social welfare benefit schemes;** and sustains their economic development by creating special safety nets.

How and when will this progress get translated into better social opportunities for the poor and downtrodden?

Where and how do people live? At what age is the mortality highest and from what disease? What sections of the area are unhealthy and what is the underlining cause of death there? In comparison with similar area is this area healthy or not? In what sections of the area is improvement is achieved? In which parts on the other hand, is disease on the increase? Are certain diseases attacking specified groups of the population more than others? To what extent are the hospital facilities staffing, drugs and equipment able to cope with the disease problem?

Is there any season at which various diseases have a tendency to break out? Is the rate at which births occur in the population the same for various socio-economic levels? What factors are associated with higher or lower birth rate? Community Health Nurse (CHN) has to study geographical set up, population, customs and beliefs, social relationships, structure and health services to know the magnitude of the health problem for purpose of making comparisons with other areas.

It will help in meaningful involvement of the community in the planning. Her responsibilities are not just giving only care but also train support and supervise basic health workers in the community. They can be instrumental in bridging the gap between preventive and curative services; adapt to the sociocultural factors and economic resources of the community. To work in the rural areas, language plays a very important role in the communication.

In rural area most of the houses are attached to cattle sheds, using firewood and cow dung as fuel. There is no proper ventilation, lighting and drainage system. Many health hazards will emerge in the human environment from fumes of firewood and dried cow dung.

The purpose of community health is to help people attain high level of health and well being through various controls/prevent in the community; for that community nurse has to take suitable measures, evaluate programs, and improve methods and techniques. She will have to mobilizing appropriate community resources. The ultimate goal is to help people to achieve self-reliance on all aspects of health. She has to be well versed to provide health care in highest possible degree.

Her role is broad, and comprehensive she is lawfully accountable for professional behavior accountability for the care of the client. She holds prominent position where she develops capacity and sharpens her ability, links people and sustains, enhances in social transformation.

She has to look at the person as a whole along with his family and community in which he lives. She has to know that people move from the villages to the industrial areas leaving their families behind. **Society is a web of various social relationships;** this gives rise to overcrowding and unhygienic environment in the slums, which causes problems like alcoholism, drug abuse, and social evils.

Economic status is closely related to health. Ignorance and high fertility is common in poor. The type of work they do; they do not perceive health as a need when condition becomes fatal they seek last minutes cure. There is poor assess to availability of health services. So poor health has financial burden to the family to make them capable of improving their health through their own effort, for that community nurse has to motivate good personal relations with on going education guide and support. Make government schemes and income generative schemes available to them. Teaching of economic and social values is important in all her program. Before launching any program the communities need to be informed of risk and benefits; so as to provide comprehensive health.

Preventive is a growing concept of social or community medicines, to prevent occurrence as well as progression of disease and disability with timely intervention to promote health is important. To make every effort for disease prevention early diagnosis, screening, notification, monitoring and surveillance to control and elimination of all that dehumanizes the community. Health cannot be considered in isolation only community nurse cannot alone promote the health of the community. She works in collaboration with the health team. **Community health team** has responsibility for health care of entire community.

Nutrition is important single factor required to maintain health and improve resistance to disease. Community nurse sees that adequate nutrition is provided in the community for the people especially venerable group of mother and child to be healthy and diseases free. To maintain their body, sufficient calories, protein, fat, carbohydrate, green leafy vegetables and nutritional education on food hygiene to be taught to prevent infection, using diet locally available to reduce the cost of a meal.

Women's health is multifaceted and forms the core crucial part of general health. If her body does not get the proper kind of food in sufficient amount for maintaining health she suffers from malnutrition and becomes anemic, lethargic, fragile, weak, have low resistance, and is unable to do any hard work. Body needs food to build and to provide energy and replaces weak tear of tissues. **Food** gives body fuels for the production of health and energy. Food is essential for the healthy skin and mucous membrane. Additional food during pregnancy and lactation needs the special attention. If the diet is inadequate body becomes physically and mentally hampered, the vitality is lowered and has a low capacity to work.

Villages could be encouraged to plan **kitchen garden**, which provide fresh vegetables and fruits; which can help to improve the diet of the family. Teach them proper cooking which makes food easy for digestion. The success of family welfare service mainly depends on well-informed individuals and couples. She must utilize and explore various means of education for progress, as it is the essential component of Community Health Nurse (CHN) services. All health services are taken to the homes and family. Community Health Nurse (CHN) is a valuable asset to the community and to the health programs.

Community Health Nurse (CHN) is important pillar forming closest contact a bridge between health service and community, where family feels free and relaxed to voice their doubts and fears and is more receptive to any health advice, encourages family to state and discuss their problem in their own words. Nurses are backbone of community health. She binds homes together. Health is most prized, treasure, valuable possession. The community is taught to treasure health as the most valued possession. In health education the community has to be aroused from its ignorance and apathy and motivated to improve their state, this gradually results in long-term change in human behaviors.

She has to advise preventive measures such as boiling water, good nutritious diet, personal hygiene, **safe clean potable water**. Simple techniques like a hot towel soaked and squeezed in warm water and wrap around, chewing neem sticks for cleansing teeth is effective method, chewing paan, betal leaves should be discouraged. Regular splashing of cold water on the eye washes away the dust and the dirt, looking at distant greenery, wearing sunglasses. Avoid digging the ear, nose and ear picking, nail-biting habits. Be careful as insects crawl into the ear sleeping on flower or outdoor at night; do not introduce hairpins, pencil, pen, and stick in the ear.

While sitting, standing, wear flat slippers, use hard chair with straight back, relax by listening to music, playing games reading, sleep in a dark well aired quiet room on a flat mattress with a thin pillow. Daily intake of sufficient water, diet with adequate calories, avoid breeding flies, mosquitoes, rats, disposal of garbage, netting doors, windows, foods covered under wire mesh, discouraging sharing of combs, clips, pillows, towels. Cattle sheds, poultry houses build away from human dwelling these entire simple advices, which cost nothing and instill good health habits in the community.

Health services start from top national level and end at sub-center level to reach the last man in the last hut in the last rural family. Essence of community development 'of the people, by the people and for the people' its members become more involved, the community strides rapidly toward social and economic progress and this is the essence of community development.

Education should be adaptable to the local culture and language, and should build upon existing channels of communication – song, drama. Why should we expect the illiterate villager to adjust to the way of thinking of the educated man? Why should he alert his perception of the world to understand us? It is we who have to simplifying medical information that is full of technical words and jargons that often tend to distance community from providers. At the same time, we need to communicate technical information in a language that even lay people can easily understand. This not only increases the comprehension of the matter quickly but also the retention of the information for a longer time. We need to communicate all this "new" information in a manner, which is easily understandable to the people and their family members in the limited time available for a public health concern.

Women constitute a sizeable section of **rural work force**. The realization of women's full potential is crucial to the overall socioeconomic development and growth of the society. With regard to the multidimensional responsibilities, it is required to strengthen the status of rural women economically to enable them to stand in society on their own with confidence. Lower fertility leads to better health outcomes for both women and children. Health risks to infants and children are worse in poor families with more children. The main reasons for a male preference are not only the avoidance of a dowry later, but also a guarantee of the lineage of the family. A lower female ratio is a fairly clear indicator of a male dominated society. No female rights to the property, low female literacy rates, poor health, and domestic violence against women seem to be prevalent in conservative, in their thinking.

The emerging and spread of sex determination clinics are early warnings signals for the distortion of sex ratios at birth in the coming decade. If the abuses of sex determination and sex selection methods are not curbed, there will be greater demographic imbalance in the country in the coming decade. Violence against surviving women will increase dramatically as women become scarce for labor and marriage.

Providing accessible primary care at low cost, preventing illnesses and promoting good health, reducing the burden on hospitals, managing many health problems economically, and utilizing the healing systems like Ayurveda, Acupressure, Yoga and Homeopathy.

Ayurveda and Yoga have tremendous insights to offer in the area of prenatal, perinatal and postnatal health of the mother. Going by the alarming decline in the sex ratio, the **girl child** in India is doomed from the womb. Female infanticide is still practiced and mothers are forced to kill their own female infants. Instances of infant girls being abused are not uncommon.

Resorting people's livelihood through **skill development** and **gainful employment** are key factors. The grit and determination of the women to move on and achieve their targets result powerful development movement. As they have a collective strength as a group. The principle of self-reliance motivates the women. The process of sustainable empowerment has begun and will take these women through a journey that will establish the unlimited capacities of their spirit. "In the voice of many lies the heart of every woman – the heart that wants to be free and strong. This spirit is the celebration of women taking the first step to overcome the shackles of economic dependency, **gender insensitivity**, poverty and illiteracy." The challenge before us is to evolve strategies to break the stereotypes of the past by empowering women; it is necessary to make women equal partners in the national development process and equip them to make choices in order to actualize their self worth.

Many a time the state government does not consult the local communities before planning to develop an area into an industrial hub. The agricultural land is acquired for industrial estate from the villagers by paying compensation and promising jobs in the proposed units. However, the villagers soon realize that the promised jobs are nowhere to be seen, as industry requires skilled personnel. With their source of livelihood gone, the villagers often end up as contract laborers in the factories. Who pays for the cost of resettlement? Many people faced economic disruption. The cost of travel to workplace increased, so also the time. Women who had been working for daily wages also stopped going for work. In many houses there was a financial crisis pushing people into debt. For many children schooling stopped, dashing the hopes of the parents. While resettlement has been difficult for all, the greatest burden has fallen on those who had lower incomes.

Are you concerned about increased commercialization in the medical field? Are there ways to cut the cost of health care? The condition of children belonging to **poor families living in vulnerable pockets such as slums, tribal areas, remote places, hilly tracts,** etc. is alarming. Health services need to be strengthened, so that every child gets proper protection against the common diseases of childhood. Those that fall sick should get timely and proper treatment.

However, the greatest impact of this resettlement has been the social disruption and its consequences ongoing social breakdown. These social groups used to provide physical emotional and frequently even financial support to each other as also social control because of years of familiarity and presence of elders. There is anger and frustration due to unemployment amongst many people. Many people feel they were better off in the slum.

Community rehabilitation options should be given priority over institutionalization of children in conflict with the law. If slum children today desire much more than they have, these desires are driven by their exposure to the 'good life'. Poverty and limited choices make this gap virtually impossible to bridge, giving rise to a host of stress, conflicts and frustration. For many children, city life is merely a transfer of rural poverty to the slum. The joint family has a very stabilizing influence on children. There are long distances we must travel and many obstacles we must overcome. No magic wand is going to banish poverty and starvation overnight, no miracle. Struggle for survival begins before birth.

This tale depicts the disruption into people's lives when evicted and resettled. Then why there is no planning for these people when Master Plans for the cities are drafted? Instead of improving their conditions of life urban planners aggravate their difficulties by invariably relocating them on the outskirts of cities, with no or very little facilities. The poor need direct action to bring them into the development process and create the conditions for them to escape from poverty. Markers are aimed at maximizing profits, not attacking poverty.

The weather wreaking havoc or the monsoon playing truant and causing draught conditions, is not a new phenomenon in India. The central question here is how well we are prepared to face such disaster. "Don't let dreams die! Otherwise life is a broken winged bird that cannot fly"

The existence of large number of poor children, women and men – elderly, destitute, disabled, including mentally challenged – with no roof of their own, is a painful reality of modern cities. It may be the worst in terms of the way the poor are treated. These homeless include the people who sleep on the pavements, rickshaws, handcarts, railway platforms, flyovers, in parks, under bridge etc. A homeless person is anyone who lives on the street or in any place not meant for human habitation or someone who lives in night shelter. A home is a place, which provides shelter and takes care of one's health, social, cultural and economic security.

Homeless people do have their right to live in peace, dignity and security. Empower and mobilize the homeless people to form a body of their own in order to assert their rights and take up their issues at all levels. Poverty in rural India is the root cause of homelessness; urges for a more **holistic approach towards homelessness.** Our aim is to do **capacity building** of the homeless so that they can move forward, on a sustainable basis.

Panchayati Raj Institutions have been made responsible for social services. It will be highly desirable to develop models to show how Panchayati Raj Institutions can take over the control of rural health care institutions like sub-centers, primary health centers and community health centers, sustain these institutions and develop them further with the active and informed participation of the people.

Public health thus involves a much wider area of health action. Diseases when they occur are detected early and treated promptly. When diseases are chronic in nature, steps are taken to prevent disability; and, when disabilities do occur, the victims are rehabilitated. A Public Health Organization has always to be on the alert to 'come before' any threat to the health of the public health promotion, specific protection, early diagnosis and prompt treatment, disability prevention and rehabilitation. Life is getting more and more difficult as days roll by.

Malnutrition is one of the most significant indicators of poverty. Malnutrition manifests itself primarily as protein energy malnutrition. Malnourished children are unable to evolve an efficient immune response. They are thus more likely to be infected by childhood diseases. Improving the nutritional and health status of children; reducing mortality, morbidity; reducing the rate at which children drop out of school due to health reasons; and providing health education to enhance the ability to the mother to make correct choices for her children's health; sufficient evidence to indicate that the status of women in any society is one of the key determinants of the general health status of its members, and specifically, of children.

Many of the tube-wells and hand pumps constructed under government programs are completely dysfunctional or have been inoperational for long period of time. **Ground water** sources are also known to **dry up**; compelling people use other unsafe, sources of water in urban areas. A large percentage of the urban population lives in areas where the quality of water is not monitored. Consequently water-borne infections such as cholera, typhoid, dysentery, hepatitis, amebiasis, etc. are common in rural as well as in urban areas. The situation is aggravated as a result of lack of personal hygiene, by poor disposal of waste, and in certain regions, even a total absence of sewage disposal facilities. Poor maintenance of these also results in contamination of water. This is especially true of urban areas.

Involving the community and women representative in the Panchayat, in particular, can play an important role in improving children's health. Community Health Workers (CHWs) help bridge the distance between communities and the public health system. Any policy for children must be holistic, practical, address ground realities, be needs-specific, and be based on objective research and knowledge; based on systematic research and data.

Children may develop symptoms of mental impairment due to environmental and social influences. Children born or living in situation of extreme physical and mental deprivation and abuse, are more likely to develop symptoms of mental impairment than others. Various health care systems have surfaced.

Public education on preventing and coping with mental impairment has to be undertaken. Programs must be designed with a view to reorienting public attitudes towards mentally challenged children, with a clear focus on their abilities, as opposed to handicaps. Have option for the poor, sick, the illiterate, the lepers, the unwanted orphans, the destitute, the handicaps, the aged and dying children of mother India.

Every child has the right to access and receive education, and to avail of rehabilitation services that promote self-reliance, and prepare the child for future employment.

Besides the feeding program, to be undertaken the **balwadis**; medical check up of the children. Health workers visit the balwadis every week, to supervise the personal hygiene in children and the hygienic surrounding of the balwadis especially the place of cooking; monthly weighing and monitoring of weight in children to keep a constant track of the progress.

Today we live in a world of wrapped values, insecurity, we have to go ahead, even if it means to challenge, take sides with the powerless. Millions live in avoidable poverty, trapped in illiteracy and diseases. Child labor thrive, bride burning, gender and cast discrimination continues to besmirch the face of India. Upholding justice, compassion, truths without side tracking real issues like poverty and oppression.

Survival is one of the greatest instincts of humankind. Nobody wants physical pain and suffering. Neither does anyone like to see his or her dear ones suffering. So the human searches for cure, healing and wholeness have been unlimited and continuous. India with its richness and diversity of traditions has contributed a great share in promoting healing and alleviating pain and suffering.

Various facilities offered by high tech medicines today are not quite relevant to the needs of the poor. Medical technology is advancing by leaps and bounds from the past few decades. New diagnostic and therapeutic discoveries are being made every year.

Integral development based on education, that the villages would develop social, cultural, and political awareness. This will enable the community to join in the main streamline of India, while, at the same time it keeps alive its culture and identity.

When people do not have enough to eat and to take care of their sick, it is clear that they cannot think of education. Sadly, children are employed at a very early age in labor. The parents need the money urgently. The employers have cheap labor. Child labor is rampant. Children cannot go to the school. There are government schools. However, the teachers are either absent or come very late to school. They are happy if the children are not present.

Lack of education is also felt in the **agriculture technology**, which would help them to increase production. Without proper fertilizers their effort to grow the crops will be of no use. In order to grow better crop they need to use the fertilizers. As the farmers of the area are very poor they cannot afford to buy the fertilizers when the season comes.

Provide to the **farmers** the better quality of fertilizers; distributed at the beginning of the seasons every year. The farmers had to pay 1/3 of the price at the beginning and then they will pay the rest of money through the small installments when the crops get ready; the needs to charge from traditional including sowing, transplanting, types of hybrid seeds and fertilizers, become imperative because the viability of agriculture will demand it. This is another scheme which helps the farmers make both ends meet. The main crops in this area are rice, jowar, wheat; pulses etc. in order to have richer crops and fodder for animals, the better quality of seeds and fertilizers have to be provided to the farmers; quality seeds as well as fertilizers.

As we know many of the rural poor have no land and whatever piece of land they have is not leveled. Due to this they cannot cultivate the crops. So the purpose of land leveling is to provide the facilities to level their land so that they can cultivate and have better nutritious food.

One of the benefits of land leveling is what the cropping patterns can be improved richer crops and fodder for the animals; the needs to charge from traditional including sowing, transplanting, types of hybrid seeds and fertilizers, become imperative because the viability of agriculture will demand it.

To develop, foster, conduct, manage, administer and carry out activities connected with agriculture, establish and maintain experimental, model and/or development farms; conduct, guide and encourage research in and implement projects connected with modern agriculture technology, scientific methods of farming, effective and optimum utilization of agricultural land, increased farm output, enhanced crop production and productivity and impart training in modern scientific methods of agriculture.

To carry out special work in the field of **agricultural education**, to provide professional training, job oriented courses, human resource development programs and to establish, endow, develop, conduct, maintain, manage, equip, administer and carry on educational and technical schools, colleges, hostels and boarding houses and thus support and promote the advancement of educational activities.

To take over, acquire, provide, establish, endow, develop, conduct, maintain, equip, carry on, improve, alter and close down or dispose of educational, scientific, technical and research institutions, community medical or educational centers, agricultural development centers, works activities to promote the primary objects.

To acquire, provide, construct, organize, maintain, improve, alter and conduct buildings, hostels, premises, research centers, facilities, equipment and means for the propagation and advancement of agriculture, formal and non-formal education, including the holding of classes, conferences, lectures and competitions and giving of prizes, awards, scholarships, freeships, diplomas, and certificates in respect there of.

We need to note that it also created problems associated with heavy and continuous irrigation, indiscriminate use of fertilizers and pesticides which led to depletion of the water-table, deterioration of the surface soil, and multiplication of pests.

Bunding and land leveling is also vital, as, the land of the fields have become like real ponds or small lakes, for paddy crops. To improve the land and to stop the run off of rainwater, to get the ground surface recharged, to stop the washing away of the topsoil and the organic bioculture; to increase and improve the food production, to provide richer crops and fodder for the animals.

Irrigation schemes like wells, water tanks, and pump sets once organized; there will be a great improvement in the quality of the crops, income of the farmers increased, control of rainwater run off, control of erosion, better percolation of surface recharge. The soil's natural bioculture will be preserved. Bunding system will create water reservoirs, which create better moisture for a second crop.

Vermi composting is the method of making organic manure by utilizing organic waste from villages and towns. Converting these wastes into vermicompost also can solve the environmental hazards due to improper garbage disposal. It is the way of processing the organic wastes into a better plant food by using earthworm. Vermicompost converts the degraded soil into the natural form and accelerates the healthy growth of plants by giving the required micronutrients. It is a good organic fertilizer for all kind of crops/plants. Vermincomposting uses earthworms for the decomposition of organic wastes. Need to promotion of vermicompost among the farmers through awareness and demonstration is very important as it has got a great contribution to the sustainable agriculture and it establishes an honorable relationship with nature. Awareness among farmers is important to encourage them the usage of vermicompost or any other organic fertilizers to reduce the use of harmful chemical fertilizers.

Vermicompost contains macro, micronutrients, also plant hormones, and antibiotics. It is good manure for all kinds of plants and trees. They improve the pore spaces in the soil and increase the water holding capacity and permeability of the soil. Hence, the recharging of groundwater can be improved. The disposal of wastes for the preparation of this manure adds to the cleanliness and purity to the environment. It will improve the quality of the crop product. Since the compost gives the plant, strength and resistance to disease, the pesticide application can be reduced or can be stopped.

The **buffalo to provide milk** for the children and pregnant women, improving food-habits, and additional income for their families; by the milk cooperative. Thus, a new source of income is being developed in this village. Veterinary doctor pays a visit at the center and examines the buffaloes. Each animal is insured with the insurance company. As slowly the people are learning to take the responsibility and to run the milk co-operative for their own development. Most of these women have learnt to keep some milk at home for their children or for themselves. For that the revolving fund was used to purchase more buffaloes. It has brought economic and social change in the villages. We can conclude that their living standard also has been improved with this income. The people of the village have completely stopped migrating into the cities to earn their livelihood due to the buffaloes at home. "Our economic condition has been improved much; before we never used to have the cash in our hand. Now the situation is not so. My husband also stopped going to the cities to earn the livelihood". To rear goats is income for their families.

Kitchen garden: To assure proper vitamins for the family and to provide vegetables at home, creating new food habits, income from the sale of vegetables.

Most of the mothers are aware of the need for an extra supplement of nutrition during pregnancy. Many a **mother are anemic** and malnourished and there is hardly a woman if not motivated and provided would go for an extra supply of food. Provision of diet helped the mothers to maintain their health during the vulnerable stage of pregnancy. Most of the mothers are aware of the need for medical examination and supplementary medicines during pregnancy. Many a mother would like a hospital delivery, but it is not possible because of poor transport facilities as well as financial stress besides the fact that the young daughter-in-law has to abide by the decision of the elders in the family. Most of the ***dais* of the village** is untrained, of which there is no choice as she is the only woman available in time of need. But the education to the young mothers and the village health workers have led to an improvement in the delivery practices specially in terms of hygiene. Mothers need to be educated more on the feeding of Colostrums to the children. Though there is elimination of maternal mortality rate to a certain extent, one needs to be alert about the child mortality rate; and the different recurring diseases in the children.

Today more than ever, we see the need to organize the rural communities, make them aware of their rights and responsibilities, and in assisting them in organizing themselves, thus gaining their status in the society. Today we can see that village community is better organized where such awareness and motivation has reached.

In a welfare state, **health and education** are the two most important areas of government intervention. The problem is far more serious owing to a poor sense of commitment on the part of doctors, lack of medicines and drugs, lack of skill and aptitude of the grass-root level public health workers and the poor utilization of the primary health centers and sub-centers; unhygienic dwellings, non-availability of safe drinking water and unsafe disposal of human excreta merely add to their obnoxious environment. Health insurance schemes are such that the poor cannot afford to have the health coverage like the privileged rich. Only one-third of the villages of the country can have easy access to medical facilities of one type or other.

It is thus clear that health care implies more than medical care. It embraces a multitude of services provided to individuals and communities by agents of the health services for the purpose of promoting, maintaining, monitoring and restoring health. **Community participation** has been recognized as major component in the approach to the whole system of health care treatment, promotion and prevention. The stress is on the services to the people representing a shift from medical care to health care and from urban population to rural population.

During the past twenty years, at least thirty new diseases have emerged to threaten the health of hundreds of millions of people. For many of these diseases there is no treatment, cure or vaccine and the possibility of preventing and controlling them is limited. The factors for **emerging and re-emerging infectious diseases** are unplanned and under planned urbanization; over crowding and rapid population growth; inadequate public health infrastructure; resistance to antibiotics; increased exposure of humans to vectors disease and reservoirs of infection in nature and rapid and intense international travel.

It is this context that various grassroots, regional, national and international **health campaigns** have emerged to generate awareness among people and to mobilize them to demand better health policy and public health care system. Right to health is a right to life; right to live with dignity and right to livelihood.

Keeping vision wherein people are assured of clean air, water and environment, where they do not suffer from any **preventable diseases**, and are able to manage their health needs. Able to uphold their dignity of human life and nurture to grow into its fullness; where they are ensured availability of health care of reasonable quality at reasonable cost. For that the paradigm shift from institutional approach to community-based approach stressed all over again. **Network** and collaborate with organizations to combat the communicable diseases; use of available resources to the maximum benefit to the poor. Achieve basic health needs to the poor by focusing area-wise could be taken as our major concern. This needs stress on interventional journey towards health movement.

Assessing the impact of the intervention—multiple measures to be taken to build identity by adapting to their food, culture and way of living to booster their self-esteems. So they feel comfortable with their way of living, which is unique. Multiple measures can be taken to promote the women where they can become assertive and acquired status not bound to household chores; conscious of their rights and duties, awareness of equal citizen and feel encouraged going ahead. By awakening their self-confidence, will able to have access to wider world of knowledge, can get better job prospects in the future; which will help them to promote and preserve their culture and heritage, to identify and compete with the mainstream for better job prospect.

This is a brief outline on the various parameters that constitute problems of development. The economic disparity: between the rich and the poor. The social inequality: structured in a hierarchical way. They are very crucial and critical issues. The government with its reforms and radical legislations is trying its best to eradicate these evils and the **NGOs** are both committed to these struggles. Whilst a lot may have been achieved, we have a long way to go.

"I expected to pass through life but once. If therefore, there can be any kindness I can show, or any good thing I can do to any fellow being, let me do it now, and not defer or neglect it, as I shall not pass this way again".

Inspired by the above saying, through community participation, mutual accountability and responsibility conditions are being created wherein people are empowered. Much is achieved; still much more is to be achieved. We hope that our united efforts will ultimately lead the community to stand on its own. The process is slow, laborious, painful, and steady. We are hopeful that with the determination, dedication and commitment of many may one day definitely bear fruits.

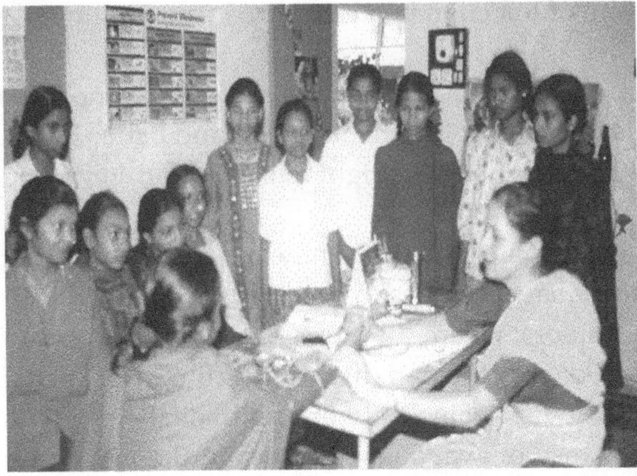

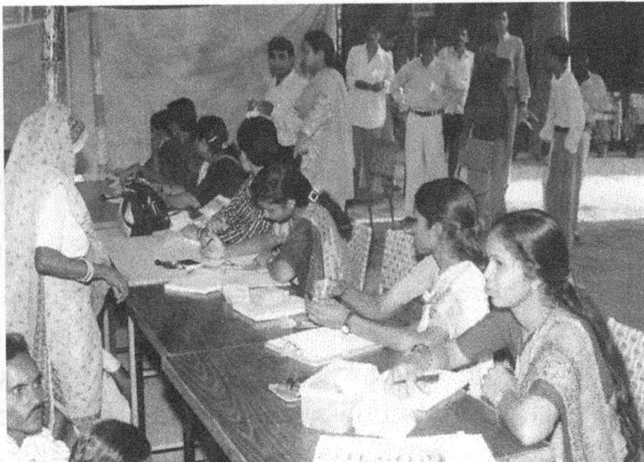

Figs 5.1 and 5.2: Preventing, promoting and curative health services through medical camps; Recognizing patients' needs and health problems. Observe record and report accurately and provide clean and safe environment

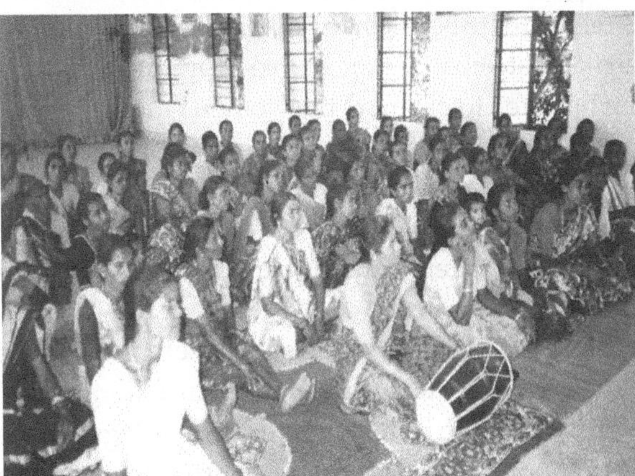

Fig. 5.3: Spiritual dimension: Common place for worship; villagers are peace loving, God-fearing people

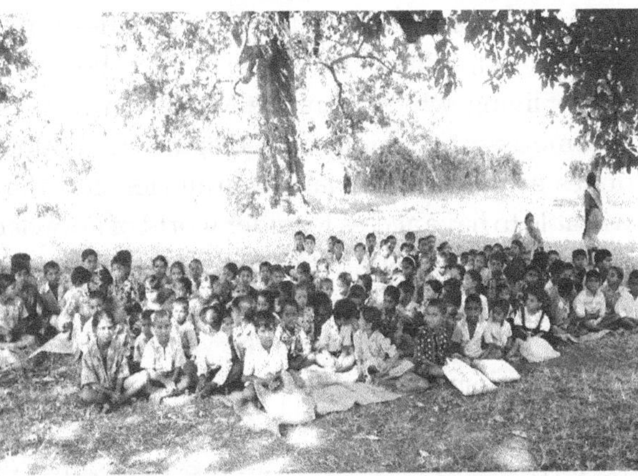

Fig. 5.4: Illiteracy through education; helps them to develop realistic view of life and help them to join the mainstream of society. Shaping and moulding the character by knowledge. Balwadis/anganwadis

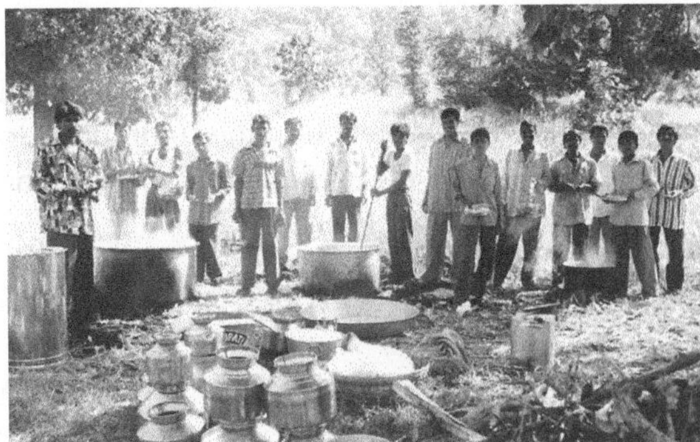

Fig. 5.5: Sharing together a community meal. Common contribution in sharing

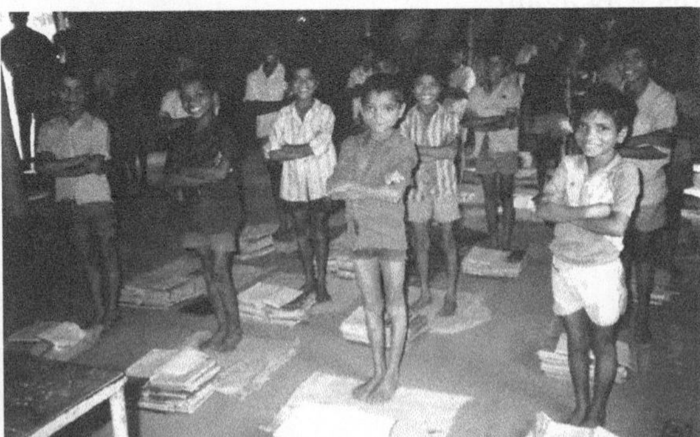

Fig. 5.6: A healthy child, sure future. Children's health, tomorrows wealth

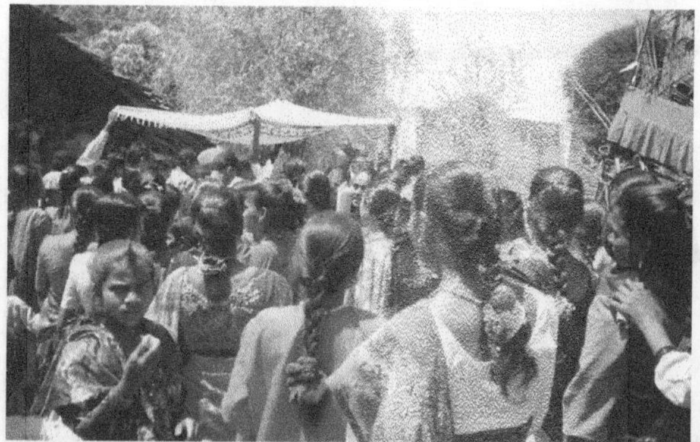

Fig. 5.7: Identifying the community health needs and problems to set priority of various age groups in conducting different programs, which help to respond to the needs of specific group

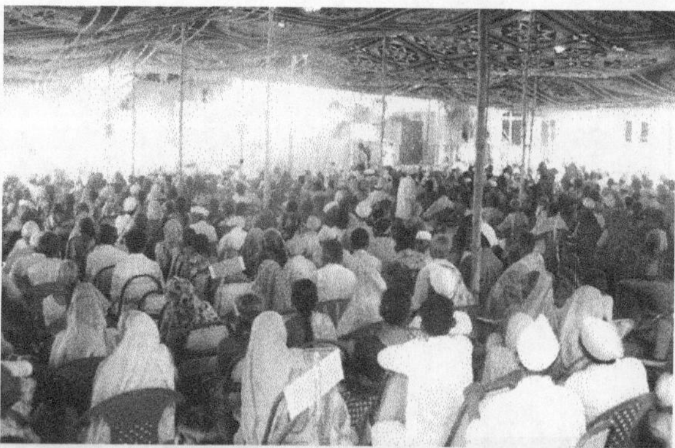

Fig. 5.8: Establish rapport and maintain cordial relationship, health promotion that help people move closer to higher levels of wellness

6 People Awakening

Health is a God given **gift** that has to be protected and conserved, by promoting a healthy lifestyle that favors, not only to take care of the body but also not to harm the spirit.

Relations between doctors and their clients if we evaluate we can see that 80% of the information needed to make a diagnosis comes from talking history, and making conversation with the client, or from physical exam and some simple test. Technology takes years to master, it is good for our progress yet Technology can come between our doctors and client and their families. Unless we find a **balance between the old arts of healing and the new technology,** we may lose as much as we gain. And the loss may be irreversible.

All the wealth of the world cannot help one little Indian village if the people are not taught to help themselves. No equal opportunity will ever be real and effective until the poorer sections of the people are given adequate facilities. We are endowed with many excellent educational institutes and the biggest stock of trained manpower in the world. But it is of no use if efforts to accelerate literacy are not supported with massive investment in social services—primarily education and health. What we lack is a human face. What is needed is a considerate analysis of the situation. As a result of incorrect education system, many young Indians lack a clear vision of their own future and ambition to excel. We should have an education system that creates an environment in which the young generation can set its own goals and take decisions for the betterment of the future.

As health is primarily an individual concern, like any other necessity in life, health transcends the individual realm to the family, the local community, the nation and the world at large. The concept of people's health in people's hands strongly points towards this shared responsibility.

Studies have shown that only about five percent of medical care requires high technical and professional skills. This means that with proper social skills, based on sound epidemiological considerations, the rest of the problems could be handled by health functionaries at the village levels. This will have advantage of demystifying medical care, cost effectiveness, cultural acceptability, early detection and prevention, sustainability and community involvement.

Such a move will give protection to the people against the costly private sector and inaccessible public sector. To show how even the marginalized and disadvantaged sections of people can make difference in the quality of their lives, in a positive atmosphere, created by catalytic agencies and individuals. People's awakening is very crucial. It is proved beyond doubt that even the poor and illiterate have the basic intelligence, giving the opportunity, to control over their own destinies.

The condition of several government hospitals in the country is appalling. Some are literally on the brink of collapse, both for want of sufficient funds and lack of management planning. Leaky rooms, rickety furniture, obsolete, inadequate, unusable equipment and paucity of essential drugs are just some of the many problems.

The presence of medical and paramedical personnel, often much less than required by the prescribed norms, coupled with the grossly inadequate facilities have been responsible for over crowding leading to a steep decoration in the quality of the service. Many public health centers and sub-centers are either not visited for months together by doctors assigned to them or medicines allocated are sold off in the market.

Private nursing homes, corporate hospitals and sophisticated medical institutes, confronting to international standards are available only in the metros and few other cities to those who can afford. But since the emphasis is largely curative rather than promoting preventive medicine, the costs are relatively high.

With issues like life expectancy at birth, infant mortality and the causes of death still remaining the most pressing health concerns in the country and our health cares system under pressure, the thrust of all effort should be on long-term plans and permanent solutions.

We nurses play a vital role in reducing the pain of a client when they approach us. The first thing we have to do is to smile, to be delicate, sensitive, and warm towards the client. While talking to a client we can hold their hand, just by this gesture we can feel how much the client is suffering. Like-wise we can communicate healing and courage. To give the client hope and respect, no matter how serious is the illness. The illness of client does not make her less human. Not to scold the client when they are sick, they tend to be more sensitive. Understand their feelings. The person includes body-mind-spirit; the sick person needs not only our medicines but also loving care, kind words and attention.

Every sickness is unique because every person is unique. Hence, it is not possible to find two identical ways of reacting to suffering. Sometimes our experience of a person who is known to be a very strong, worry about any minor indisposition, while other person who seems to be weak is able to bear great pain with admirable courage. Besides physical sickness there are suppressed, internal, moral, spiritual sufferings, Death, separation of a person we love, to feel despised and rejected by others etc. Sometimes extreme sickness has caused to loose very meaning of life and existence of God, our role here is of great value.

Difficulties faced by community health personnel are many; working with minimum facilities and scarcity of medicines, not able to meet all the needs of the client's. We may have limitation because of language. In spite of all the education and guidance given, there are times when you experience lack of cooperation from people. Their strong belief in the influence of the evil spirit in all events of life still remains as a big drawback in the developmental and health work.

You may at times feel isolated, tense, and anxious alone and lack of professional qualification, and up-to-date knowledge, so it is quiet natural to feel that you lack moral, spiritual and material support in your community area. In spite of the continuous attention, clients discontinue the medicine and come back when they are worse. In case of urgent needs inability to treat serious client due to lack of facilities and knowledge. High cost of drugs and lack of access to investigating facilities leaves health worker handicapped in rural medical ministry. No follow-up of the treatment once they get all right and lack of interest and initiatives from the people to arrange any health programs.

Effective communication is crucial to any kind of health action. Motivating people is not making them do what you want to do, but making them understand their own potential. People are not objects of decisions made by others. They are the agents and subjects of decisions and planning. When people are strong no evil force can overpower them. Meetings must be organized at convenient times. Unless people are involved in decision-making, they are less likely to commit themselves to the course of action. Cultural and religious practices are very much part of the life of the people. It is difficult for them to come out of some of their age-old customs. Go to the people live among them, love them, learn from them, start from where they are, and build upon what they know.

The secret of national health lies in the homes of the people. Man is a social animal; no man can live on Island. Health cannot be isolated from its social context, so many factors responsible for it. Advanced scientific knowledge increased enormously.

The acute communicable diseases brought under control. Good medical care is available to more people than before early detection and treatment. Notification, isolation, reports the cases to the health authorities' at once active mass immunization. Proper disposal and disinfections of urine, faeces, milk pasteurization, avoid over crowding, education on diseases and consequences, strict avoidance of close contact, precautionary measures, sprays, survey, prevention of disabilities, rehabilitation, counseling, vocational training, social measure, community nurse to be always remain vigilant and treatment stares without waiting, increase public awareness as many ill health is due to all these factors.

Practice makes man perfect and leads to the development of routine that help in building skills. Discover new facts about known phenomenon, find answers to problems which are partially solved, improve existing techniques, discover pathway of action, design method for the study, find new knowledge and scientific answer, scrutinize, gather new date for new purpose which is reliable and valid. It demands accurate observation, which is logical and objective.

You have to gain knowledge about the functioning of primary health center, sub-center, with its physical and administrative set up. And can acquire knowledge about various rural development schemes required for **uplifting villagers like ICDS, Anganwadi, Mahila Mandal,** and **Gram Panchayat** etc. She also can find out the functioning of various rural health services and scope of rural health services in India.

Identify the community health needs and problems through **house visits** in their respective families; which will in return help her to develop an ability to set a priority according to the health needs of the community. And develop a skill in planning or organizing nursing activities in a given community. Acquire an ability to communicate with the group through health education in prevention of health problems. Develop an ability to assess the health problems of various age groups by conducting school health programs.

Plan nursing care by using nursing process; and co-relates theory and practice while carrying out care. Use all opportunities for health teaching. Communicate effectively. Observe record and report accurately. Find out what are common diseases treated? Are X-ray facilities available? Is laboratory attached with PHC? Is the stock of medicines adequate? Is the PHC adequately equipped? Are maternal and child health services carried out? New antenatal mothers registered? Number of antenatal referred from sub-centers? How many domiciliary deliveries conducted? How many total deliveries, live births, still births, number of abortion, number of children 0 – 6 years. registered and immunized?

Utilize proper approach, develop and maintain good rapport. Utilize stable methods to collect relevant data related to health of clients, individual, family and community. Conduct interview with individual family and other key persons. Make clinical observations and examination. Accurately identifies the problems, which requires nursing care. State the problem scientific, rational on the basis of subjective data and objective data; formulates the objectives relevant to problems on priority. Write out standard nursing care plan in clear and measurable terms in congruent with other planned therapies; involves the client and other key person in planning care.

Demonstrate the clinical skills necessary to carry out the nursing interactions. Elicit participations and cooperation of clients or other key persons in delivery of care. Utilize opportunities to teach health care concepts to clients or other key persons. Follow-up of the nursing care plan developed and make referral services. Routinely evaluate the effects of the nursing care provided. Communication of ideas, information and health messages effectively. Know the meaning of Important Terms Used in Community Nursing.

What is a brief history of the situation? Who is involved in the situation? Who is the decision maker? How do you own this challenge? Who needs to be a part of the solution? Who might gain if the situation is resolved? What successes have you achieved so far? What are things that have helped you? What are some obstacles you've encountered? Where have you found help? When is the situation occurring or reoccurring? When would you like to have action taken? How long has this been a concern?

Why is it a concern for you? Why might this be an opportunity for you? What's been thought of or tried already? What are your gut feelings about this challenge? What are your feelings affecting your behavior? What might be your ideal outcome or goal? Is the matter relevant to the group? Is the knowledge up-to-date? Is the matter reliable? Does she communicate the idea correctly? Is the language used appropriate? Is the response of the participants positive? Does she involve participants?

Develop art and skills of community assessment: Survey the community and families. Identify the community needs. Identify the available resources to meet the needs. Provide comprehensive health and nursing care to families: identify the health needs. Create awareness of health and help them to take care of themselves. Use problem-solving approach while providing care. Understand the organization of peripheral health service. Study the structure and functions of PHC. Study the roles and responsibilities of peripheral level workers. Take active part in involving PHC activities. Identify the problems existed in the peripheral health center.

A community nurse must have wider knowledge of social services. Unique functions of the nurse are to assist the sick or well, in the performance of those activities contributing to health or its recovery or to peaceful death. Develop pride in your profession besides keeping abreast with current knowledge and professional trends for a successful career ahead. Function as efficient member of the health team, to keep pace with latest professional and technical developments and use these for providing nursing care services, use of ethical values in personal and professional life.

Community Health Nurse (CHN) should have respect to her own calling, because precious lives are placed in her hands: she should have a sympathetic heart and willing hands. To have scientific knowledge and principal for better care provider, and utilization of specialized skills and techniques for the care of the client as a whole person: Meaning physical, psychological, spiritual, social, economical, and intellectual needs of the client. It is a service promoted to the promotion of social welfare. To observe clients illness and prevent complication and provide comprehensive health care, have sense of moral duty and obligation towards the lives entrusted to her hands. The fundamental responsibility is to conserve life and to promote health.

Respect authority, report unusual symptoms to the doctor, respect the client's beliefs, and hold all the information entrusted to you. Work with cooperation and harmony in care of client. Polite in your talk, address them with respect, work in team and in cooperation. There is an interpersonal relationship between client and nurse. Treat every client as an individual person. Avoid medical negligence and keep the knowledge up-to-date in order to maintain highest standard public care. Its functions is to care the sick and injured, prevent communicable and non-communicable diseases, promotion of health, diagnosis and treatment, rehabilitation, research, medical education.

Health service should be closer to people. Health functionaries should involve the people. Should inform and take them into confidence while implementing programs. How is it going to benefit people, what sort of cooperation is necessary from people should be clear to the village community. If people take the lead for certain activities, the government health services become supportive. Every village should have access to basic health services. For this, a person residing in the village needs to be trained, who can treat minor ailments and refer serious ailments in time. They can dialogue with people in their own language, and can work together in the village for preventive activities. So they get support from government and community. Community conscious is much bigger in rural community than in urban community. Animals have herds not community, community has community sentiments, and have feelings, sense of sharing belonging. It is not mechanical or artificial but natural, spontaneous phenomenon. Their interests are common.

Landless laborers fighting for land-rights and fair wages, finding ways of surviving, and living in subhuman conditions where they too breath the same polluted air and impact of a depleted ozone layer. We have to reaffirm them for sustainable development peoples right to life with dignity, we are committed to fight poverty, loss livelihood, unemployment, we oppose all policies that exclude people, derive and prevent their human potential to contribute to live with dignity and without fear. We are to be people oriented, build up local community, vital areas of health, education, communication, media, public system, and environment.

Human beings and nature have a unique relation. Natural resources are our life support; we relate to nature as a giver of life and own its endowment to future generation. We value conservation of our natural wealth—air, land, water, and mineral. Human and all forms of life are depended on nature and part of larger universe. Uphold human dignity and equality in all respect. We strive for protection and equal participation and motivate people to be free of addiction. People's agenda and people's politics, selfless and creativity valued, promote on the basis of equality and justice, to attain a truly prosperous and human life for all.

People need education, medical care, protection from evil elements in society and someone to listen to their concerns and problems. It is often easy to forget that the poor are not an object for our pity, but our own brothers and sisters. Identify the need of the community and work to fulfill these needs. Build self-esteem and self-confidence among women, raise the status of the women in their communities, build individual and collective capital and promote assets creation.

In spite of 50 years of independence and a number of schemes meant especially for the rural communities do not reach to the needy; hence a majority of them have more or less in the same primitive condition. Many families possess little piece of land and cultivate but as the land is not fertile and in the absence of irrigation facility, only one crop is cultivated. With good irrigation facility and with the help of subsidized fertilizers they can grow cash crops. To improve the food security situation by an increase in the food production through education, land leveling, seeds and fertilizers distribution and milk cooperatives.

This can be done by good linkage well-established structure with good infrastructure facilities; well-trained vibrant enthusiastic and committed staff supervising and monitoring the program. Good coordination regarding the implementation, a high degree of community involvement and participation in the planning, implementation and evaluation of the various programs.

To organize families into occupation-based self-help groups; sensitize, motivate, empower and enable them with knowledge and awareness and skill through appropriate capacity-building trainings so that they are enabled to take "lead role and interface role" for the development of their villages and Gram Panchayats in a sustained manner; to instill and foster social and human values of justice, equality, cooperation, solidarity and communitarian spirit of collective reflection, collective decision and collective action. To build up sustainable systems with sincere and reliable cadres with social concern so that the development process is continued and sustained after phasing out.

All livelihood programs are to be implemented through self-help-groups right from the beginning so that group's active participation and ownership is assured. Initiation of process of group empowerment through regular group meetings, identification of problems, analysis, reflection, decision, action etc. study, market survey, analysis, economic viability and technical feasibility of every livelihood package. Only trainings can empower and enable group leaders with knowledge and skill and motivate for action. Particularly vulnerable categories of workers are migrant workers; frequently separated from their families. They are often denied equality of rights and condition, without access to adequate accommodation, health care, or legal protection.

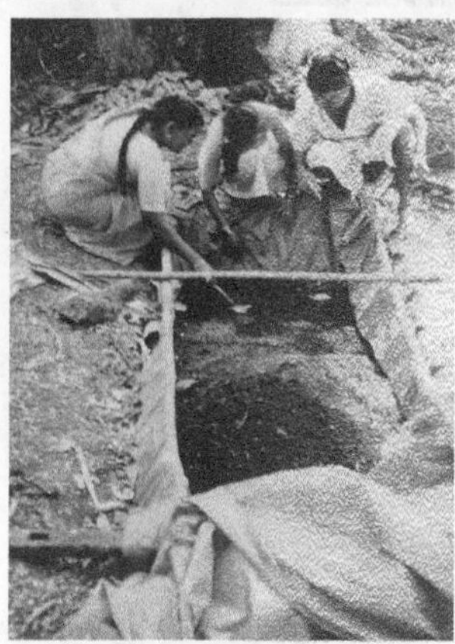

Fig. 6.1: Vermi composting:Training village team in the process of demonstrating change due to scientific and technological innovation

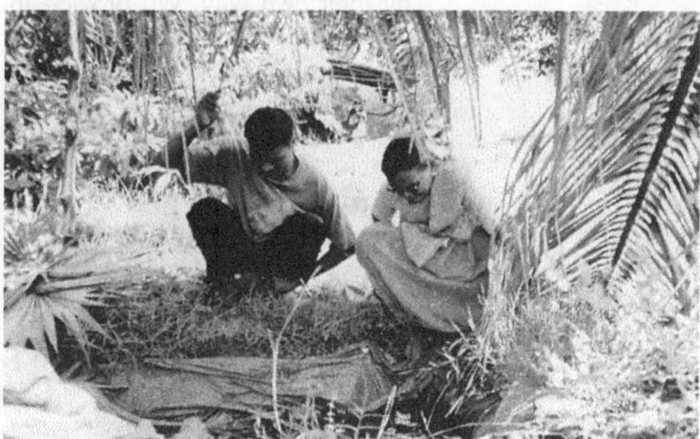

Fig. 6.2: Process of vermi composting

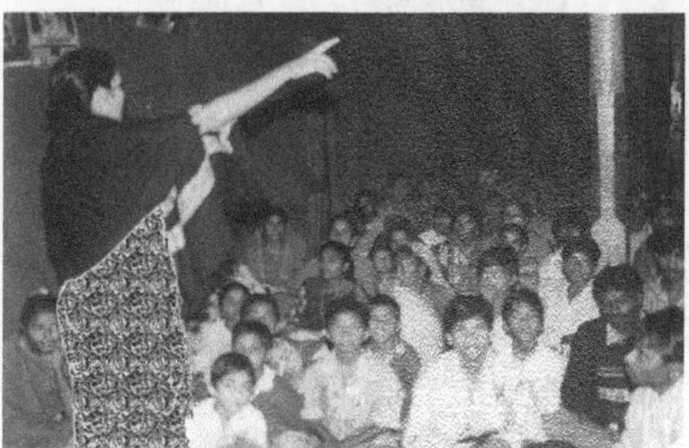

Fig. 6.3: To awaken the community and seek their active involvement and cooperation. Health education is a process, which affects change in the attitudes of people. It is necessary for building a strong power basis of community. People arise out of their own needs, their resources and capabilities

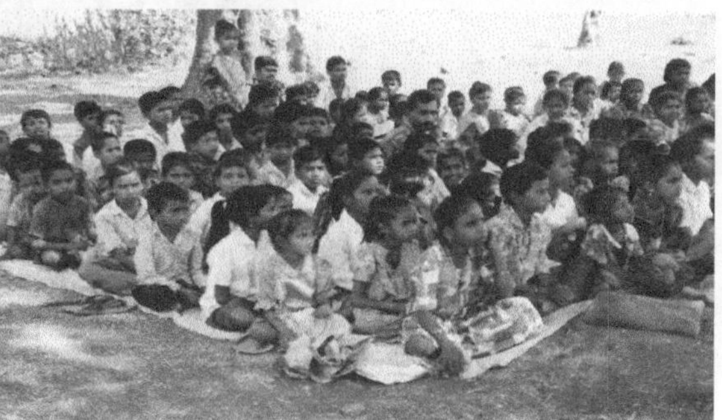

Fig. 6.4: Anganwadi and school health program through ICDS

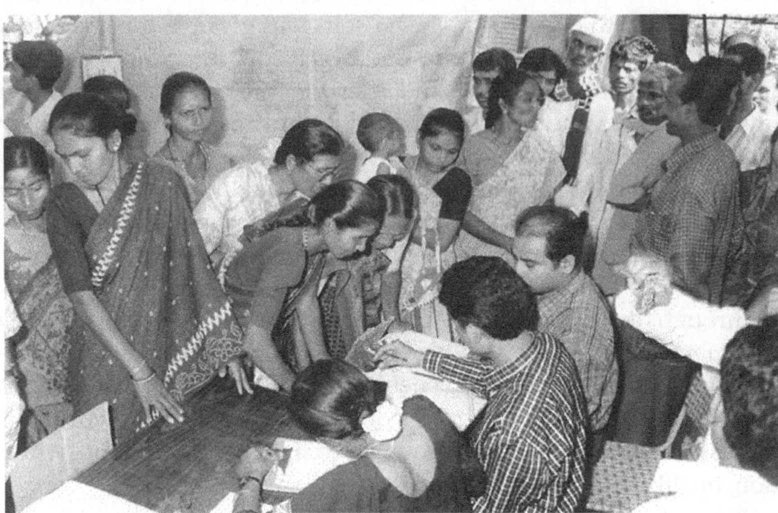

Fig. 6.5: Health is an asset; it has value, which helps people to solve their problem by their own way. We provide them information and create awareness through campaign and medical camps

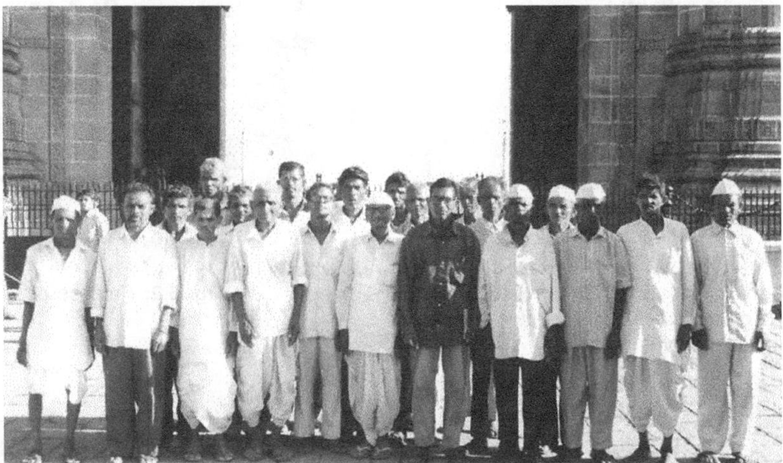

Fig. 6.6: Recognizing existing leadership, they are representatives of the community health education is as wide as the community is. The elders of the villagers are motivated and taken into confidence before launching any program for change in the village to get their cooperation and involvement. Leaders are the right channels of communication, through them health activities can be achieved easily. Meeting them and explaining the purpose of the field visit. They are the agents of change and they are decision makers of the needs of the group

7 Comprehensive Health Care

PHC is essential health care made universally accessible to individuals and acceptable to them through their full participation and at a cost that the community and country can afford. It is an institution, which provides comprehensive health care, Preventive, promotive and curative services to the people living in a defined geographic area. It provides these services under one roof, under the direction of a medical health officer who coordinates the health work of the area.

Making curative services available at the PHC; usually two doctors, lab-technicians, pharmacist and supportive staff are available with 112 essential drugs kept in adequate quantity. Admission facilities for serious clients and women in labor with functional vehicle for transfer of serious patients to a referral hospital kept present.

At the sub-center one ANM and one MPW available to provide treatment for minor ailments with 27 essential medications available; regularly once a week doctor visits the sub-center. Preventive services like immunization, examination of pregnant women who are given iron supplements and immunization.

A person who is ill is in distressed and vulnerable. Such a person treated with sympathy. Clients are not made to wait unnecessarily. They are examined properly and relevant facts explained.

Programs to prevent disease regular well-chlorination, insecticidal spraying where necessary is done. **Anganwadi to give supplementary foods** other services carried out. Kitchen gardens and plantation of medicinal plants be encouraged with health education. People's experience shows that certain traditional and herbal remedies are effective, which the villagers themselves know, which do not cost anything, and they are available nearby.

Locations of the PHC make it difficult for women to avail of health services. Often state transport buses do not reach the PHC village in advance for clients to receive medical treatment as OPD of most PHCs functions between 8.00 am and 12.00 noon and reopens from 4.00 to 6.00 pm. So the delivery of health care suffers. Short supply of health personnel and the drugs, makes the journey to the PHC futile. Cuts in the health budget are squeezing out the poor from access to ordinary health services.

In PHCs variety of clients with multiple diseases come for treatments. They have to accept and treat all types of clients who come to them. No one must go without medicines or medical advice even the chronic clients who need to be treated. All the medical facilities available which are supposed to be rendered at the service of the clients. They have to try to send clients satisfied and in peace. They must feel happy and free to come to our PHCs. Many clients who come to them are sometimes from the very far, remote unknown villages. Among these clients who need special care could be admitted and given complete treatment. The serious clients are to be shifted to hospitals for specialized treatment and latter the follow-up is to be done in PHC. They have to try to avoid unnecessary check ups and costly drugs. In interior villages there is non-availability of quality services at reasonable cost. A doctor's services at PHCs are required when dealing with diseases that need special expertise and technical facilities, so the cases that cannot be dealt with health workers, nurses, and the assistance of the doctors and the facilities of the hospital are made use of. Together with curative service health awareness, preventive and promotive aspect of health is to be stressed.

Gain knowledge about the functioning of health center, various rural development schemes for uplifting villages, set priority according to the health needs of the community. Find out the immunization status of the less than five age group, assess school health programs, and develop a skill in planning and organizing activities in the community through health education.

All the people in the villages who are sick can take benefit from **Mobile service**. If anyone needs special treatment, could be brought along with them in ambulance to the PHCs for the needful action. Thus, they can avail medical services available to the people in the remote villages at the minimum or free of cost. During planned visit people can come to get medical advice. This will help village people to build confidence in them and also to build up close rapport with their health team. And by their mobile services all the age groups can get the first aid at their doorpost. Here the health workers can take active part and do the follow-up during month and report at the center of the progress. In this way health workers can get more confidence in people, and can become efficient and capable, by this way in any emergency they are able to act promptly.

In clinic under nutrition mothers whose weight is less than 40 kg, anemic with hemoglobin less than 8 gm, age less than 20 years, history of difficult delivery, abortion, stillbirth, death of newborn baby and low birth weight is generally observed. They are provided with injections, TT. Tablet iron, folic, calcium and nutritional food grain is provided. Regular weight record is kept and any observation of abnormalities detected is sought medical help.

Health is a vicious circle. If the mother has good food during antenatal period, less risk of health, more strength and stamina, better blood hemoglobin healthy baby, good lactation, more vitality to work and less infections, better quality of life and more chances of survival. As village women belong to the lower socioeconomic status and are under nourished. Women continue hard physical labor till last stage of pregnancy. In addition to their household works, working beyond the limits of physical tolerance, their bodies are depleted of essential resources thus resulting in low baby weight.

Family counseling is also an important aspect where community health nurse must focus. She will have to strive to help troubled families; crisis in the life of married partners, trauma that the children undergo, the impact of broken families in society. There is a need to prevent a family from being broken. What can be done? How? Patch up their broken relationship; after the marriage has gone apart beyond repair. During the visit, have a good rapport with the family members. Listen to what family says and does not say – such as one of the partners looking sad / not talking/ laughing artificially. During such, regular visits the problem may surface. She can assess the problem. What is happening; Physical fight, verbal fight, non-verbal fight. Who are involved?

What is the degree of the severity of the problem? How are you going to approach it? According to problem give counseling and guidance. Need for other-centeredness unrealistic expectations are sources of unhappiness and separations; acceptance of limitations in self and others. Family adaptability requires a balance, stability. Living in the past carrying guilt and sadness for what happened and worrying over the future with tensions. Make a kind of family map – who relates with whom. Maintain total confidentiality. Only an initial guideline, your work for forming healthy families is very important because without healthy families we cannot have healthy society.

What do we hope for, from this? We will together chalk out our plan for the future. What we have learnt from this experience? What should be our strategy for the future? Their wisdom and experience is an immense help. They are the guiding force in many of our communities. "By the fruits you will know the tree!" there is scope however for plenty of improvement.

Comprehensive health in all dimension and all round all people involved including rural youth. We are living in the world among human community. As if one eye is weeping can the other sleep! When our brothers and sisters of rural community suffer, then it is our moral responsibility and task to create an atmosphere or situation, where they feel comfortable through providing them the facilities available in the cities and live happy life.

As we know that 72.2% people of total population of our country is living in rural area and the existing system and situation deprive them of advanced technology and modern facilities: advanced technology in many fields like information, science, industries, engineering, agriculture, including health.

When we talk about the development of the country, we cannot avoid, rather we have to consider rural population and include them in the main stream of the country. Many times when we talk about development, we exclude rural population, for we mean the development of the city population. Today when we talk about the development of the country, it should mean the development of rural population as well.

The advanced technology and modern facilities reach to the cities and the big towns and they are the immediate beneficiaries of development; and rural villages remain as they were. These advances do not make any difference in their lives. For example, mobile phones have reached not only in the cities but in the villages as well. However, the fact is that most of the time there is no network because all the towers that receive and send the signals are situated in the cities or close to the cities, thus the network rarely reaches to the villages. Yes, we say that mobile phones have reached even in the villages, but what extend?

The youths of the rural area are victims of deprivation especially of education. Even for the higher education and technical education, they have to take the admissions in city colleges, and often they are not able because of financial, social or cultural problems; thus, they are deprived of higher education and technical education resulting in unemployment and even frustration.

There are enormous numbers of rural youth drop out from the school because of various reasons. Those who do not get the admission in the city colleges are also considered as dropouts. If we want to get away with unemployment from the rural population and want to offer the employment, we need to provide them with advanced technology and modern facilities. To achieve this we have to build the capacity of the youth by giving them knowledge and skills; higher education and technical education like polytechnics, engineering colleges; and ITI for the youth. Even existing polytechnics, engineering colleges and ITI should start their extension centers in the rural area to give skill training and short courses like tailoring, embroidery, jewelry making, purse making, hand work, cooking, glass painting, computer, wireman, welding and fabrication, secretary course etc for the youth so that they would be able to get self/wage employment.

Therefore, it should be our vision and mission to build up the human community that is broken and torn apart for various social, economical, political, and environmental reasons. However, our vision is not only promoting the economic status but to build up a new society, formation of life and to inculcate human values and dignity. It is possible when people are motivated towards the development of the community and most effective approach for the development is community organization. The participation of the people is important factor for the community organization.

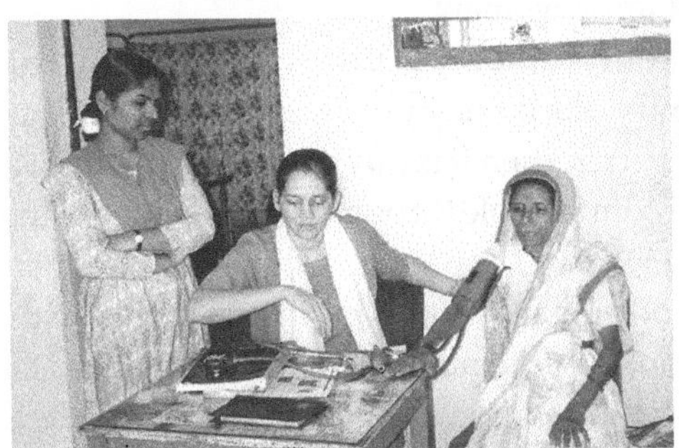

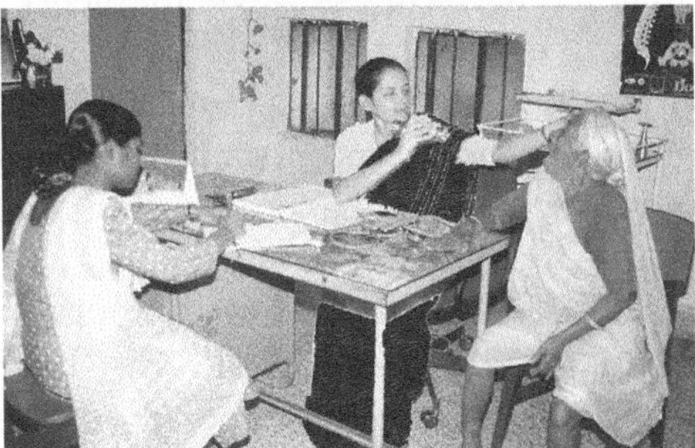

Figs 7.1 and 7.2: Every individual is a part of family and of wider community. Well-being of whole person. Health care delivery system; assessing health needs. Community Health Nurses' role in health care services

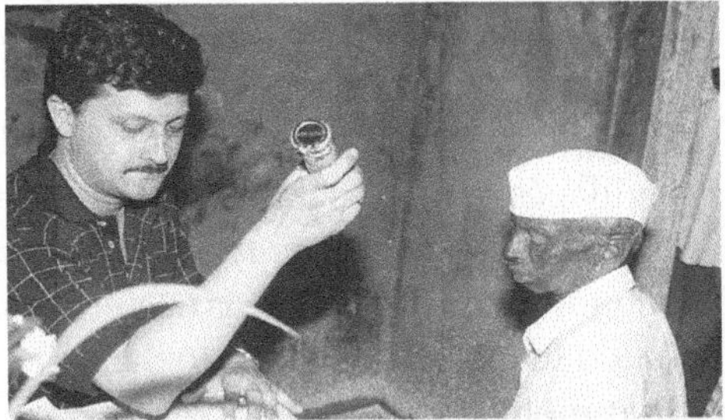

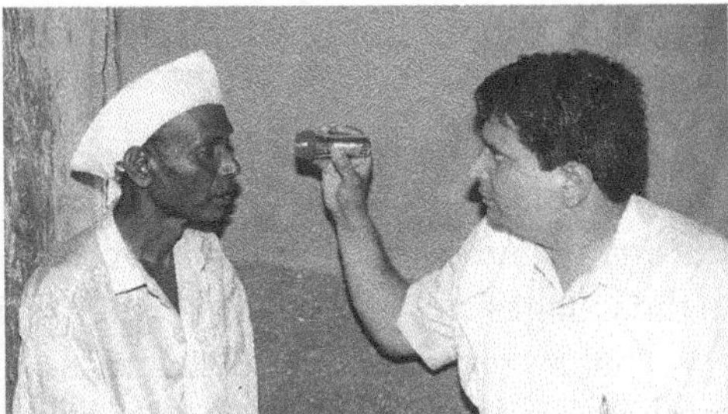

Figs 7.3 and 7.4: Talking the health services to the doors of the people. Eye care and detection of cataract; Reaching to the public through the rural programs

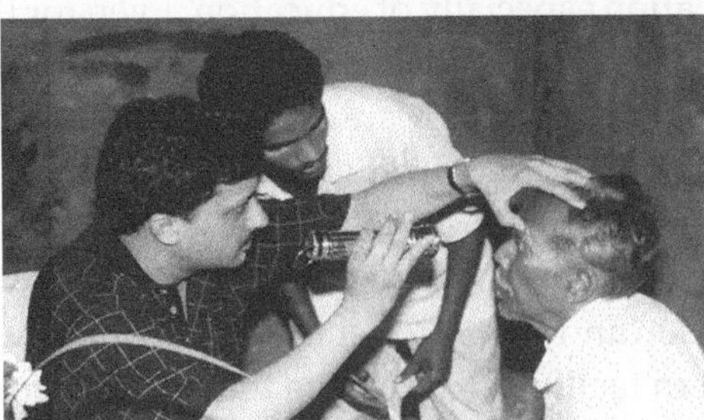

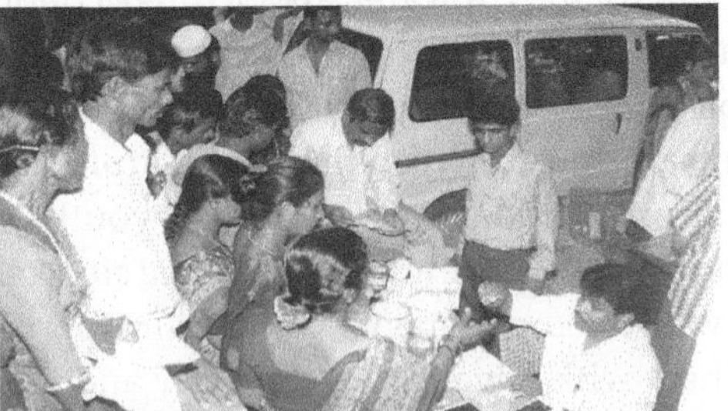

Figs 7.5 and 7.6: Voluntary health agencies, which are helping to uplift the health status of nation. The health personnel and community nurse should be oriented with other groups of people working in the community

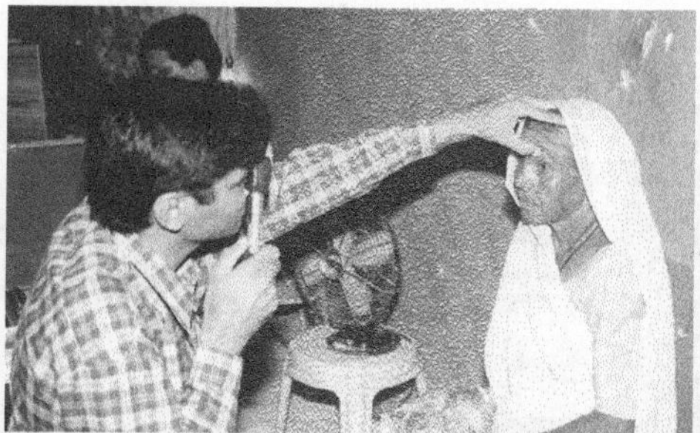

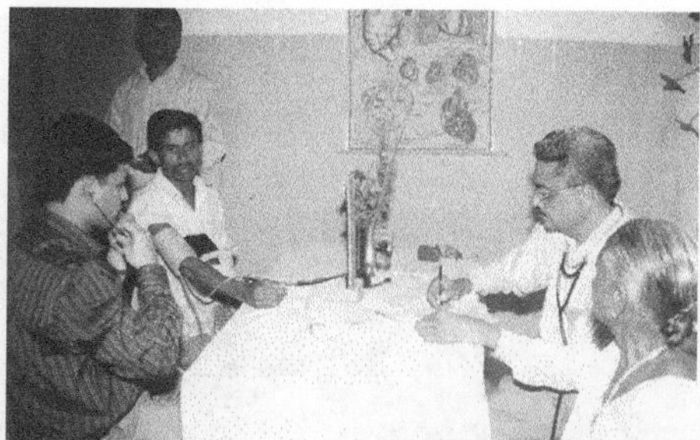

Figs 7.7 and 7.8: Control of communicable and infectious diseases; due to rising costs of medicines and diagnosis; and failure to reach to bigger hospital set up, specialist doctors' team and volunteers are giving their specialized services in remote areas at free of cost

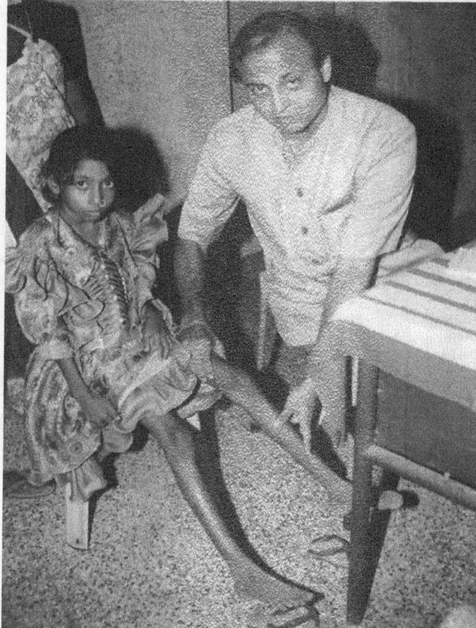

Fig. 7.9: Specialist doctor in community setting. Malnutrition and lack of calcium and vitamin D deficiency

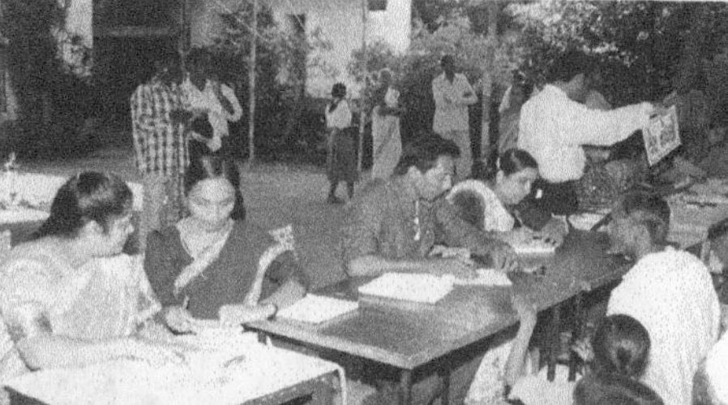

Fig. 7.10: Medical camps: The secret of health lies in the homes of the people. Health care delivery system in community setting

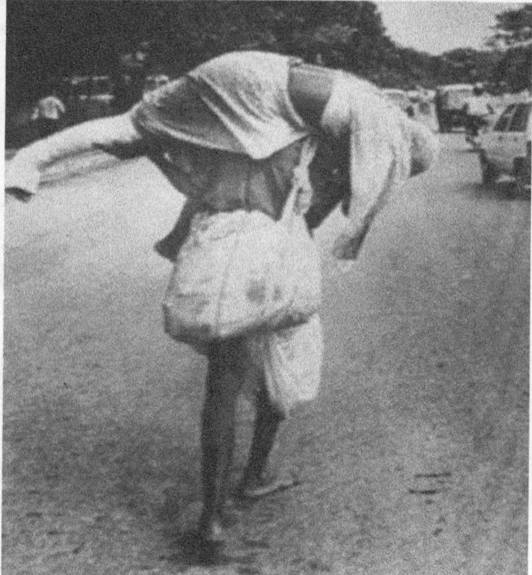

Fig. 7.12: Plight of the rural poor. When one eye weeps, can the other eye rest? A powerful photo gives the explanation of rural poverty and the plight of the poor that makes health team to work harder to reach to the voiceless mass. Do unto others what you want to do unto yourself. What so ever you do to the as least as this little one you do unto God. Very deep meaning and powerful inspirational photo

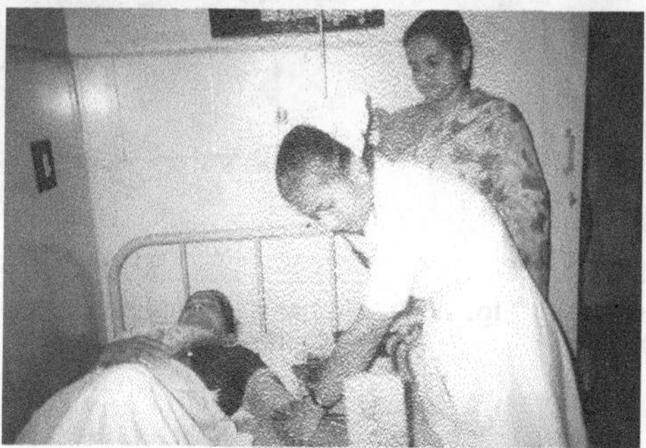

Fig. 7.11: Curative aspect of community health

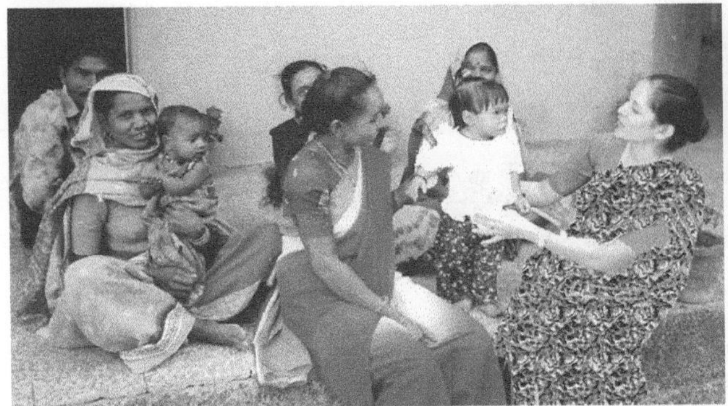

Fig. 7.13: Health of vulnerable group, mother and child program

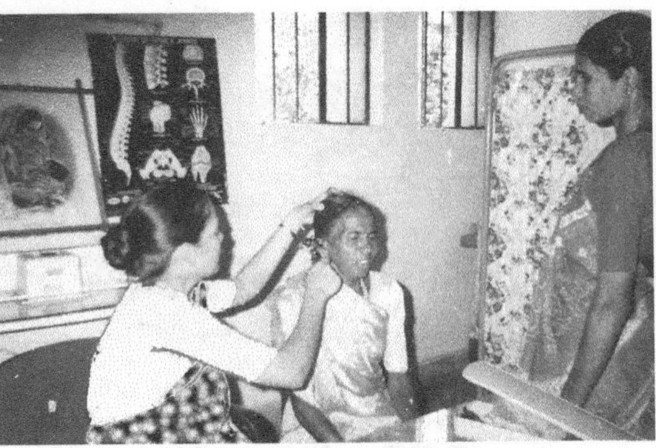

Fig. 7.14: Expensive illness. Comprehensive health care of rural poor

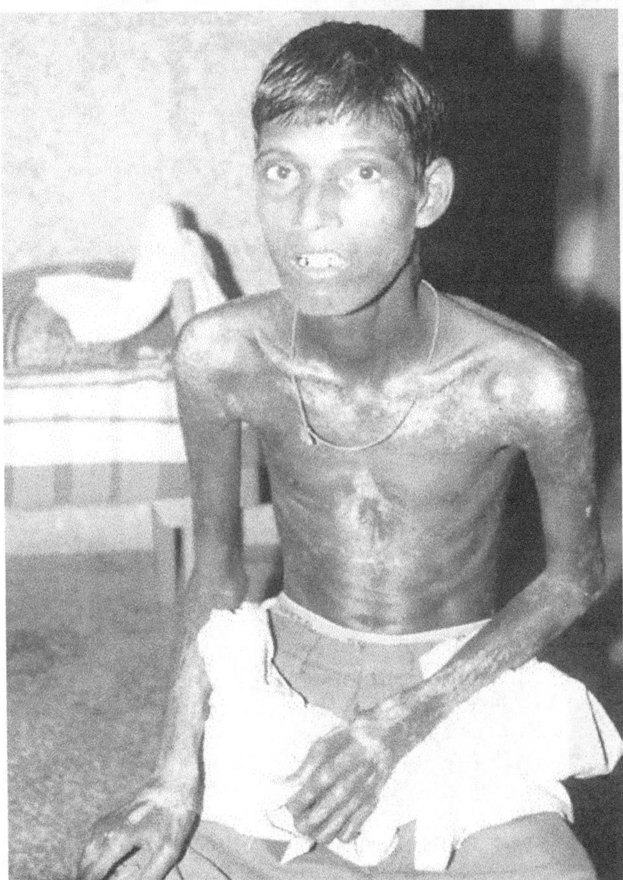

Fig. 7.15: Nurses' role in 'National Health Program'. Early detection and notification of diseases *(For color version see Plate1)*

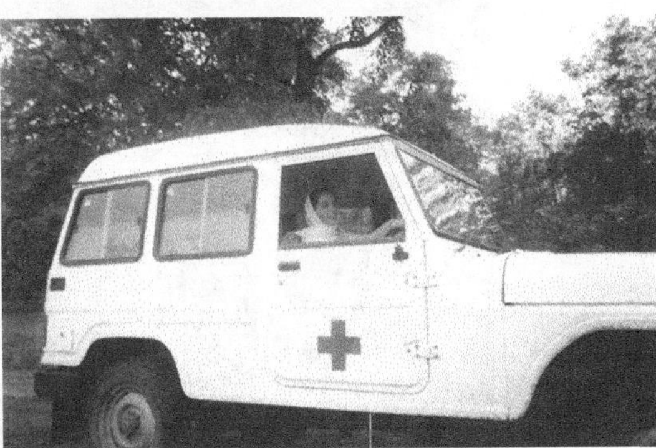

Fig. 7.16: Mobile clinics: Regular medical check-up and follow-up. Detect early malnutrition, tuberculosis, skin diseases of the rural poor who are living in subhuman condition due to poverty and lower socioeconomic condition, and not able to reach to the center

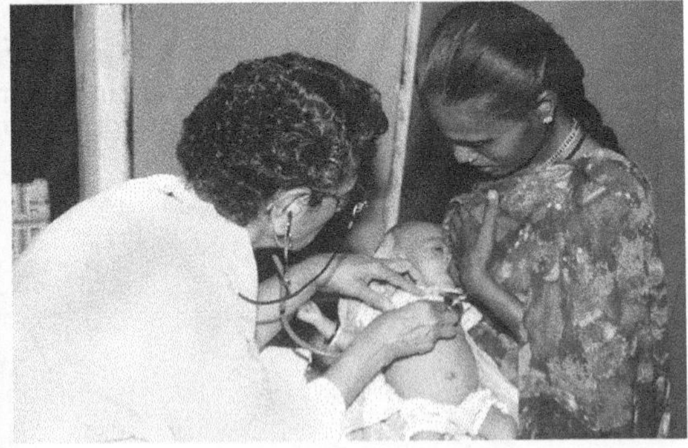

Fig. 7.17: Mother and child health care. A healthy mother, bouncing baby

8 Community Based Health Worker

In India 72.2% of people, live in rural areas. They are hardly covered by the health services. It is now realized that a wide range of sickness can be treated or prevented at the village level by a person with simple training. A community oriented health movement is the role of the village voluntary health worker. They are normally women from the village who have passed a childbearing age and have some good leadership qualities. They are selected by the local community and well accepted and welcomed by the villagers. They are trained and given a simple manual, which gives those detailed instructions and a medical kit containing essential first aid medicines.

With basic first aid training, knowledge, abilities and personalities community health worker shares the common goal of the village health; and provides the first contact between community and the center. They refer cases to the nearest center; and are important person who forms a link between families to the health center; as she has contact with every family and its needs.

Voluntary community health workers can easily handled illnesses that do not require medical specialized intervention. Such work that is carried out by them are balwadi and homes visits, provision of first aid medicines, health education, supervision of the nutritional intake of children, pregnant and lactating mothers, identification of communicable diseases, home deliveries, immunization, assess the growth and the development of the infants and take necessary actions, build rapport with village leaders and motivate them for promoting family welfare programs, participate in camps and campaigns, construction of latrines, garbage disposal, and disinfections of wells etc together with village *dais* they give emphasis on child survival and provide domiciliary mother and child health. Assist various national health programs such as control of tuberculosis, malaria, and leprosy. Over all she has to do the work her authority orders.

After the initial training there is also an on going health education and some technical instructions with that they are able to treat minor sicknesses like cold, diarrhea, stomach illness, wounds, fevers etc. A Medical officer alone cannot meet the health needs of the people in the community so using their services people can provide more and better health services. They are attached to the health center and guided for welfare programs.

They are trained to ask basic questions such as to ask the mother what the young infants problem are. Determine if this is an initial follow-up visit, weather the infant had any convulsion, fast breathing, nasal flaring, look for the infants movements if are they less than normal, is there blood in the stool, is there any difficulty in feeding, does the child vomit everything, has he had measles now or within the last 3 months, is there ear pain, is there any ear discharge, what is urgent and when to need to refer hospital she is being taught.

Therefore with their co-operation they can try in the area of work to avoid unnecessary check ups and costly drugs, which poor villagers cannot afford. Only cases that cannot be dealt by them could be brought to the PHCs clinic and assistants of doctors and hospital facilities made use of. They play a crucial role in building and forming good network.

They bridge the gap between villages to the center. They become more responsible and effective. People in the rural count and depend on them for medical assistance much more than before. Now they know when to rush with certain cases to the hospitals. Thus, many lives are saved due to their timely intervention. The progress is noticeable as the years go by. As they aim to promote harmony and efficiency and helps to improve the quality of life. They have direct approach to the public health service to the individual and group. As they are very well accepted by the villagers and are respected by them as their own.

Educational outings are taken so that they are exposed to a world beyond their narrow village boundaries. Initially they did not value education because they were living in an isolated world, where they had lack of exposure to the world. They do passive domestic role and they have no significant role to make. Therefore, there is the poor literacy rate among women. So these exposures can give an opportunity to just see another outside world that is somehow affecting their lives and their lifestyles.

Literacy and health education for the women is to be stressed. As women remain oppressed and ignorant do not leave the confines of their houses when they are outside village thus finding themselves lost in public. They are dependent on the men folk to catch a bus, they are dependent on the shopkeepers for the prices of essential commodities and they are dependent on their self-images as being useless and unintelligent.

During regular training deal with new topics and revised the known ones; as health education too can motivate and help them see that diseases have a cause beyond magical reasons and can be controlled and prevented by simple methods. Seeing the new reality in a true-life exposure situation makes what was once impossible into the all possible.

Knowledge too is power. Organizing demands dedication consistency and regularity, visit to the villages, meeting women personally, explaining to them the aims and needs. Women are on the move they are awakening slowly they are gaining courage, are capable of greater things. Feel motivated. Relive of their tensions, anxieties, and burdens. See a lot of improvements in relations between mother-in-law and daughter-in-law. They are more aware of social setups and problems.

Many women standing as candidates for the seat Sarpanch as well as Panchayat members; proves that the women are aware of their legal and political rights; better organized and have improved their status in the community/society.

The community health worker as symbol of the community organizing itself is crucial. Strong educational component to build an awareness of what, why and how sickness and health happen. The mud and water-borne diseases can proliferate due to the very structure of the environment–common wells, common small playgrounds, open areas and fields where morning ablutions are done. Diarrhea and worms; ignorance of the severity of diseases that can easily be transmitted, e.g. TB that can cause a multiplier effect as the bacillus spreads on an already malnourished population.

Delivery kits are small-prepackaged units of sterile cotton, gauze, thread, fresh blade etc. to promote a hygienic and safe delivery. These are given to women in the antenatal care, mainly dealing with primary health care.

Crucial factor in a community-oriented health movement is to identify and organize children for the under 5 clinic. Identify and organize pregnant women. Help in handling referral cases. Educating mothers help the medical staff understand cultural practices, early detection, right regimens of treatment, supplementary food for digestion of the medicines, regular visit to balwadi, medical check up of the balwadi children.

Provision of first aid medicines, preventive medicines to children up to 5 years of age helping the women folk for the vaccination of their children, form Mahila Mandal and village committee, maintains morbidity and mortality record, supervision of the nutritional intake in children as well as pregnant and lactating mothers, identification of infectious disease, chronic infirmities referring them to the PHC.

This will help the village community to get better organized. More awareness will be created among the people as to the personal responsibility of each one for their own health and the health of the community. Awareness will be created among the people regarding AIDS. Awareness regarding 'Panchayati Raj' and the people's rights could reach to the people. People can start using herbal medicines at home, a sort of self-help at the first stage of sickness, awareness for immunization coverage; a closer net works in all functioning with the village community will improve health status of mother and children.

The health status of a community is very much dependent on the mother, the housewife, the woman, for it is she who nurtures the children, cooks the food, washes the cloths, and cleans the house. If she has no status at all, her health is not taken care than the health systems suffer. Most of the women suffer from anemia and malnutrition, because of insufficient availability of food in terms of quantity and quality. Spending more time in the villages and with the wholistic health approach, can build an awareness of sicknesses.

As people are still in darkness due to ignorance; and therefore they go to Bhagats the witch doctor a village medicine man that interprets the sign's sent by the spirit and invoke powers from the spirits to heal the sick. So myths and superstitious beliefs affect; even to this day they go to Bhagats, they have explanations of every illness that they get - for instance, Measles is supposed to be a visit of the Ori Mata (goddess) who is going to bless the village.

Health workers are like small lamps, becoming like a big torch as the days pass, crucial role in bringing together the whole area under one umbrella. It is worth giving them a chance to look after their family and their village health. As they are taking a keen interest in learning and listening, and removing many health taboos related to health thus able to diagnose simple illnesses, and restoring people to health and wholeness. They try to be like little lamps that break through the thick darkness of the heart and mind of the people bringing them to enjoy fullness of health.

Their continuous efforts, regular personal touch, and close contact with people have changed the situation. Now they can see and feel the changes in themselves and in their own children, the result is mothers have good health and the children's malnutrition level has decreased.

Malaria and tuberculosis is coming back to society with force. Malaria fever with other clinical manifestations and resistance to chloroquine treatment makes management difficult. This is an issue of worry and concern. Since they are professionally not qualified we need to update them with ongoing training programs.

Antinatal mothers come in only when they are in their fourth/fifth month. Sometimes it is due to shyness that they hide the fact of their pregnancy. So with constant visits and awareness a significant move in becoming women more sociable have changed families bringing about better understanding and co-operation. They move around with added self-confidence, they feel efficient and effective in their work in community as animators and promoters of health.

They keep the **records** of morbidity pattern, home visits, health education, daily records of the patient's sicknesses, first aid medicines received and given, monthly training, monthly meetings, have been taught the habit of saving money for their future, personal saving which makes them self-sufficient and increases confidence, they know now how to manage with the finance of their family.

They are a means of dialogue between the people and health team. Periodically reviewing, evaluating and on going training, and living in the same areas helps them to arrest infection at its on set, medical facilities not available and villages are fairly remote which makes there intervention viable.

The **balwadis visit** and the house visits of the balwadis teachers have been a very positive step ahead. They have come closer to their own people of the village and it has given them respect and status in the community as leaders who are sincere in their efforts for the development of their community.

The health of any community is the sum total of the health of its members. They spend a great deal of time on activities related to supplementary nutrition program, immunization, health check-ups, referral services and non-formal health education.

Supplementary Nutritional Program has made a great impact on the nutrition status of the children in the villages. They make great efforts in educating the mothers in preparing the supplementary food, use of home remedies in diseases like diarrhea and vomiting, fever, common cold and in the treatment of simple respiratory tract infection.

The nutritional status of women in the villages is comparatively poorer than men, due to poverty biased and social structures. It has a negative impact on women during pregnancy. Normally, village women do not take advantage or approach any health centers for check-ups during pregnancy, make them aware of the need of regular check-ups, lactating mothers are encouraged to breastfeed the children because of its nutritive and immunizing value; all parents do not seem to understand the necessity to educate children. They are still sending the children to the cattle grazing and for child labor. Still there is a need for the village community to be better organized with more awareness to be created among them for the personal responsibility as well as that of the community.

Encourage all the parents to make use of **National Pulse Polio Campaign,** continue convincing every woman to take antitetanus injection for promotion of a safe delivery. Home deliveries are very much prevalent in the villages. Often there are complications during delivery, intervene to shift them to the nearby health centers, which often save the lives of the mother and child. From the very beginning of pregnancy the women are brought to the nutrition program and are given antenatal benefits. Infant mortality rate has continued to decline due to their services.

Cooperation and coordination is a powerful tool in the hands of health workers who work towards social change and social justice in health care, aim to help people to achieve health by their own actions and efforts, developing a sense of responsibility for their won health betterment as individuals, and as members of families, communities.

Health is one of the elements in the general welfare of the people, and health education is only one of the factors in improving health and social conditions. It is, however, an indispensable factor and should therefore be integrated with other social, economic, health and educational efforts.

Health education has to be with proper relevant topic, up-to-date knowledge, reliable matter, given with interest, proper method, to communicate ideas correctly, with appropriate language used, effective matter well prepared, clarity, and using visual aids aptly, to get positive response from the participant, help to develop rapport and understand the health needs and problems. Provide comprehensive health care and act like a postage stamp, stick to one thing until you get there.

As a result superstitions, ill practices and ignorance regarding health and sickness have given way to better awareness and healthy practices in curing and preventing illnesses, at the grassroots which has enhanced life and promoted health and sensitized the public towards a scientific attitude. Start low, go slow, but do so, act as umbilical cord-link, build good network with village committee, removing many health taboos. They are slowly learning the art of discussions and sharing.

We realize that they have greater incentive and motivations for further learning; they move around with added confidence and are more efficient in their work; and strive to make health as a reality for all, especially the unreached and the oppressed. We are far behind the developed world standers. Thus, what has been achieved leaves no place for complacency. We need to go many miles ahead.

To become a sign of hope and love to the world, a true reflection of God's love to the sick, crippled paralytic, and dying. Our way of proceeding has to combine with love for the poor, serenity at work, and professionalism in medicine. Give to the client's human dignity. Promote, defend, develop, and protect the health and life of every client till he or she reaches the plenitude of life.

Make serious efforts to help the sick to accept sickness, backed by unconditional love, and selfless service, defend the right to live denounce openly, the structures that lead to unjust suffering, pain, sorrow, sickness and death. Work with the weakest section of the community.

Health is more a socio-economic-political problem than a merely a medical one. It is a trap of a vicious cycle. Mothers overworked and under weighed leads to mal-nutrition, poor birth weight, low resistance and high susceptibility to infection. The child gets less energy that is required for, results in failure of growth, vicious cycle all infections have nutritional impact, it can depress appetite, decrease body's absorption, can reject food, results in diarrhea, RTI, this is big set back on child's growth – who later becomes malnourished parents.

The major share of progress in our country is passed on to the cities. 72.2% of our population lives in the villages, which are still in underdeveloped or semi-developed. Therefore, we have to give power to the poor, to integrate their sufferings and instill hope in their lives, liberate them from forces of evil in order to give fuller life, and to heal the unhealthy tendencies that hide in our human condition such as selfishness, ego, ambitions, individualism, and lack of solidarity.

It is universal truth that failure in health systems hit the poor people the hardest. They are forced to live in the vicious circle of poverty, indebted and ill health. The sign of the times are frightening. Many parts of the country are under the grip of severe drought and floods, natural calamities, global warming. Failure in the monsoon or heavy rainfalls and rise cost of essential commodities will mean further hardships for the poor who are living below the magical line.

The private sector in the medical care and diagnostic services has mushroomed in large cities giving rise to unethical practices and negligence.

These coming years are not going to be easy. Income is less and expenses are increasing .We have already begun to sip the bitter cup that awaits those who dare squarely to face injustice. Obstruction and objections may have to be faced, but they are the challenge and this is the task ahead of us, March ahead in love to build a better community. India has the second largest child labor population in the world; where children work in miserable conditions.

How do we see these above-mentioned challenges around us? How do we respond?

We have made progress in the field of health, positive indicators such as falling IMR, and fall in fertility rate, and rising life expectancy at birth, is a sign of hope.

Health is beyond sickness and walls of hospital. Early detection of any diseases is very important and crucial. People need to be made aware, motivated and awaken for self and family health.

When it is ideal to have all deliveries in a hospital, why talk about home-based newborn care? Equipping of family members and parents with adequate knowledge of 'home-based newborn care' becomes important. If they are knowledgeable, they will ensure that the person conducting the home delivery will follow the minimum essential procedures to ensure the survival of the newborn. This knowledge also helps them to recognize complications at the earliest, and to seek care of a specialist immediately.

Often, the lack of "sense of urgency" on the part of family members and the delay caused thereby in seeking expert care are what kill thousands of newborns. Neighborhood solidarity in helping a family to rush to a hospital with money and transport is so crucial in the survival of a newborn. Can an Anganwadi worker be trained to meet this challenge? Increasing the knowledge level of family members and community leaders on newborn care is a must in order to change behavior at household and village levels.

Significant reduction in newborn mortality can be achieved through training and equipping community health workers, Anganwadi workers. Life expectancy in India has increased during the last century. It is higher in villages and urban slums among economically disadvantaged groups.

Community health workers, providers if trained, equipped, supervised and supported by sensitive health care personal in newborn care, significant reduction in newborn mortality can occur. Special emphasis must be given to maintenance of hygiene at the time of delivery in homes, cutting the umbilical cord with adequate aseptic precautions, cleaning baby's mouth-to mask respiration and feeding the premature baby, not giving bath on the same day, weighing the baby immediately, heating the room, (burning coals/1000 W lamp), increasing the humidity (water boiling /drying wet cloths in the room), encouraging breastfeeding and minimal handling of the baby to prevent infection. Giving expressed breast milk by spoon to babies who are unable to suckle and adopting risk management strategy for LBWs, small size, preterm births, feeding problems, illness and difficult labor, referring the sick neonates, if more than one risk factors are present, are some of the practical points in reducing neonatal mortality rate at primary care level of newborn. What is needed is awareness, energizing at the grassroot level and making it functional with limited resources. Newborn week is celebrated in November 15, 'give a breath, save a life'.

Improved survival of **low birth weight babies** can be achieved through educating mothers and family members on home-based neonatal care. Survival of the low birth weight babies can be strengthened by training of persons involved in the health care delivery system, i.e. medical officers, nurses, community health workers. Reorientation of the medical education at undergraduate and postgraduate levels, together with strengthening of the neonatal units (level II) will definitely help in achieving this goal. The programmes of Government of India "Child survival and safe motherhood (CSSM)" and "Reproductive child health (RCH)" emphasize the need for involving mothers and family members in the 'essential newborn care'.

If the delivery is going to take place in the house, the family members should ensure the presence of a well-trained birth attendant or a nurse-midwife. A pre-packed delivery kit obtained from the nearest ANM/AWW should be handed over to the trained person conducting the delivery. Also, clean clothes to wipe dry and wrap the baby.

Low birth weight babies between 2 kg to 2.5 kg can be managed at home. Such babies should be provided warmth, ensured adequate and frequent feeding, prevented from infections, the baby should be wrapped well with thin layers of soft clothes and blankets, head should be covered to the mother's abdomen or chest.

More than half of the child deaths could be prevented if a new model – home-based neonatal care – is tried. What can be done to prevent these deaths? Malnutrition, which starts in the uterus, and infections occurring after birth due to dirty environment are the main causes of these deaths. Thus, these neonates are born, cared for, and they survive or die inside these rooms without the knowledge of the outside world. Neither health services nor free economy reach them. How can these be reached, and saved? Every mother has the right to have proper health and nutritional education during pregnancy; her child has the right to survive like many others.

Drugs should be used to the minimum because they are foreign agents in the body and have lot of side effect. Real healing takes place only when the person is brought back to the purpose for which God created her/him. Human life is significant and it is dear to us. The precious life entrusted into our hands needs to be cared, nourished and nurtured in all sense of the word. To uphold the human dignity and quality of life for which God has created one and all. May that person be a poor or rich, rural or urban all dealt with equality and held the life as dear as mine and yours, as children of mother India.

It is heartening to watch India's quest for becoming an information technology upper power getting realized slowly but steadily. Lot of importance is being given to this area, with huge investments in human and material resources. But a major concern exists as to how far these developments will help the nation surge forward in other directions as well. Will the country accord similar attention to the social development sector also?

These are very pertinent questions because; ultimately this progress has to be instrumental in improving the quality of life of the people, not a handful, but everyone. Do our current national priorities oriented towards this goal? Do the present measures ensure a good, accessible and affordable Medicare and disease prevention and control mechanism, the cumulative effect of which will boost the health status of people?

Available health indicators are, unfortunately, not too affirmative. It may be an indication of further deterioration in public health care standards, despite massive efforts, may have dangerous portents for future. Changes in policies, concepts and practices, habits and customs leading to a fresh mind set are necessary to drive home the point that health is every body's business. We need policies to spur the nation to break the shackles of the vicious circle that exists between poverty, inequity, poor health and the precarious access to health services.

Major problem we will face in working with them could be difficult to make them to give up their false beliefs and practices, difficult to elicit full co-operation due to fights and disagreement, they have constant recourse to alcohol, poverty, too easily give up the struggle. Various myths like belief in life after death, God as the creator of the universe, closeness and dependence on nature. Unclean habits excessive drinking by parents leads to neglect the children, parents are not sufficiently motivated. Unemployment, addiction to alcohol, smoking, gambling and they do not see need to change this habit.

Always at the receiving end, Strong will power to work with them is needed, to make serious effort to understand them by learning and speaking in their own language, accepting their culture, adapting to their way of living will only help us in community building and that can be done by becoming supportive system to them; creating awareness on the evils, training leaders at various levels to motivate people to pick up good value and stand firm. We have to make our intervention.

Walking to the village, reaching out to the poor and sick, spending time listening to them, being friendly, simple, and loving nature you will be accepted by them. They are simple and happy in spite of being poor, they share readily what they have with others, they live for today; their simplicity and love for nature, dance, respect for life; their celebration bring the whole village together, their structure, house, lifestyle, food habits of their own. Acknowledge that they too have knowledge skill and intelligence.

Community Health Nurse (CHN) can help to change the health behavior of people, as she will see the real situation and surrounding in actual field, which will help the people also to be relaxed, mood atmosphere to accept changes that she suggests with convictions as socioeconomic factors affect the health. She can notice if any **superstitious beliefs** exist that affect the family health. Certain diseases are caused due to the wrath of god and goddess such as sitla Devi mata- they do puja to appease the gods like nagdev, magurdev, dungerdev. Some people they consider are responsible for disease, evil eye affects, some ghost intrusion into the body and they drive away evil spirit do certain ceremonies and do not take treatment in time.

Tongue examination is an important in medical care as it yields valuable information about patient's indicators of underlying diseases and thus helps in diagnosis of the condition such as discoloration or a pale smooth and bald tongue indicates iron deficiency, anemia, etc and dry tongue sign of dehydration, white patches thrust.

A health from all dimensions of human person one has to believe and be convinced the importance and challenge of Medical Care. Thus in short to point out the progress made and to be made in the field of Health and the challenges the 3rd Millennium is forcing us to face, People's health in peoples hands base into grassroots.

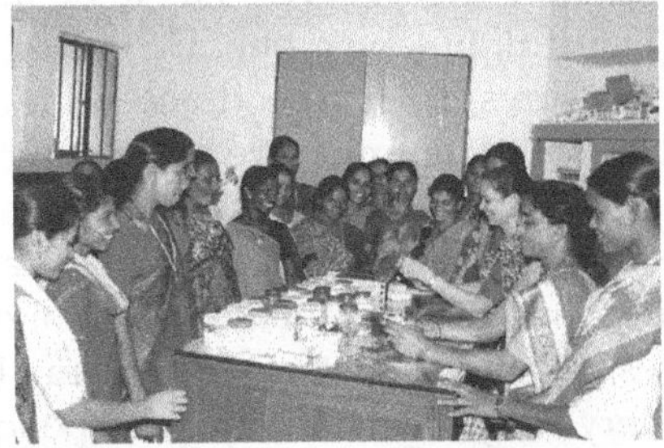

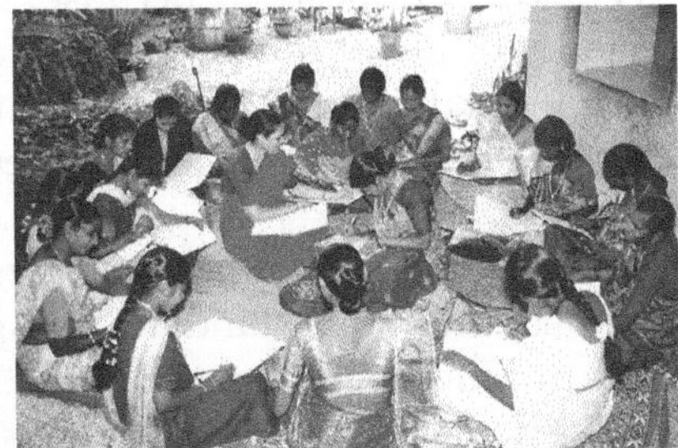

Figs 8.1 and 8.2: Demonstration and teaching the health education on how to handle first aid kits. Health education and communication skills. Scope of health education is very wide and vital. Emerging women as leaders to take up responsibility of their own community with guidance. Health functionaries, health team helping in integral development of whole community

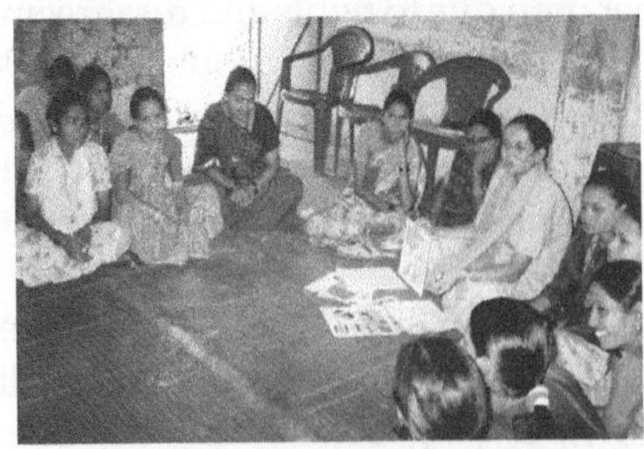

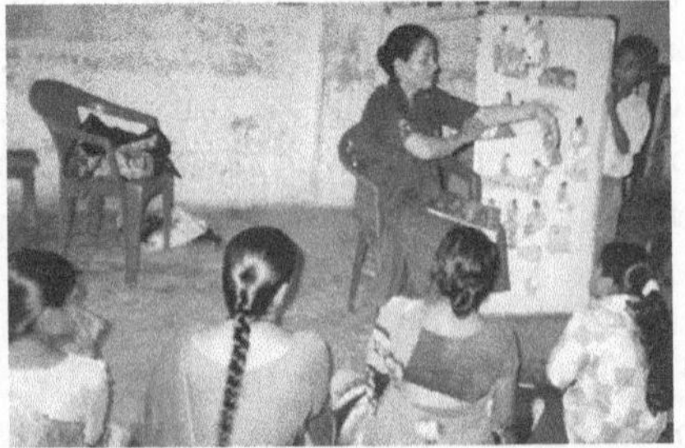

Figs 8.3 and 8.4: Communicate effectively with the group. Modification of behaviors is the aim and objectives of health education. Take away misconception and harmful blind beliefs

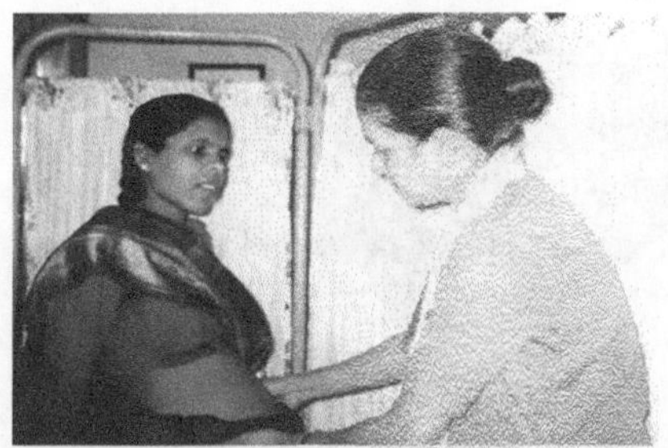

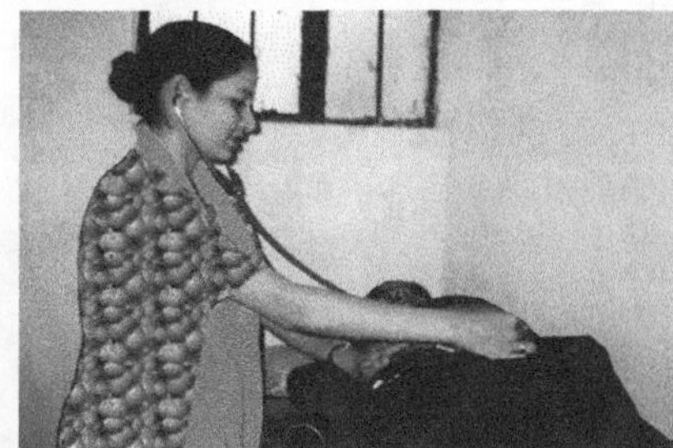

Figs 8.5 and 8.6: Visits to the clinic that saves lives. To promote and maintain antenatal care, find out high risk pregnancies and ensure safe motherhood. Promoting institutional deliveries

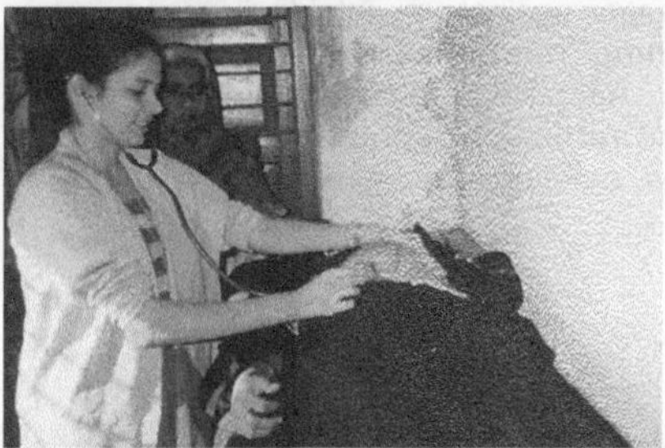

Fig. 8.7: Dimension of health care. Auscultation for fetal heart sounds with stethoscope, making motherhood safe

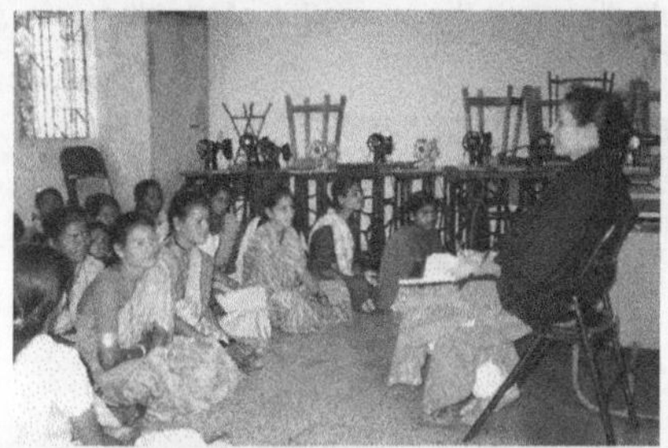

Fig. 8.8: Community participation and levels of health care through health awareness

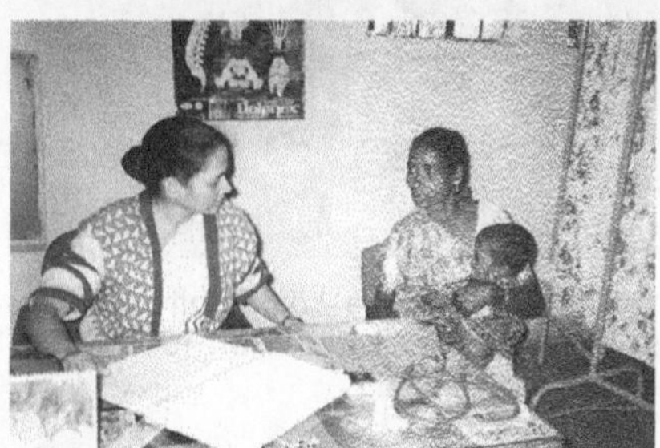

Fig. 8.9: Population explosion as social problem, urgent steps towards MCH and family planning counseling

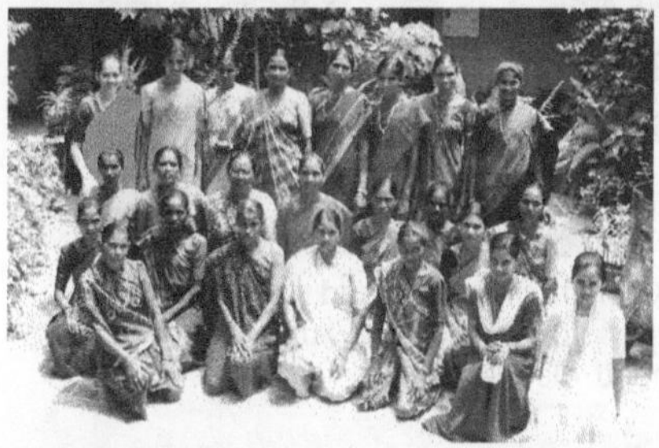

Fig. 8.10: Roles and functions of field functionaries: Health team, the spinal cord of the health care delivery system

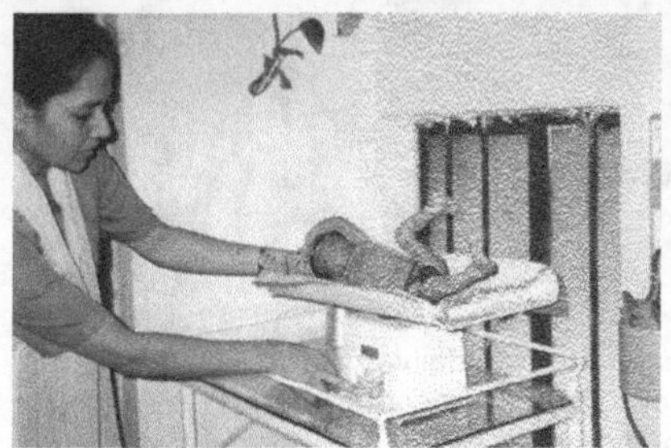

Fig. 8.11: Indicators of health. Recording birth weight using infant weighing scale

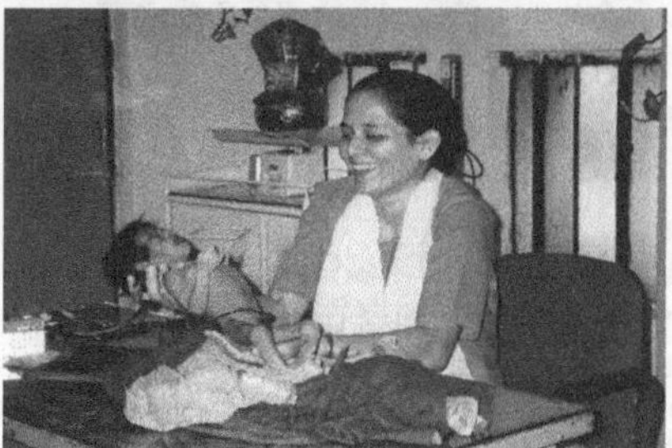

Fig. 8.12: CSSM—Child Survival and Safe Motherhood. Physical examination and management of program. Prevention of IMR. CMR, i.e. 'Child Mortality Rate' through efficient MCH services, low birth weight, breastfeeding, growth monitoring, in order to attain total well-being

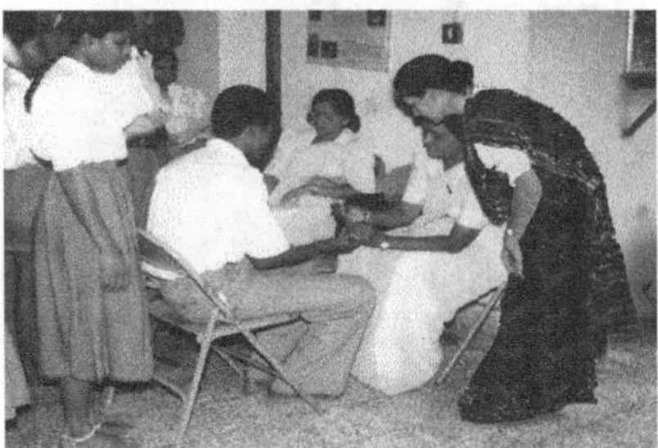

Fig. 8.13: Regular health check ups in school. School health services. Detection of early diagnosis the promotion of positive health

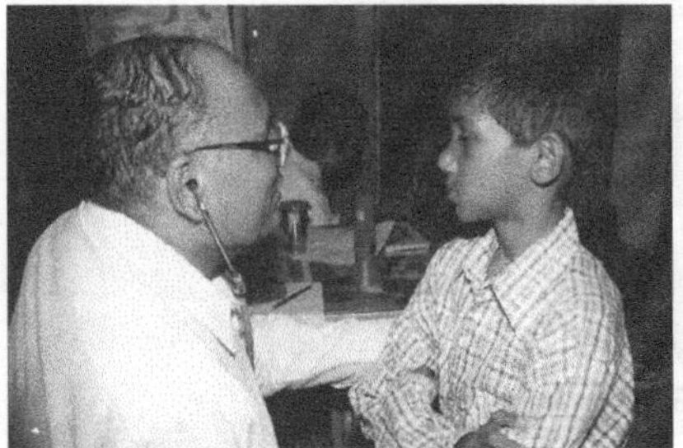

Fig. 8.14: Regular medical check ups of school children, by medical officer, immunization against preventable diseases. Awakening health consciousness in children. Attention to remedial defects like errors of refraction, dental caries, skin diseases, emotional problems

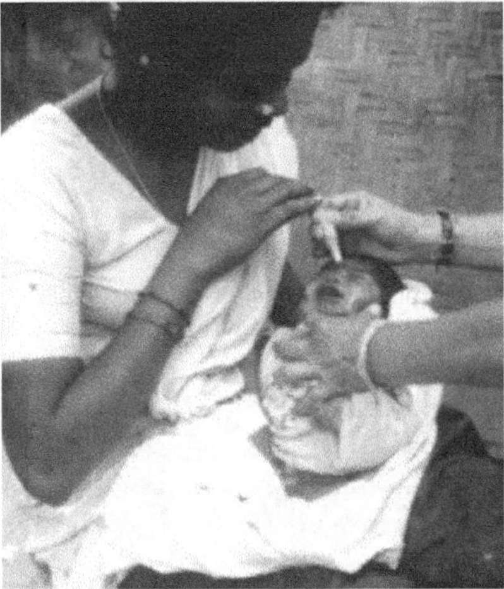

Fig. 8.15: Immunization and recommended vaccines for prevention and control of childhood diseases

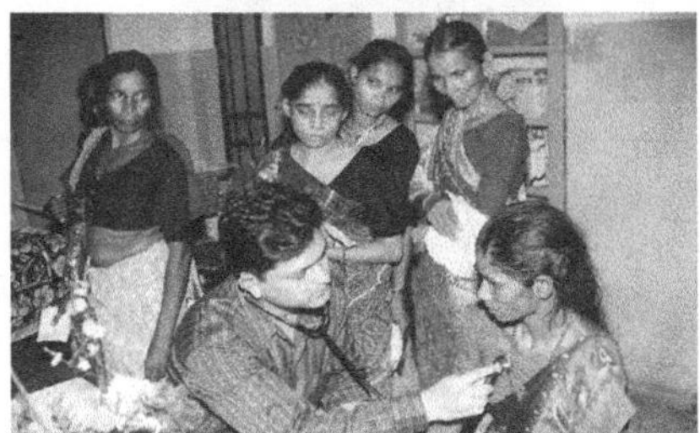

Fig. 8.16: Comprehensive community services. Prevention and detection for early diagnosis

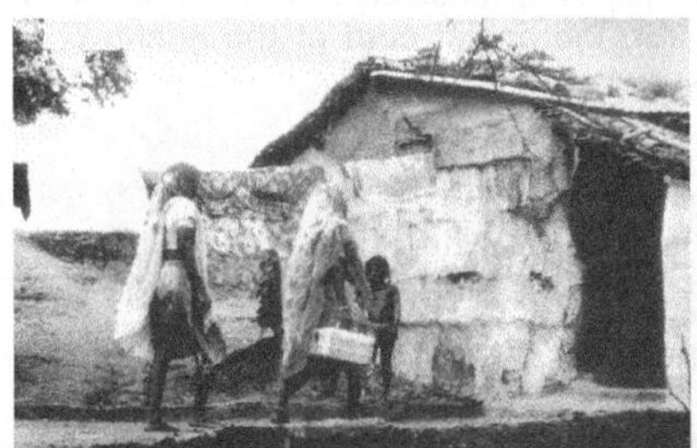

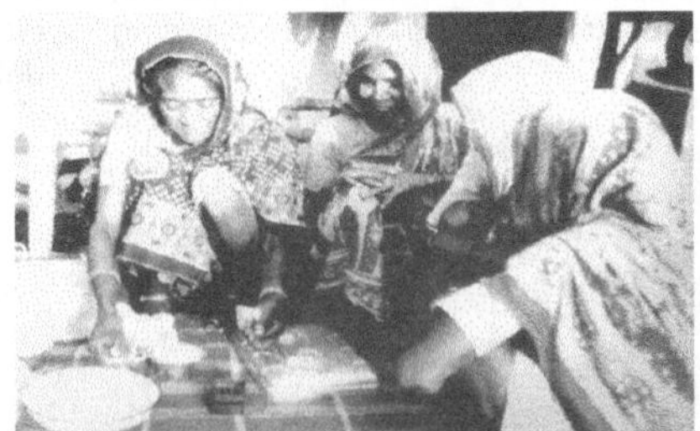

Figs 8.17 and 8.18: Door to door visit of *dais*, traditional *dais* with safe delivery kit visiting the homes of pregnant mothers. Techniques of clean delivery kit and procedure carried out. Health is a vicious circle. Good antenatal care, healthy baby, better family

9 Indigenous Alternative System of Medicines

Human body is the nature's highest evolution. It is a machine unmatched in its design, unparalleled in the integrity of its functional systems and unfathomable in the depth of subtle and natural emotions. Human body keeps working day and night for 70-80 years. The man has so far not devised such as efficient machine, which can work so effectively and for such a length of time. It has its own devices to make and break and healing phenomenon.

The human body is a perfect machine, which can regulate itself, provided the natural rules of food, work and rest are observed. When we transgress natural rules, we create toxins in the body, which the body attempts to get rid of. This attempt is considered as disease and is given different names according to different symptoms.

Of all kinds of happiness the best happiness is good health. The greatest wonder in this cosmos is the human body. Nature has provided in our body an inbuilt mechanism to maintain and to repair.

For centuries, traditional healers have taken care of the health needs of their own community as a part of their social responsibility. They have used the knowledge that has been passed down the generations regarding the medicinal value for locally available herbs and plants. This tradition still continues, particularly in the rural pockets of the country.

People choose, prefer some times the natural alternative therapies to synthetic medications and their desire to control the allopathic toxicities. Also to control undesirable side effects that the drugs have they want to lessen them, there are times they feel sick and there is failure to determine diagnosis in spite of many tests, some times they are suffering from chronic illness with poor prognosis, other times cannot afford and want to reduce insurance coverage, at times due to healing system that is part of a clients cultural or identify group heritage, increased interest in preventive strategies and holistic approaches to health, are some of the reasons clients turn to the different alternative systems of medicines and find solace.

Some times just following healthy eating with a more nutritionally sound diet, which helps them to maintaining fitness and reducing stress. We have to provide information to teach healthy life style, modification behaviors, weight loss strategies, stress reduction strategies, exercise and fitness, ask what else are you doing to cure for your health, become familiar with local patterns restore the client back to total health open and guide them and refer them to right practitioner.

The allopathic system tends to view people as composed of distinct mechanistic organ systems like the gastro-intestinal tract the cardiorespiratory system, the urogenital tract, the nervous system, etc. The Indian indigenous and homeopathic systems, in contrast, see human health more in terms of balances and flows of "doshas" and energies. They are less concerned with the physical boundaries and connections of organs.

The allopathic approach to medical treatment is characterized by attempts to fight, remove or eradicate causative agents that are germs, allergens, and defective parts and to suppress symptoms. On the other hand, the indigenous and homeopathic systems aim towards restoring balances and flows in the person without considering the parts separately. The latter approach is called holistic.

Realistically speaking, each approach has certain strengths and weaknesses. The golden rule is to test everything in the light of reasons and experience, no matter from whom it comes. It must complement it and which can be used profitably for the benefit of wellness and healing.

Whatever the particular health system, the healer doctor, vaidya, hakims, vaidu can exploit his power over the sick person and relatives. It is doubly so with women, who are sick. In this respect there is little difference between practitioners of the holistic and non-holistic systems.

Complementary Health treatment has been rapidly growing in popularity over recent years. As a group of diverse medical and health care systems, practices and products that are not presently considered part of conventional medicine- homeopathic and naturopathic medicines are examples. One can do fasting and dieting properly; using magnets to cure illness. Every person can use any one of the methods according to his conviction and convenience. What is required is faith in the treatment adopted. Through the natural treatment he can be his own doctor of health. The life battery is capable of controlling and keeping fine and fit but when it has overwork it gets weak and the body becomes prone to disease.

Ayurveda, Siddha, Unani, Yoga, Homeopathy, Naturopathy, color therapy, Acupressure, Acupuncture, Reflexology, Pranic Healing, Home and Herbal Medicines, Hydrotherapy, Cold – Mud Packs, Massage-exercise, Fasting, Prayer-meditations, home and herbal medicines are some of the system of medicines. These provide the bulk of medical care to the rural people. The use of indigenous systems of medicines is widespread and growing. Co-ordination between is to be established yet. Allopathic physicians do not refer most of the patients who avail this therapy, yet most of the patients self-referred themselves. There is the increasing popularity worldwide of complementary medicines reflects the changing attitudes and needs of the population.

You can live hundred years a healthy life if you follow the laws of nature. The nature will teach you how to live what to eat and what to avoid and if you do not follow the law of nature it will be shown into ill health. Where do the animal's birds go for medicines if you watch you will see them eating some kind of grass that has medicinal values and importance? They never over eat. They take sufficient rest. Tips to live healthy life are in our hand once we have awareness and control. We are what we eat. The food we take shows in everything from our stamina and strength to the glow of the cheeks. It helps us live well and look well. Changing life style has altered our eating habits, instead of traditional patterns, which contributes many nutrients and good health.

Medicine causes overuse, disuse or misuse of faculties; errors in judgment; and influence of seasonal changes. According to ayurveda all human diseases can be classified into the seven broad categories namely: Genetic, congenital, constitutional, traumatic, seasonal, infectious and spiritual, natural. In ayurveda, physicians try to assess the symptoms of these diseases as much as the nature of ailment and its root causes.

Exercise is essential and must be done regularly to promote good health. It helps in body functioning and maintains and restores strength and helps to maintain proper weight under control. Exercise is good for improvement of health or correction of physical deformity. It maintains the muscle tone, helps in joints mobility and stiffness. It maintains the born density and prevents osteoporosis, stimulates the blood circulation and prevents venous stasis. Assists in the exchange of oxygen and nutrients into the tissues and waste products from the tissues, prevents varicose veins, helps to reduce edema, and reduces the workload from the heart. It also prevents venous thrombosis and pulmonary embolism. Prevents obesity, regulates body temperature, improves appetite and digestion, and prevents constipation and flatulence. Promotes elimination from the skin, improves the lung ventilation, promotes physical and mental well-being, prevents depression and boredom, improves memory and provides an outlet from emotional tension. Exercise should be planned according to age and physical condition. Avoid over fatigue, chills and draught should be repeated daily if possible at same time.

Oil bath— Vegetable oil such as groundnut or mustard is applied and massaged into the skin. It is the Indian custom to apply oil over body to keep the body cool and skin soft.

Rest and sleep, relaxation— By which body recovers rapidly back to normal gives good night sleep after busy day, it relives fatigue, it is essential for good health, it is a natural process to recuperate the energy sound sleep and vigor.

Ayurvedic physicians alone are estimated to be about 3.37 lakhs. Studies indicate that nearly 90% of Ayurvedic physicians serve the rural areas. Most of them are local residents and remain very close to the people socially and culturally. In resent years there has been considerable state patronage to foster these systems of medicine. Many Ayurvedic dispensaries are run by the states. Indigenous system of medicine could best be utilized for more effective or total health coverage. In indigenous folk medicines patients and relatives can talk freely to these practitioners, who is the part of the total way of life of the people, treatment is bared on charity. Medicines are prepared from ordinary plants common to region. It is not alien to culture patterns of the real folk.

Geneva has reported that 60% of the Australians use 17,000 herbal products. In Belgium, almost 40% population use this 59% doctors use alternative medicines. In France, 49% people have used herbal and homeopathy. In Germany, there are 10,000 – 13,000 alternative medicines practitioner and 75% of the physicians use complementary; in United Kingdom, 90% people use and 8,000 non-allopathies practitioners. United States, a National follow-up survey has shown that – use of alternative therapies have increased from 40 to 42% and expected to increase and grow up to 60%. In India at present there are about 587,536 practitioners. There are 3,862 hospitals and 22,104 dispensaries in the government sector. In addition, there is a large number run by NGOs. There are 300 colleges of ISM with five and a half years degree courses. Fourty-five Ayurveda colleges impart postgraduate training.

Each tribe has its own socio-religious life; but money, hunger, power that have displaced them from their original habitat and lose touch with the wealth of experiential knowledge handed down orally by their forebears. To make effort and future attempts to collect and preserve the knowledge that exists. The use of indigenous system of medicines is widespread and growing. Yet coordination between both is not established. Increasing popularity worldwide of complementary medicines reflects the changing attitudes and needs of the population.

In **Indian culture, heritage indigenous medicines** were used but due to industrialization, globalization natural herbs and herbal medicines are in verge of extinctions. Local villages that have still knowledge about this have to be kept alive by encouraging and preserving it. God has created the earth with many medicinal plants. At the village level this medicines should be propagated so that this important heritage does not die. Sixty percent of illness is said caused by virus, medicines given for it are not scientific, therefore one has to know the useful vanaspati. It is gift of God given to mankind, so one has to develop in people faith in these medicines. In ancient times when science was not developed like today; people lived healthy life. Are we living better / healthier life than our ancestral? Today alternative system of medicine is becoming popular in western countries.

Home remedies which are available in our kitchen such as turmeric, ginger, garlic, pepper, onion, honey. Many people who get tired of allopathic medicines they find outlet in such medicines, when sudden illness sticks doctors are unreachable and if Community Health Nurse (CHN) have knowledge of these medicine can save life. It is natural hidden treasure in the forest, fields, and around our houses. Herbal health is viable low-cost and self-supporting.

The use of **cucumber** (*khira*) juice is an excellent remedy for bladder infection. It is a very effective diuretic. A glass of this juice, mixed with two teaspoons of honey and tablespoon of fresh limejuice, should be given three times daily.

Spinach is a cheap vegetable, which contains the same amount of protein one gets from the same quality of meat, fish, egg and chicken. It is a remedy for many ailments. Regular use of spinach during pregnancy will help prevent the deficiency of folic acid. It will also prevent threatened abortion and accidental hemorrhage, temperate-sprue associated with lassitude, shortness of breath, loss of weight and diarrhea.

Being a rich source of vitamin A, spinach promotes growth and health, especially the health of the eyes. Lack of this vitamin may lead to night blindness. Spinach is thus an effective food remedy for the prevention and treatment of night blindness.

Two garlic pods a day for good health. It kills viruses responsible for colds. Eat a garlic when you feel a sore throat coming on, acts as decongested; it has immune functioning by stimulating infection fitting. Eating one or two cloves of raw garlic a day is recommended to people with chronic or recurrent infections. Natural health natural medicines eat raw cloves into small piece and swallow then like pills. Garlic has said to have thinning effect on the blood and it claims to prevent or cure cancer boils, cyst, cuts, food poisoning and many more ailments. It helps in arteriosclerosis, diabetes, common cold and influenza. It has healing benefits and it contains super.

Few tips to treat asthma—Asthma is an allergic condition resulting from the reaction of the body to one or more allergies. **Using honey**— Honey is one of the most common home remedies for asthma. It is said that if a jug of honey is held under the nose of an asthma client and he inhales the air that meets it, he stars breathing easier and deeper. **Using lemon-** Lemon is another fruit found beneficial in the treatment of asthma. The juice of one lemon, diluted in a glass of water and taken with meals, will bring good results. **Using Indian gooseberry-** Five grams of gooseberry mixed with one tablespoon of honey forms an effective medicinal tonic for the asthma. It should be taken every morning. **Ten garlic cloves** boiled in 30 ml of milk taken once daily helps to keep asthma under control. A soup prepared from **drumstick leaves**, taken once daily add handful of leaves to 180 ml of water boiling it for five minutes allow it to cool, add little salt, pepper and lime juice may be added to the soup is good remedy in asthma.

The cactus plants rough thorny exterior hides in its core medicinal nutritious elements. The plant has multiple uses. It has important medical properties. This plant is a neglected crop in our country. It has biochemical and molecular botanic and psychogenetic aspects. It is a vegetable and staple food in desert of Mexico; which has high content of fiber, which decreases gastric acidity.

Margosa/Nim healer and air purifier, a juice helpful in controlling diabetes, 5 ml early morning for 3 nights or 10 leaves chewed daily. Malian, piles and ointment prepared from nim leaves also useful in healing ulcers of wounds.

Ginger has a tonic effect on the heart. It is antibacterial, anticonvulsion, antiulcer, antisecretory, antifungal, antispasmodic and antiallergic. It is valued world over as a culinary herb, spice, and home remedy and medical curb. It works as a painkiller.

Guava pear is regarded as best laxative fruits for easing constipation.

Raw vegetable juices, carrot juice with the combination with spinach juice has proved beneficial in ringworm.

Plants cure the clients from their illness; they are tested for efficacy of the plants used in treatment. They are effective, have no side effect and are nontoxic, e.g. tulsi.

Alfalfa seeds- a leguminous herb-it is said that Arabs discovered it and promptly cherished it. The father of all foods; being an excellent source of energy and has been used by the Chinese since the 6th century to treat kidney stones, fluid retention, swelling and to correct digestive problems, menopause and good source of vitamins and calcium, potassium, iron and zinc. One can sprout seeds and eat sprouts raw.

Black cumin/onion seeds (Kalonji)—Hailed as the seeds of blessing in Unani medicines. Used for cure of many ailments such as allergies, asthma, immune disorders and skin conditions. It is bitter to test and taken with warm water for better absorption.

Fenugreek seeds (Methi)—To increase the flow of mothers milk tea can be taken made of the seeds. It stimulates breast growth; it has ancient and modern reputation. One of the oldest medicinal plants and it has been ancient remedy in respiratory congestion. The seeds of good health and the storehouse of nutrients. One can derive many health benefits from spices and seeds.

Peel nutrition—The skin of most fruits and vegetables are rich in fiber if you cook a peel-based dish you are bound to get all the benefits of a high-fiber content recipe, like getting rid of constipation. Peels are also rich in antioxidants, which help strengthen one's immune system and protect against pollution. Some peels or the skin of fruits and vegetables are also rich in beta-carotenes, which is a precursor to vitamin A. many peels are rich in potassium as well. Gourd or dudhi peels is believed to be a good source of vitamin K, which is supposed to be good for heart. As for the seeds of fruits and vegetables, most of them have higher protein content than the fruit or vegetables itself and is always a good nutrition source.

Watermelon beats the heat in hot summer thirst quencher and contributes to conditions like asthma, diabetes, colon cancer and arthritis. Sweet, juicy watermelon important antioxidants and excellent source of vitamin C and A, it has higher water content and lower calorie content then many other fruits and has outstanding health benefits.

Mind body medicine uses a variety of technique designed to enhance the minds capacity, which affects the bodily function and its manifestations. Help sort including meditation, prayer, mental healing and therapies that use creative outlet such as art, music and dance. Biological-based therapies use substances found in nature, herbs, foods and vitamins. Manipulation and body based methods— massage, meditation-vipassana-deep relaxation. When natural balance or harmony is disturbed illness results. Holistic practitioners advocate the use of lifestyle modification skills such as meditation, exercise, relaxation that alleviate stress. Meditation is a way to tune and train our mind that leads to greater efficiency in everyday life, guided imagery, a form of relaxation technique. Therapeutic touch ancient practice of laying on hands. Client experience relaxation, breathing becomes deeper, decreases muscles tension and warms hands and feet.

Human body heals itself if people take responsibility for their own health. To have better health nurture your faith dimension, develop useful hobbies that are constructive, love life and love people, have self-esteem, build positive outlook towards life and its happenings, use your creativity and ability to the maximum levels, live with harmony with universe, eat well, exercise daily, do not hold grudges, be at peace, find satisfaction in work and be contented in what life has offered you, you feel fresh, happy and will have holistic health.

Acupressure is nature's health science inbuilt in our body. Based on Bioelectricity-bioenergy, it operates on same principle as acupuncture. Acupressure is an ancient healing art that uses the fingers to press potent points on the whole body surface. It works by stimulating the body's self-curative abilities. Acupressure mainly focuses on relieving pain and discomfort as well as on responding to tension before it develops onto a disease.

When the keypoints of the body are pressed they promote the circulation of the blood and release muscular tension. In acupressure, it is said that pain is the cry for hungry nerve for the want of better blood supply. There are no side effects from drugs because there are no drugs and the basic equipment needed for it is individuals own two hands. Thus, acupressure therapy can be practiced anywhere and any time.

Everyone at one time or the other has used our hands spontaneously to hold tense or painful places on the body. More than 5000 years ago, the Chinese discovered that pressing certain points on the body relieved pain where it occurred and also benefited other parts of the body more remote from the pain and pressure points. Gradually other locations were found that not only relieved pain but also influenced the functioning of certain internal organs.

Acupuncture and acupressure uses the same points but acupuncture employs needles while acupressure uses the gentle but firm pressure of fingers of hand and some modern scientific devices. It is a nature cure system originated in ancient India for treatment in which pressure is applied on points to the ailment of body without any medicines, whenever any organ of the body goes out of order, we start feeling pain on the particular point. Several diseases can be cured at a time by treating concerning reflex centers. Acupressure instruments can activate and stimulate blood circulation and regular flow of bioenergy to develop immunity against disease in the body.

Acupuncture in china practiced for more than 250 years; the theory of acupuncture exposures belief that there is a pathway of energy flow Qi throughout the body that is vital for health. A trained acupuncturist can correct inadequate Qi at various sits with the insertion of needles or applying heat or electrical stimulation at a number of acupuncture points. It is a Chinese form of medicine.

Reflexology use specific pressure techniques on the reflex points of the feet and hands are able to remove the energy blocks. The energy currents flow freely again and the body is returned to harmony. Reflexology is based on concept of the zone system. Every zone an organ or gland is located; a corresponding reflex area is found on the feet and hands in the same zone. The base of the big toes or thumbs is the reflex areas to the neck; the rotation of the big toe or thumb that is equivalent to rotation of the neck.

These reflex areas are important when a person suffers from headaches or migraines, sight problems. Man is a single whole unit and it is to be learnt that the feet and hands are a corresponding projected whole. For every complaint of the individual there is a disturbed balance, which can be found out on the relative reflex point on his feet. Reflexology is not alternative form of medicine. It can be combined with other forms of medicines like hydrotherapy, homeopathy, herbal medicines, but all these different methods cannot be applied together.

Too much stimulation from too many different directions can have bad effect. The switchboard of the electric current flowing in our body is located in the two palms and sloes. Ten minutes a day to keep the disease away. Mind has a great control on our body. A happy mind in a healthy body is the target to achieve. In nature nobody worries for future. To give is divine. To earn a living honestly is human. To snatch others property is a sin. We all are born as humans. Let us try to be Divine. When mother nature has provided us with such cure, let us not forget nature in our pursuit of science.

Ayurveda practiced in India 5000 years includes diet, herbal remedies and message emphasizes the use of body, mind and spirit in diseases prevent and treatment.

Fasting is a way of knowing your body. The two important pillars of health are good nutrition and moderate exercise. Diet control has lot to do with mind control, self-discipline.

Hydrotherapy—Water the giver of life has become a scarce commodity today. As soon as you get up before brushing your teeth drink half liter of water at a time. 45 minutes do not eat or drink anything. After breakfast, after two hours drink two glasses of water. This is useful for all well and ill people. If daily routinely you follow you will not become ill.

Waters, the liquid of life; nothing ever can take its place. Water enters into every action within the human body. More than two-thirds of our body is composed of water in some form. If you require a glowing skin drinks plenty of water in the morning. Water is very essential to keep ourselves healthy. At least minimum eight to ten glasses of water one must consume. It helps to flush out the toxic from the body and purifies and makes you fresh. It will relieve you from constipation and headaches and other digestive complains, kidney stones, urinary tract infections. The person who does not drink soon has trouble with his internal organs. Everyday our kidneys filter between fifteen and twenty gallons of water. All who desire to remain healthy must drink abundance of pure water each day. Purify your own drinking water.

Nature's pharmacy— If you are going for a walk in the garden or lawn, walk barefooted and the grass in the morning till the dew dries. Touch the rough trunk with your hands. All forests, fields, meadows, are sacred. These are the temples of nature, without them we cannot live; fresh air for healthy living, ancient medicines were combined with super natural belief, religion, magical reties, superstitious, mysticism prevailed. Animals and birds have instinctive drive to choose right medicine for their disorder. Survival is one of the greatest instincts of humankind. Nobody does anyone like to see their dear ones suffering. So, the human searches for cure, healing and wholeness have been unlimited and continuous. India with its riches and diversity of traditions has contributed a great share in promoting healing and alleviating pain and suffering. Faith and healing too has tremendous effect on body mind related illness, psychosomatic etc.

A number of plants grow wild in the forest, wastelands and around the villages every year and die without being used of there ingredients, many plants are important from a medical point of view. Naturopathy system of healing that does not use drug or other unnatural treatment. It relieves on cleansing and restoration of the body through the use of natural forces such as air, light, heat, water and message.

Folk remedies for heatstroke is application of oil and ghee or glycerin, caster oil on the soles of feet is cooling specially when one has a hand and let burning syndrome and graying hair, eyes burning.

Naturopathic medicine practitioners work with natural healing forces within the body with a goal of helping the body heal from disease and attain better health. Practices may include dietary modifications, exercise, acupuncture, minor surgery and various other interventions. Curanswrismo system of beliefs or folk medicines include a variety of techniques such as healing rituals, spirituality, herbal medicines and psychic healing. Special heating, intercessory prayer, faith healing, therapeutic touch, promotion for wholeness; More than 40 alternative diets claim to prevent or treat a variety of conditions. Macrobiotic diets based on belief that disease is caused by an imbalance of yin and yang. More than 20.000 herbal and dietary supplements are sold in US.

Homeopathy is a system of medicine whose principles are older than Hippocrates. It seeks to cure in accordance with natural laws of healing and uses medicines made from natural substances; animal, vegetable and mineral. A German physician, Samuel Christian Friedrich Hahnemann, discovered homeopathy in the early 1800s.

The homeopathic medicines believe that like cures like meaning that small highly diluted quantities of medicinal substances are given to cure manifestations; when the same substances given at higher or more concentrated doses would actually cause those manifestations. It believes that body is always striving to keep healthy, or in balance. When harmful external forces threaten the body, the vital force produces symptoms such as pain, fever, and cough. Pain is warning that something is wrong. Its aim is to strengthen the body so it can resist the harmful organism. We believe that all parts of the body are interdependent, and therefore we treat the client as a whole person, rather than concentrating on one organ or one part of the body.

Homeopaths do not attempt to separate mental from physical illness; all are symptoms of the individual, and see him from holistic approach point of views, and therefore it is on the rise all over the world of its use. A homeopath spends more time with each client and sees fewer clients. Its treatment is less expensive, involving fewer doctors' visits. It involves fewer diagnostic studies. It is less expensive and does not have side effects.

Homeopathic remedies are derived from animal, vegetable, and mineral sources. Some of these sources, in their crude state, are highly toxic. Belladonna is made from a plant, deadly nightshade that is accurately named; its red berries are poisonous. Arsenicum album is made from the metal arsenic a deadly poison. Strange as it may seem, the most noxious substances make the most potent healing agents when prepared homeopathically. The process of preparing homeopathic medicine, potentization (diluting and shaking, or grinding, the substance at each stage of dilution) produces a medicine that contains only trace amounts of the original substance. What is left is the medicinal essence of the substance, so that all homeopathic medicines, regardless of source, are harmless.

The best time the talking the remedy is in the morning before breakfast and before brushing the teeth; putting nothing in the mouth except water fifteen minutes after or before the dose. When opening the bottle, make certain that nothing touches the inside portion of the cork to the cap, and close the bottle as soon as possible. To take a remedy, tip the dose onto your clean palm or onto a spoon, and transfer to the tongue. Eliminate the coffee, which might neutralize the action of the remedy. Drugs are available in various forms, such as mother tincture, globules, pillules, sugar of milk etc. the benefits of homeopathy are being widely recognized the world over.

Healing illness through mind power—In today's times most of us are facing stress, tension, fears, phobias, and diseases. Everyone wants to know the different ways of healing diseases. Yes, this can be achieved. Our mind specially the subconscious mind is a miraculous tool. In addition, we must understand that any disturbance in the mind causes disturbance in the body. So stop talking, stop thinking about your illness, think and live, as you are healthy. Affirmation of positive therapeutic mind set such as I have very high level of energy, I am at peace, and I forgive everyone. Morning and evening do 20 minutes of meditation to increase the power of mind. Research has proved how meditation is beneficial in lowering down your blood pressure, stress, tension and any other illness. Mastermind meditation increases the power of mind. Sit comfortably, loosen your body, with complete backrest, close your eyes, clasp your fingers, and put it on your lap as comfortable position. Focus on your breath. I am going to heal myself with the power of my mind. Moreover, follow the guided meditation. You will feel the inner force of energy and feel light, fresh and at peace with self and around; feel total well being of body and soul.

Yoga applied for integral health—Today the world is full of stress due to lack of leisureliness and fast lifestyle resulting in the absence of mental peace. Psychosomatic illness has increased in urban populations in India and all over the world. Mental health appears to be fast deteriorating not only in adults but in adolescents and children as well. Usage of tranquilizers and antidepressants to induce sleep and reduce tension and depression seems to be the order of the day.

Drug culture has increased and consumption of alcohol and tobacco to reduce stress is common in both men and women. In this type of alarming scenario the message of yoga is like a fresh healing breeze bringing joyful and healthy tiding and optimistic message for the entire humanity.

Just as the musk of deer runs after the source of the perfume not knowing it is within him. Yoga helps us to rediscover within ourselves that lost happiness which so many search for in vain in a thousand different ways and places and never seem to find.

Yoga is one of the greatest gifts of India to humankind. Having discovered this divine path to happiness through their constant meditation and through their reflection on their experience the Indian masters shared this wisdom with other to bring about harmony and peace in individual persons and in the society at large.

Yoga helps people who are yoked under trials, tribulations, tensions, and conflicts and confused of the world, to reach the serene shores of the Divine. The body is purified by water; the mind is purified by positive thoughts and truthfulness. Contemplation is the fruit of accepting God's will in our life. The yogi has to discipline his body and mind for God realization. The yogi is a person who has surrendered himself completely before God; all his actions aims at fulfilling God's designs in his life.

Controlling the mind is not an easy task but we are able to train the mind through constant practice. Our mind is a tool, which we train, use in any way we wish. There is tremendous power and intelligence within us constantly responding to our thoughts and our words. When we start to control our mind a conscious choice of thoughts we are on the way to achieve these powers.

Positive thoughts foster integral growth while negative thoughts crush our life. Therefore to attain happiness one should fill ones mind with positive and creative thinking. It means evaluating ones thoughts from all distracting mental activates and centering them on the supreme reality. This helps us to become one with God. The aim of this mental discipline is to free the mind from all the external belonging and to bind it together with the supreme reality.

It is through breathing that this life-giving energy flows spontaneously into the living beings. Our life begins with the arrival of prana, our heart. We will be able to pray and meditate.

This type **exercise** teaches specific postures and breathing exercises. This form of therapy has been shown at least to improve quality of life for some clients by leading to relaxation and reduced stress levels. A way of life that combines mental, physical exercising to bring the mind and body into balance and prepare the person for union with the higher spiritual power in an ultimate state of being.

It is a method for the integration of human nature as a whole. It is a means for higher life. Yoga means union. Union with oneself, we have body, mind, intellect, will, senses and their activities, emotions, feelings, desires, thoughts and so on. If we look at ourselves we see that inner harmony. Yoga teaches us to develop this inner harmony. It teaches us Union of man with nature. Yoga means union between man and man.

Our body is part of the nature. Yoga means union with the creator. Life today is full of stress and strain of tension and nervous irritability, of hurry and excitement. Non-violence is not only on action but also in speech and thought. Our attitude must be always non-violence. Think and speak and act what is good. Be true in everything. Do not claim a thing that is not yours. Do not keep with you more than your minimum need. Accept what you have. Man is so greedy; even if we give the whole world to one man, he won't be satisfied. He will desire more. We should not multiply our needs.

Focus is purity of the body and mind. Keep the mind with good thoughts. Be constant with what comes to you, good or bad, pleasant or unpleasant; experience God the master of the universe. In yoga there are Asana and pranayama. Once we sit in one posture, there should not be any disturbance from any part of the body. Be at ease. Our life is a movement from our source to us and from us to the source where we experience the movement of the spirit.

When you breath our mind wanders around and it is difficult to focus and keep steady. But when the breath is clamed the mind, too, will be still, and the yogi achieves long life. Therefore learn to control the breath. Every breath of life is a precious jewel, which can buy eternal treasures; breath is the bridge, which connects life to consciousness, which unites your body to your thoughts.

Awakening the chakras, the energy centers of your body through yoga—Chakras are powerful energy centers in the body. Although they are invisible to the eye, these spinning wheels of spiritual energy keep our bodies and spirits in balance. They store dynamic energy known to the Yogis in India *kundalini*, to the Chinese as Chi and to the Japanese as Ki.

Chakras mean 'wheel' or 'ring' in sanskrit. There are seven chakras (wheels of energy). Six of them are found along the spine and the seventh is located at the crown of the head. Chakras store *prana* or vital energy.

Yoga and the awakening of chakras, the practice of yoga are directed at awakening the divine energy in every human being. Asanas play an important role in awakening of this vital energy. This energy, when awakened has a powerful and regenerating effect. It can be channellize for self-development and healing of the body and mind.

Practice of asanas, the following asanas help awaken each chakra, from the most basic, the muldhara to the highest, the sahasrara. These yoga postures direct energy to each chakra center.

Seven asanas to awaken chakras:

1. **Muladhara chakra**—*Upavista Kanasana (seated wide-angle pose):* Sit against a wall and keep your shoulders and spine upright. Place your palms on the floor behind your hips and open your legs wide into a split.

   Chakra activation— This pose stimulates energy of the organs of the reproductive system and the ovaries.

2. **Swadishtana chakra**—*Salabhasana (locust pose):* Lie on your stomach with legs extended out. Place your hands below your thighs. Lift both legs up, off the floor, as high as possible without bending your knees.

   Chakra activation— This pose stimulates energy flow into the stomach, liver, small intestine and bladder thereby increasing the bodies' digestive fire.

3. **Manipura chakra—Ardha matsyendrasana** (spinal twist): Sit on your heels with your back tall. Lift the right knee off the floor and place it on the floor outside the left thigh. Raise the left arm and bring it over the right side of the right knee; reach your arm around to hold your ankle. Turn your head to look over your right shoulder and wrap your right hand around your waist.

   Chakra activation—This pose stimulates energy flow into the liver, spleen, bowels, kidney and gallbladder.

4. **Anahata chakra**—*Bhujangasana (the cobra):* Lie on your stomach with legs extended out. Place your palms downwards, directly below your shoulders. Keeping your shoulders relaxed and elbows slightly bent lift your spine off the floor.

   Chakra activation—This pose stimulates energy flow into the back, chest and lungs.

5. **Vishudhi chakra**—*Sarvangasana (shoulder stand):* Lie on your back and raise both legs bringing them up at a 90-degree angle. Place your hands below your hips and lift the body off the floor. Continue this movement until your body is resting on your shoulders. Point your toes and straighten your back as much as possible.

   Chakra activation—This pose stimulates energy flow into the neck and throat region. The focus is on the psychic energy center of this chakra, in the throat region.

6. **Ajna chakra**—*Padmasana (lotus):* Sit cross-legged on the floor. Place your right foot on your left thigh and your left foot on your right thigh. Place your hands on your thighs in chin mudra (first finger and thumb should touch each other). Close your eyes and focus on the point in between your eyebrows (the spiritual eye).

   Chakra activation—This meditation pose awakens cosmic energy and develops intuitive powers.

7. **Sahasrara chakra**—*Sirasana (headstand):* Sit backs and keeps your elbows on the floor and clasp your hands. Place the back of your head on your firmly clasped hands. Slowly walk your feet towards your elbows and take your feet up towards the ceiling.

   Chakra activation—This directs flow of energy to the crown of the head, where highest chakra is located. When this awakens there is oneness with spirit.

Massage—Involves rubbing, manipulation of body's muscle and soft tissues. It may reduce stress, anxiety, pain and depression. We get oxygen via nostrils as well as through skin, to keep the skin clean helps by message with oil. Start your massage from leg and come to the head after that have hot water bath. It brings untold freshness and energy. It takes away tiredness and fills the body with renewed charged vitality. Skin stares shinning, you feel active and alive. Regular massage improves eyesight and develops your intelligent. Helps you maintain your body weight. Skin disease disappears, hair stops falling, and body gets exercise.

Magnetic therapy involves the use of variety of different sizes and shapes and individual magnets of the body to reduce pain and treat disease.

Therapeutic touch derived from ancient technique called laying on of hands and based on a premise that it is the healing force of the therapist than affects the clients' recovery. Healing is promoted when the body's energies are in balance and by passing their hands over the client, healers can identify energy imbalances. In Bible, we see Jesus healing by laying of hands; Jesus did not study medicine nor had medical science studies. It is the person that heals. His person generates health. Jesus does not analyze blood, nor has electromagnetic test. He only analyzes the faith of the person. He diagnoses all sickness as possibility that the work of God is manifested. He does not treat with pills, chemotherapy, his therapy is love, and he cures out of compassion. He heals the whole person; he liberates fear, sins, sinful structure and proclaiming the truth.

Coping with stress- essentially, coping with stress involves a change of lifestyle. In the way you think, act and react, and feel. Make it a practice to scan your body in stressful situation. Check pulse, breathing, temperature, and muscular tension. If you observe you are under stress, take a deep breathes, as you exhale, feel tension leaving your body. Daily exercise at least 10 minutes yoga, jogging, walking in the safest exercise. Get adequate sleep. Learn to relax totally. Get a hold on negative, stress provoking thoughts and filter them out of your mind. Meditation of 20 minutes will have the profoundest effect on your ability to handle stress. Develop control over oneself ones thoughts, emotions and desires. The better your self-image, the better you will be able to cope with stress. Build your own self-esteems. Reinforce your self-confidence. Talk assertively. Clarify values and goals what you wish to accomplish in life. Do some forms of social work; develop a sense of humor. Look at the lighter side of things. Learn to laugh at yourself.

Physical and **mental signs of stress**, which may place the body under high risk, would be excess weight for your age and height. High blood pressure, lack of appetite, desire to eat as soon as problem arises, frequent heart burn, chronic diarrhea or constipation, inability to sleep, feeling of constant fatigue, frequent headache, muscle spasms, feeling of fullness although you have not eaten, shortness of breath, tendency towards fainting or nausea, inability to cry, excessive nervous energy that prevents sitting still and relaxing.

Mental symptoms such as a constant feeling of uneasiness; constant irritability with family and work associates; boredom with life; feeling of being unable to cope with life; anxiety about money; morbid fear of disease, especially cancer and heart disease; fear of death of your own and others; a sense of suppressed anger; a feeling of being rejected; a sense of despair at being unsuccessful as parents, teacher; an inability to concentrate for any length of time or to finish one job before beginning another one.

To overcome stress, note any change of routine, work, climate, way of doing a task take note in your life where you are facing change. If your job casts on you the responsibility of producing certain results but denies you the authority to take certain decisions, the stress is even greeter; conflicts pulls between job requirements and family life, disagreements, open hostility or suppressed aggression, conflicting loyalties. The relationship between husband and wife is an indicator of stress level. Discord in marriage has been found to be one of the most dangerous of stressors. Review how you get on with your parents, children close relative. Job insecurity is one of the worst. Stress generated by internal and external factors.

Recognize it and deal with it constructively. Practice yoga, meditation, relaxation. Be assertive, you feel good. You feel respected by others. Your self-confidence improves. You make your own choices. You are in touch with your own feelings. You feel valued, so break though, you will feel confident and successful; you feel controlled and self respected and you are goal oriented. Way to transformation; my relationships are my opportunity to express myself as a loving person. Any difficulty or painful moment in my relationship is a new opportunity for me to develop as a loving person. At the moment of conflict choose not to blame others but willing to earn from experience. In the infinity of life where I am, all is perfect, whole and complete. I live in harmony and balance with everyone I know.

Reiki is a Japanese word representing universal life energy. Reiki is based on the belief that when spiritual energy is channeled through a Reiki practitioner, the client's spirit is healed, which in turn heals the physical body. It is a system of natural healing by laying on off hands/ transmitting a special form of subtle non-polar life energy. Reiki is a Japanese word prana-cosmic bioplasmic energy universal life force. There are 360 alternative therapies available. Reiki is not forced on anyone. It is always given on asking and on request. They follow 5 percepts—such as Just for today I will not fear, Just for today I will not get angry, Just for today I will earn my living honestly, Just for today I will show gratitude towards everything.

The ancient science and art of healing— Give to every other human being every right that you claim for yourself. Yoga nidra, yogic sleep which makes you feel as fit as a fiddle; these techniques are extensively used in treating cancer by doctors of UK and Europe; turning pain into gain; transforms lives, inner peace, winning over wrong, and a motivational strategy. Patient is helped to cope up with pain adequately.

Spiritual healing—The use of prayer or other religious rituals such as laying on of hands, visiting of shrines or bathing in holy waters to promote healing.

Nurses should be aware that there are other alternative health care practices may be being practiced by individual who are at the same time using the biomedical treatment offered by their physician. According to the needs curative, palliative, radical, rational, specific, symptomatic treatments are given. The ultimate goal of nursing is to help individuals regain and maintain psycho-physiological, socio-cultural equilibrium. To practice holistic nursing, appreciates each person as a total individual. Take time to appreciate and recognize basic needs so that people can function as integrated systems; helping people with unmet needs. One needs to understand the self during health and illness. Adequate self-esteem and self-respect are necessary for health. Establish satisfactory living. Coordination bridges the gap between acute care and home care services.

Pranic healing is the ancient science and art of healing. It is a distinct system of healing based on its own philosophy of life and the supreme realization that there is a basic vital energy in the human body, which is responsible for the maintenance of health. Breath of life, which holds the very key to human existence, a mysterious force that animates and sustains life. All that we needs is the willingness to heal. The unearthly must be removed from fear and superstition. Relaxing the mind helps the body to heal itself. Pray for few minutes. Then the pranic healer must sensitize his fingertips and eyes so he can feel and scan the aura of the client and thus verify where the sickness or energy leak is.

The more we know about our body, the more it becomes mystified at its wonderful working machine. The body repairs its own broken parts through the vital energy by water he drinks and the food that he consumes. We get most of our vital energy from the air we breathe.

Pranic healing is based on structure of the human body, the visible body is that part that we see, touch, and the invisible body luminous energy body, which interpenetrates the visible physical body and extends beyond it by four inches.

Pranic healing involves the transference of vital energy to the client; vital energy the life force which keeps the body alive and healthy. The healer projects prana or vital energy the breath of life to the client thereby healing the client. There are three sources of prana solar, air, and ground prana. Solar prana from sunlight, air prana absorbed by deep slow rhythmic breathing and ground prana absorbed through the soles of the feet. Certain areas tend to have more prana, during bad weather many get ill due to decrease in solar vital energy. Tired and sick people benefit much by lying down or resting underneath trees and tree helps the sick person to get well. Persons who are depleted tend to absorb prana from another person; this is why you may have encounter persons who tend to make you feel tired or drained for no apparent reason.

The intimate relationship between the bioplasmic body and the physical body are closely related and what affects one affect the other. Diseases first appear in the bioplasmic body and can be prevented from manifesting. These areas when scanned can be felt as hollows in the inner aura. Unless the client is treated, the disease will inevitably manifest on the visible physical body. The disease must be treated as early as possible to insure speedy recovery.

Sensitizing the hands, scanning the inner aura, and sweeping, (cleansing) general and localized, increasing the receptivity of the client, and energizing by removing the diseased energy, stabilizing the projected pranic energy, releasing the projected pranic energy; with pranic healing; common simple ailments such as gastrointestinal ailments, respiratory ailments, urinary ailments and minor arthritis and others. For this the healer has to be open-minded and in good health. There is self-Pranic healing; there is also distant pranic healing and invocative pranic healing. To graduate must self study and practice for at least three months or more to gain proficiency in basic pranic healing.

Invocation—Lord, make me thy healing instrument, let thy entire being be filled with compassion for other who are suffering. Lord, let your healing and regenerating power flow through this body; giving thanks and in full faith. Then mentally recite and invoke- divine merciful father, thank you for healing this client, in full faith, so be it. Prayer begins when human capacity ends.

Laughter is the best medicine, when laughter therapy is practiced regularly, overtime ones concentration level increases. The more you laugh the more your mind and body work together; this results in better performance at the work place. Practice at least for 40 minutes every day. With some warm up exercise, the oxygen level in the body increases drastically. This improves the blood flow in the body and the persons don't feel fatigue as early as he normally would. It helps you to maintain good interpersonal relationships, to maintain pleasant atmosphere. It is a stress reliever. Some workers have no other option than to go through such stress relievers with the working schedules. It provides some outlet for relieving stress. The therapy has to be continually practiced, join in laughter club; you will feel your stress level going down.

Color therapy: What is color therapy? How does it work? Which problems can it help? Is it safe: color has such a subtle effect on our lives that we rarely give it a second thought, so it is often a surprise to learn that color can heal. Color comes from daylight, which contains all eight colors of the spectrum; red, orange, yellow, green, turquoise, blue, violet and magenta. It is also a form of radiation and while we accept that other forms such as X-rays and ultraviolet light have their part to play in health; we are often reluctant to accept that color can also maintain and restore health; importance of color in treating disease. For example, looking at the blue light has been shown to lower blood pressure by calming the autonomic nervous system, while red light causes it to rise.

Color therapy uses color to treat mental, emotional and physical problems and restore the whole person to health and harmony. Color can be used in many different ways. Some therapists combine it with reflexology, aromatherapy and acupuncture.

Many therapists treat people with colored light. For this treatment you will be given a white robe to wear and be asked to sit or lie under a light machine. Light is shone through stain glass filters and focused on the body parts, which require treating. The therapist will set the machine so that it delivers the colors and complementary colors in the correct amounts. These are beamed onto your body for precisely 19 ¼ minutes. Some practitioners use a color crystal torch, an instrument that transmits colored light through a quartz crystal tip. Alternatively, therapists drape colored silks around your body or they are used with a lamp to flood the room with your required color for 20 minutes. Afterward, you will be left to bask for several minutes in the complementary color.

At the end you are given homework. This is essential and involves wearing particular colors, eating foods of those colors, and visualizing with the color two or three times a day.

Practitioners believe that color therapy can help people with mental, emotional and physical problems including insomnia, asthma, depression, pain, anxiety, stress-related disorders and behavioral problems. It can also speed recovery from disease or after an operation.

Color therapy is safe for everyone provided you receive treatment from a qualified practitioner. Too much of one color can adversely affect your health. Red, in particular should be used with caution. It can lower your resistance to pain and raise blood pressure causing changes in heart and brain function. It is also important to be careful during pregnancy as color can affect the embryonic cell structure. Most therapists will use silks rather than lights during this time.

Medicines have certain desirable and undesirable effects called adverse reaction. Some side effects are expected and unavoidable, but others may surprise the doctors as well as the patient; some may be due to an individual's specific response to the drugs. Most excepted side effects are temporary and need not cause alarm. You will merely experience discomfort, inconvenience for a short time – yet it is very important that you take your medicine exactly as it has been prescribed. Don't stop taking medicines just because you think that it does not "suit" you. Some obvious side effects include blurred vision, a dry mouth, heartburn, nausea, vomiting, diarrhea, and constipation, loss of appetite, drowsiness, dizziness, stuffy nose, skin rash, and swelling, itching, and upset stomach. Remember, that these side effects do not mean that you are "allergic" to the drug. It can be one of the reactions of your body to the drugs. Consult your doctor when minor side effects becoming persistent or particularly bothersome.

Common minor side effects management like constipation you can increase the amount of fiber in your diet; drink plenty of fluids, exercise regularly. In diarrhea, drink lots of water to replace lost fluids; symptoms last for longer than three days; consult a doctor; in dizziness avoid operating machinery or driving a vehicle. In dry mouth, suck on candy or ice chips, headache remain tranquil; take aspirin or paracetamol. In case of insomnia, take the last dose of the drug earlier in the day; drink a glass of warm milk at bedtime; request your doctor to draw up an exercise program. In condition of **itching, take frequents bath, shower, or use-wet soaks; also; calamine lotion or antihistamines may help. Nasal congestion if necessary, use nose drops. Upset stomach, take the drug with milk or food.**

Telemedicine or medicine by wire, treatment over distance; to spread health care services the doctors are casting their net far and wide to bring solace to millions through telemedicine. The process of diagnosing and treating clients without physically seeing them has gained acceptance the world over, including India. Recognized by WHO as cost-effective and practical methods to deliver quality health care, it reduces the need to transfer clients to major hospitals with high medical expertise. It also plays a significant role in disaster management. Many lives can be saved due to this. Client monitoring from report area is also an emerging area in telemedicine. Rural clients in rural areas can avoid traveling to hospital in the cities and can avail of the treatment right there in the village. This will ensure considerable monetary saving. It will prevent all the inconveniences of traveling and accommodation problem. It has made a difference in the rural pockets of India. Technology has advanced and now that is needed is a high-end computer and a dedicated channel for the interaction to take place. The system can also be linked to other medical equipment like ECG machine et al, and can thus transfer data in real time. Telemedicine in India is still in the emerging mode and has grown to become an important tool in rural health care services.

Telemedicine, or medicine by wire, is short for 'treatment over distance'. With the current technologies, it is now possible to connect rural areas and link them to super-specialty hospital in urban centers. Known widely as telemedicine, the process of diagnosing and treating patients without physically seeing them has gained acceptance the world over, including India; Telemedicine also plays a significant role in disaster management. With infrastructure in place, patients in rural areas can avoid traveling to hospitals in the cities and can avail of the treatment right there in the village. This will ensure considerable monetary savings. Also, it will prevent all the hassles related to traveling and accommodation. Telemedicine has made a difference in the rural pockets of India. Technology has advanced and now all that is needed is a high-end computer and a dedicated channel for the interaction to take place. The system can also be linked to other medical equipment like ECG machine et al, and can thus transfer data in real time. Telemedicine in India is still in the emerging mode and has grown to become an important tool in rural health care services.

Patient monitoring from remote area is also an emerging area in telemedicine. Medical tele-diagnostic research has important implications not only for the space program, but also for delivery of efficient medical care in small rural hospitals where access to radiologists is limited or in situations where second opinions are needed. The information could then be sent to a remote health-monitoring center using the existing telephone network. The device works by monitoring the microwaves transmitted by a mobile phone, some of which bounce back to the phone from the chest, heart and lungs of the person using.

Community nurse is a promoter of health. Consider health as a good, as a gift that has to be protected and conserved and preserved for the benefit of others. Life is a God given gift and human life is most sublime gift of all. Wealth is wellness. Self-motivating experience towards achieving a purposeful and vibrant lifestyle; healing is ultimately is divine and comes from God above. Faith and healing touch can do wonderful things. You as a community nurse give clients courage and hope to live. It is important to realize that we can never cure everything. You will never find homes for all the homeless, or food for all the hunger, or cure for all diseases. But as medical we can care for everyone and care will heal the spirit. Make a commitment to health and develop your own healing program, make a positive contribution to your community, through some form of work or service that you value and enjoy.

Prayer meditation is language of the heart, which has a wonderful effect not only in the spirit but also in the body. It is the only power in the world that seems to overcome. Prayer supplies us with steady flow of sustaining power on our daily life. Prayer is a secret of all success and happiness. Prayer gladdens our heart, purifies our conscious, elevates our thoughts and expressions, gives us a sense of security, and brings all work to a joyous ending. Prayer should be the key of the day and lock of the night. Prayer is the wing where with the soul flies to heaven; meditation, the eye where with we see god. Where the balance the center of gravity and will feel our fears and worries disappear in the deepest peace of the soul. A never failing eye watches us that an almighty hand protects and guides us. May all be interested in helping others; diseases and misery may perish; and may all the people be healthy and happy.

Administration of drug energy medicine from a distance: Through hair by Dr Bandhu Sahni successfully transmitted energy to the client at a distance. Everything in the world has life within. It has consciousness latent in it. As cosmic rays can be transmitted, soundwaves can be transmitted and thought waves can be transmitted in the case of tele therapy. Homeopathic dynamic medicine is now transmitted to a client in any corner of the world just like a radio broadcast system, now distance id no bar.

Method of administration: One globule of selected medicine is put into one-gram phial containing water. This phial is given 10 strokes to enhance the action of the drug. One hair is taken out from the client's body and its one end is inserted into that phial serving as an antenna. The phial containing medicine in water and hair is called transmitting set. The process of administration of drug is transmission of drug through hair.

The question arises how the drug energy affects the client through a hair already separated from his body. A selected remedy is brought in contact with one of his hairs taken from his body. Drug energy can be transmitted through any natural belonging of the client that is hair, skin, blood, sputum and it has been already proved scientifically basis. Action is quicker, method is cheaper, used in clients suffering from cancer, epilepsy, paralysis, insanity, and rheumatism has been cured by this method. The invention has international importance. This will be a great boon to the suffering humanity particularly to the poor mass of the world. A ray of hope in HIV/AIDS.

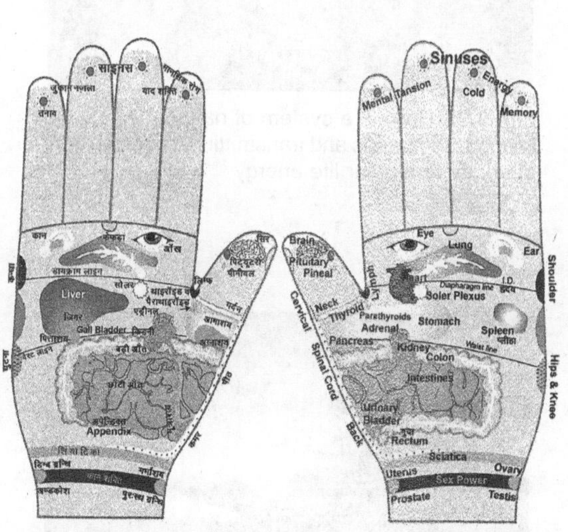

Fig. 9.1: Acupressure. It is a nature cure system originated in ancient India for treatment in which pressure is applied on points to the ailment of body without any medicines *(For color version see Plate 1)*

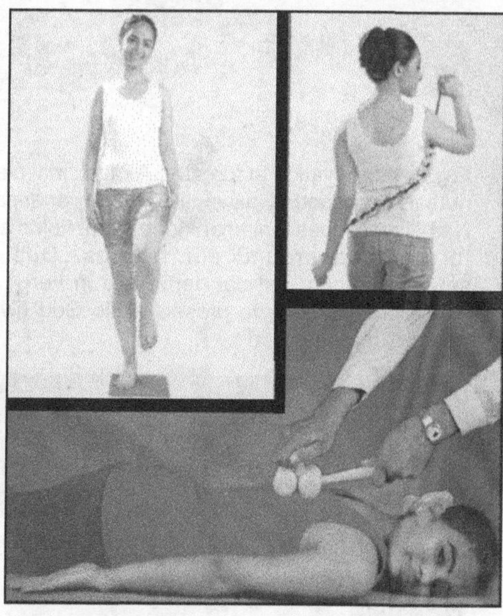

Fig. 9.2: Acupressure instruments can activate and stimulate blood circulation and regular flow of bioenergy to develop immunity against disease in the body

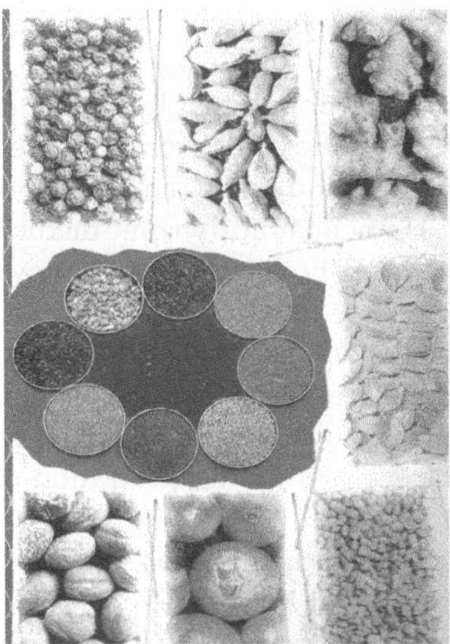

Fig. 9.3: Home remedies which are available in our kitchen such as ginger, peeper

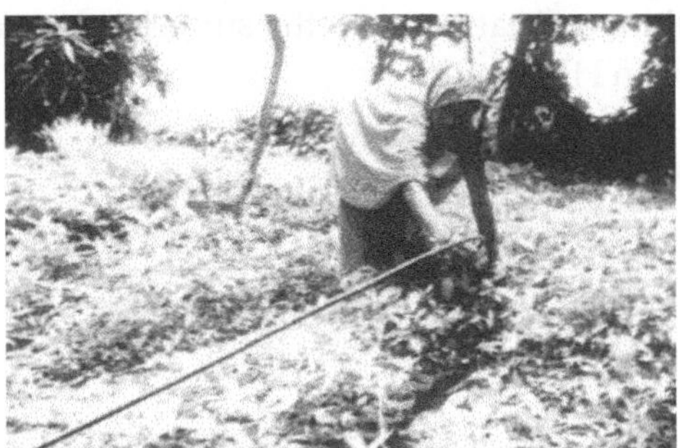

Fig. 9.4: Innovation in forestry: A medicinal plant nursery managed by a woman. Useful vanaspati/ Herbal medicines that are hidden in our fields and forests and around our houses. Due to industrialization, natural herbs are in verge of extinction, we have to preserve this God given free gift to humankind

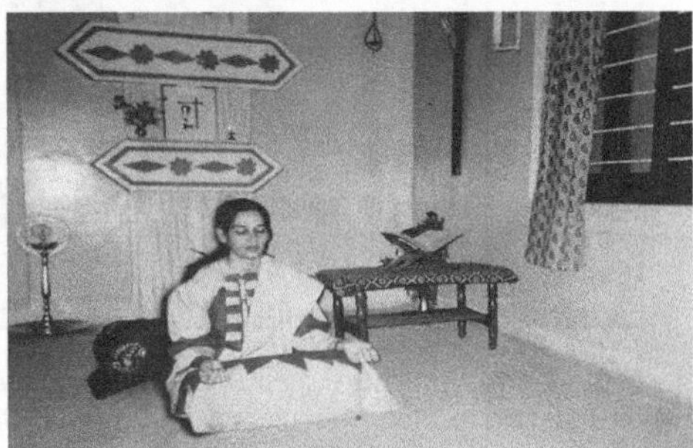

Fig. 9.5: Wholistic health approach: Meditation that leads to inner peace and harmony

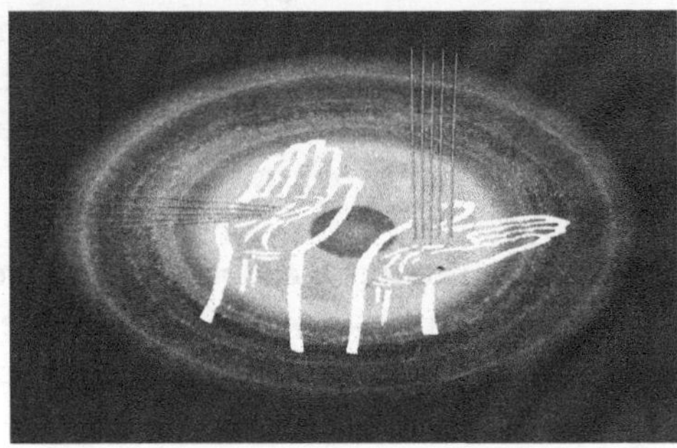

Fig. 9.6: Pranic healing is a basic vital energy in the human body, which is responsible for the maintenance of health. Presence of aura- breath of life that holds the very key to human existence, mysterious force that is sustainable non-physical component within the physical or maternal dimension

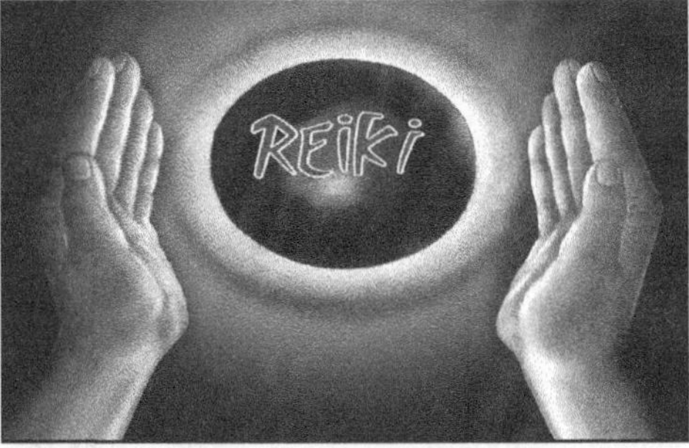

Fig. 9.7: Reiki is a system of natural healing by laying on off hands and transmitting a special form of subtle non-polar life energy

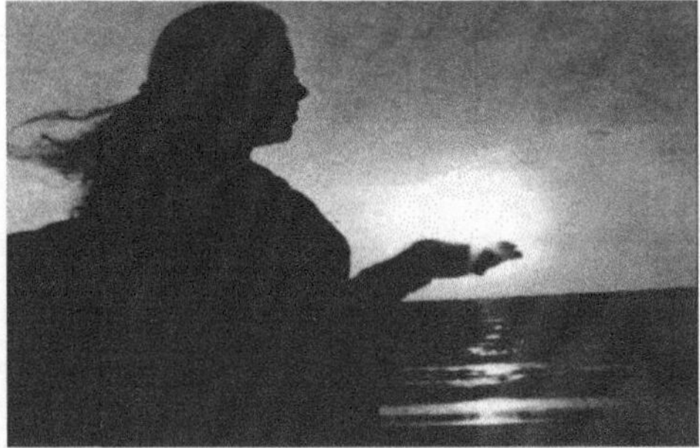

Fig. 9.8: Health in your hands. Precious life placed in our hands to preserve it and care for it

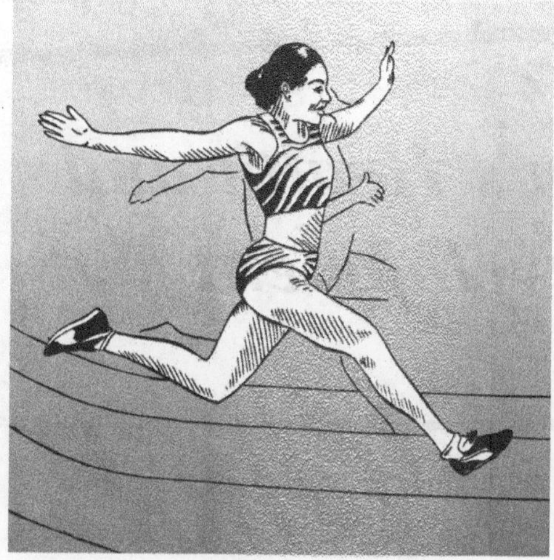

Fig. 9.9: Regular exercise to keep oneself fit and fine

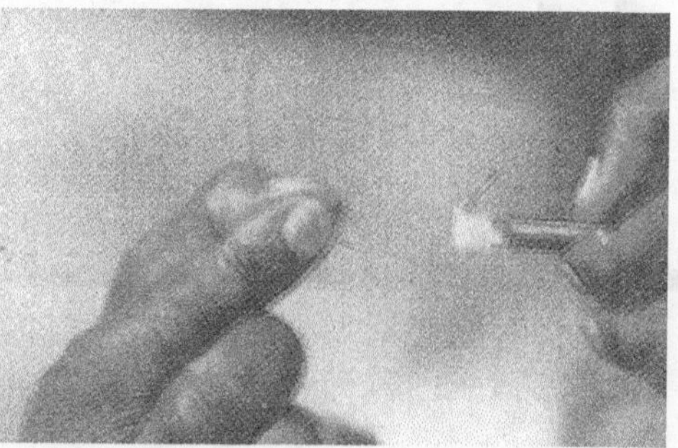

Fig. 9.10: Administration of drug energy through hair. A form of distance healing

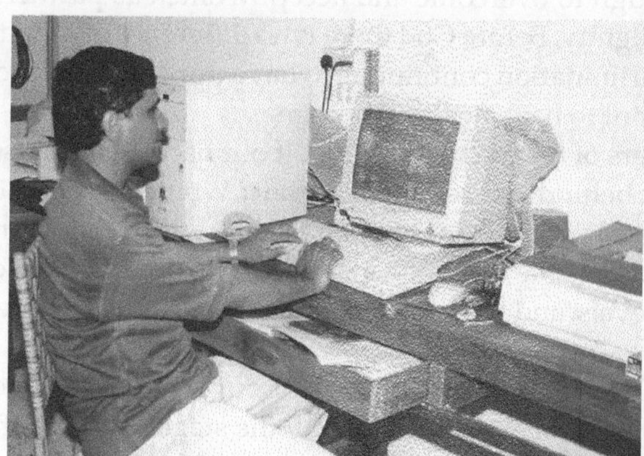

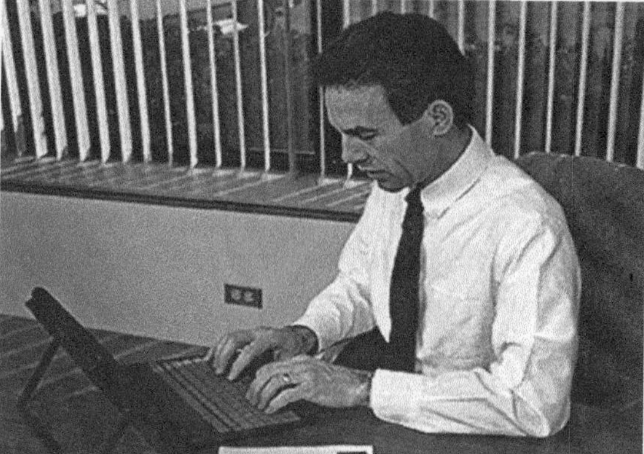

Figs 9.11 and 9.12: Significant development of new technology that is Tele Network, Internet and Web that has brought medical conferences to every living room, which can be downloaded, for future use

Distance telemedicines help to reach medical knowledge to the remote areas. As specialist and super-specialist doctors share valuable help through this—is a bliss.

10 *Women's Health and Development*

Care and treatment of a sick child at community level providing of quality care continuity through ICDS, mother and child bonding.

Without health, there is no development. The human species have made a significant progress in several sphere of life, but man has not grown enough to overcome and accept women as partners, companions, equals with same human values and dignity. Before God there is no difference of dignity and sex. Male domination, injustice and social discrimination continuous to have upper hand hence we have to put an end to this vicious circle if we want to have healthy mothers.

Women have role in national life; they are mothers of the next generation. If our nation has to rise, how can it do so if half of women of the nation lack behind and remain ignorant? Women's task is to recognize and arrest all her physical and psychological violence done to herself that, which condemns her to live a sub-human existence. The attitude towards the birth of a girl child, one down image of women in all spheres, structure of patriarchy at all levels, and the situation of deprived and victimized women will have to still change.

Discrimination against women seems to be embedded in the structures of our society. Violence against them starts the very moment of conception and is experienced at all the stages of their life. Psychological, sexual, physical, violence practiced against them is the result of inhuman and uncherished attitude. This must start in the home; women must have free and equal access to literacy and education.

Bride burning still continues and most of them are dowry, which is alarming. Wife biting is perhaps most frequent committed and socially accepted crime and women have to stay silent at all cost and due to social stigma attached to them, they remain submissive and accept it religiously. Rape is most dehumanizing forms of oppression, where guilt and shame is attached to the victim for the rest of her life. Society looks at the victim with suspicion and if she is unwed, she remains unfit for an honorable marriage bond. Instead of accepting and understanding her situation the so- called social and religious values make her outcast and untouchable.

Moved in to 21st century, how much have these advances improved the life of average women? Despite the growing evidence that investments in women have an enormous impact on society as a whole, no one can deny that women continue to face discrimination in social, economic, political and cultural spheres.

The majority of women are poor, lacking in education, health and other support services. In order to achieve meaningful equitable partnership between women and men much more will have to be done to change, to improve the condition and to promote and defend their human rights, action for equality, development and peace so that they make rightful contribution to a new world order.

Looking straight into vast horizons to new era with multidimensional opportunity and challenges ahead yet to be born; education is the surest way to ensure and overcome social discontentment and bring stability without hutting growth process. To give financial support to working women maternity benefit (that was 1961 was 250 is now raised upto 1000 rupees in 2008 is a good sign).

Today women's health status has shown improvement in recent decades. Women contribute extensively through their social involvement. Death rate has decreased to some extent but the question is not so much how many people die, but who dies? IMR, MMR varies from developed in to developing countries. Deaths due to maternal causes have virtually disappeared in the developed industrialized countries.

Women suffer serious health damage and die even before they have reached adulthood. People in the west not only live much longer, but the majority of them live until old age. Death rates of Indian women are higher than those for men till their reproductive ages are over. It is observed that until the age 35; women experience higher death rate and beyond 35, that is, after the completion of women's reproductive career is over, women have lower death rates. Age group-wise the number goes on decreasing as the age advances. So women have higher death rate in younger age. Women are significantly neglected; denial of adequate nutrition and medical attention, that has resulted in higher mortality among women.

The number of women per 1000 men in the population is low. The girl infants are more likely to die by neglect or unwanted. Women suffer critical nutrient deficits from girlhood onwards, and women work harder than men, they do life supporting task like fetching water or gathering firewood, cooking and looking after children and old people in the family besides perform seasonal activities like transplanting, weeding, harvesting. The expenditure of energy by women on a day-to-day basis may be higher than that of men. Thus, women faced deprivation in comparison with men. Women have no energy reserved for emergencies such as illness. As slum women besides their household work they go to work in the houses of other people to make their hand to mouth living, often they go walking from place to place and consume much of the energy in walking and standing.

Where is the women's health due to poor social status? The catchwords of today's economic policy, like globalization, liberalization, and open market economy are setting the blueprint for tomorrow's agenda for social change and economic growth. The danger of this blueprint, however, is that development is equated with economic growth, based on values of individualism, fierce competition, and an aggressive self-interest. The myth of the economically independent woman; 70% of girls in the rural area do not attend school. Prescribed roles for female deny them a right to an education, and do passive domestic role. Health is more of a socioeconomic problem then a technical one.

To organize women as a group certain factors hinder they are, economic disparity which divides them, religiously, and ethnic factors keep them apart. It is this context that one has to understand that the demographic factor is heavily influenced by social evils of caste and male domination. Dowries are still the typical forms of harassing women and that includes bride burning which the media like the newspapers conveniently sometimes call, "kitchen accidents". Sexual violence takes many forms including rape; and eve teasing. Physical violence, physical abuse, drunken husband, all these aspects need to be looked into and it is the need of the hour.

Women in political and social life, whether it is in the home or in the village, they are not given a say, when it comes to planning and decision-making. This is partly because they lack political consciousness. She is meant to be a good housewife. This confines her to motherhood and the house where her whole world rotates like a frog in the well.

In the cities, women's movement, women's cells where legal, counseling and medical support is made available. Special study courses for women on women related issues are becoming an accepted part. The thrust of the movement includes overcoming oppression, exploitation and indiscrimination perpetuated by women against other women. Need for women to organize themselves independently. Now women can dial 103 for help, 24 hours help-line made available for those women facing harassment of any sort, physical or mental, domestic violence be it physical, mental, sexual or financial harassment, dowry harassment, abuse by family, eve teasing, molestation, stalking, rape, buying and selling of women/girls, forced prostitution, confinement and sexual harassment. Through different help-line can get in touch with women activist who can come to her aid. Only they can tackle their own problems, as they see things from a very different perspective. They will direct and guide them to act correctly and make proper decisions and actions against such discrimination and violence. This is a good move to bring women to the mainstream of the world slandered.

Rural women are more sensitive, inward looking and God fearing, not exposed to the outer world, they are submissive. They respond and cooperate easily, overburden with household responsibilities and also forced to go out to work. Women find inner spiritual strength, observe better hygiene at home and are open to change when they are motivated and educated in non-formal way. As they are aware only of local needs they are made to imagine the global world. For these educational outgoing trips now and again to different important sports expose women to a world beyond their narrow village boundaries. Since the village world is innocent and beautiful as such, one of the drawbacks is that the people never get an opportunity to just see another outside world that is somehow affecting their lives and their lifestyles.

One of the ways in which women remain oppressed is illiteracy. They are dependent on the men folk to catch a bus, they are dependent on the shopkeepers for the prices of essential commodities and they are dependent on their self-images as being useless and unintelligent. Health education too can help them see that diseases have a cause beyond medical reasons and can be controlled and prevented by simple methods.

The healthier a community is, the more it can increase its productivity. Inter Mahila Mandal meetings between groups help them to mingle and share common needs such as agricultural and animal husbandry camps, and income generating.

Women's empowerment urges women to come together to question various forms of socio-economic oppression and to access information, training, knowledge and skill to be able to change the circumstances in their community. Banning alcohol, education and training on environmental issues, savings and credit issues. Main aim and interest is poverty alleviation, health and sanitation and community education. Community-based rehabilitation of the aged and disabled, aids and appliances by acting as stimulant by offering support, expertise and experience, training and exchange of information.

The social inequality; preference of male child, the purdah system, no female rights to the property, low female literacy rate, and poor health, domestic violence, hierarchy of caste in terms of political power some of the clear indicator of a male dominated society.

Multiple responsibility workloads, like working, cooking, child bearing, all this is considered insignificance when wages are considered. The reasons for poor literacy rates in rural set up among females/women; the education system does not awaken students to real issues. The education system caters to the urban mentality where technology and industry may be major motivations for education. The community may see no reason why a functional woman needs education when her main function is a passive domestic role; the perception that a woman cannot be a professional; the perception that a woman has no significant role to make. Confinement to domestic obligations hinders reflection and time and energy about this issue.

Health is more of a socioeconomic problem than a medical or technical one, Women's health due to poor social status. The stigma of becoming a widow is something we still have to confront ourselves with as a society. Sexual violence takes many forms including rape. Women prisoners are quite often raped by policemen under the pretext of extracting information about related accomplices in a crime. Communal violence, when it does rear its ugly head also leads to rape humiliate women. Female in trains and buses or other public transport systems are the constant targets of male sexual harassment and in some cities it is even understood that a woman is "asking for it".

Indian women play an insignificant role in political and social life. Powerful men handle the political process; women can tag on to such figures, losing their identity and voice. For those women who make it to political posts on merit their struggle is immense. Socially a woman's role in the rural areas is clearly defined. Being single is looked at askance. She is liable to be labeled as prostitute. The process of gender socialization is itself a violation of basic human rights as it attempts to control women's autonomy and their independence of thought and action, labeling them as meek.

The pain and struggle experienced by women, they are pictured as ritually impure and polluting on the grounds of menstruation and childbearing. No surplus energy could result in early wearing out the cells, and early aging. Inadequate medical care takes greater toll of these women of poor health. The first childbirth is particularly hazardous. Neglect of girls in the early ages is reflected in the high incidence of low birth weight babies for the survivors among these girls. Survival chances of girls invariably show rise in age at marriage of girls. Women are producer and reproducers and their access to health care is extremely poor. It is crucial years of pregnancy and childbirth and early prevention of pelvic inflammatory diseases, under-nourishment and complications from hazardous contraceptives is to be considered. Personnel in public services have little patience to listen to the stories of side effects of contraceptives or of women's husbands' impotence.

Women who are single, disabled, widowed, deserted, and mentally handicapped is a concern of the public health services. Thus, women suffer silently of depression, anxiety because they have not received either physical or emotional support from medical personnel at the required time. Reproductive tract infections or injury and mental trauma, are not treated seriously enough. Infertility resulting from the illness can cause untold misery. Women need quality services, and bring them out from gloomy situation talking into account the sexual rights and reproductive health.

Women need regular meetings without any bar to create platform for interaction and rapport building initiate discussions, problem solving strategies to become capable, as every opportunity is a stepping stone. Create and build confidence to create new atmosphere and break the vicious circle of poverty related sicknesses, which are the root cause of all ill health.

The village community gets better organized as the women get opportunity to be leaders and animators. They take personal responsibility in the health of the community. They start enjoying certain amount of dignity and well being. Given them chance women can excel. For this we have to move with space of the people, convince them, regularity and constancy, as their present economic condition does not allow them to look beyond. Give them the importance.

Community Health Nurse (CHN) needs to believe in the people and appealed by the poor, accepting them just as they are, respond to their demands, and to work for empowerment and liberation of people by enhancing their sense of self-esteem and dignity. Organize different activities like saving and credit scheme, literacy classes, tailoring classes, social awareness camps, income generation activities, exposure programs so as to help them to live their lives with greater dignity and freedom. For that CHN have to work hard to keep no stone unturned for women's promotion to improve their status in the society, to help them to be eligible for government schemes by reaching to the helpless, and economically constrain poor and try in small way to reduce pain and suffering; developing economic self-reliance among rural women; and providing skill training.

Oppression of women takes many forms discrimination in both public and private spheres. Women should be given the full right to control their sexual and reproductive health; women are now being infected with the HIV virus at a faster rate than men. Human security safety threats of daily life in homes, work places and the community. Among the worst personal threats women are the targeted lot. The indicators for women development show a pathetic picture. Although women constitute half of electorate they hold only 10% of parliament seats in the developing countries and 12% in the industrial countries.

The world is fast developing. There are numberless government schemes. CHN has to encourage the women to get all the rights allotted to them. Educate a woman and you will educate a nation.

Inspite of the fact that women are producers and reproducers, their access to health care is poor. Women are seen either as mothers 'or potential mothers by the public health services. Any problem related beyond that such as mental health or marital violence, are not seen as a priority by the health services. On the other hand, invasive reproductive technologies are peddled in the name of giving infertile women choice. The question of reducing potential infertility among women through the prevention or early treatment of TB, pelvic inflammatory diseases, under-nourishment and complications from hazardous contraceptives, is not considered.

The state's undue emphasis on population control also reduces the access of women to health care services, especially in the crucial years of pregnancy and childbirth. When health workers are busy, cultivating family planning cases, it is difficult to imagine that women will feel comfortable seeking antenatal or postnatal care from them. The watered-down program of maternal and child health suffers a major obstacle. Cuts in the health budget are squeezing out the poor from access to ordinary health services. This changed situation will further increase the burden of women in sickness.

Low self-perception the culture of silence in which they are brought up makes them endure the physical and mental suffering taught to believe that menstruation is dirty, a woman is hardly in a position to seek medical intervention for white discharge or for menstrual disorders. In the same light, sexuality of women is never addressed. The health of single, disabled, widowed, deserted, lesbian, mentally handicapped is a matter of negligible concern to the public health services. The system does not locate the health problems of women in the real context and ignores the need to change the ill effects to women's health arising out of such relations.

Instead of increasing the access of women to health care and to reproductive rights, the move to withdraw maternity benefits for women beyond the second child or of advocating hormonal implants and injectables, as contraceptives should be seen in the same light. On the one hand there are women who have little or no access to trained medical supervision at the time of childbirth, in spite of high gestational risk; on the other hand, urban middle class women frequently undergo repeated cesareans during childbirth. We have to view prenatal sex-determination, hormonal replacement therapy and the indiscriminate use of tranquillizers for women in this light.

The fact that the same illness for a woman very often poses quite a different problem than it does for a man; tuberculosis for a man is bad enough, but for women not only does the continued treatment or stigma, reduces her status at home, the possible infertility resulting from the illness can cause untold misery. Marital violence, desertion and death become real possibilities for this woman.

It takes many years for a girl to become a healthy mature woman, if she is healthy she can give a healthy child to family and society it is essential care to women prior to conception during pregnancy, labor, management of obstetric emergencies and after delivery. This group is vulnerable to diseases of childhood and accidents of labor, which are largely preventable healthy children to healthy mother healthy community and productive citizens.

Early identification of risk factors, prompt management of complication; all pregnant women need additional care; nutrition, periodic check ups, and rest during pregnancy and these should be stared as early as women discover that she is pregnant will improve the health status of young women and children. Teach the mother to maintain nutritional status and to look after herself.

The mother giving the child is a miracle of life intended by God, she as a co-creator, has to safeguard the life of the mother and child and make the motherhood safe. Because pregnancy and childbirth are special events in mother's lives and in the lives of the families, it is a time of great hope and joyful anticipation and also a time of fear a journey into the unknown from which many women never return.

The risks that women face in bringing life into the world are not mere misfortunes but injustices that society has a duty to remedy. Every pregnancy faces risk and life-threatening complications. The child must be wanted and planned, if the child is not wanted, their unhappiness and rejection will be transmitted to the child through the attitudes and behavior towards the child. According to Indian culture, parents treat their children as an old age security needs to protect the children from womb to the tomb.

Privatization would only reduce women's right to existing health services' We can demand good quality services from the public sector because they are funded through the indirect taxes that the people including the poor pay. The private sector is kept in some check because of the mere existence of the public health services. Once the private sector takes control over the public area, there will be no end to the greed of profit-motivated personnel. Women are especially affected by these policies given that their health status has shown little improvement in recent decades.

Since poverty does not merely deprive individuals of the basic needs for survival, but makes them powerless to even take advantage of the available resources, the plight of the deprived sections has become more miserable over years. In turn, those in power continue planning such that small sections of the advantaged continue to reap benefits at the cost of the majority of Indian people especially women's.

Marginalization of rural people, women not only continues unabated, but also vested interests are promoting social and cultural practices. Selective abortion of female fetus, female infanticide, sati, crimes against women, religious fundamentalism, and so on, are examples of this regression. The New Economic Policy encouraging structural adjustment programs, liberalization and export oriented policies, are expected to benefit those who already have a larger share in the nation's resources whereas they will push the deprived into lives that will be more miserable.

It is now widely accepted that women contribute extensively to social processes yet women's access to resources is low; lower than that of men. State policies moulded by class and gender bias adversely affect women's access to resources. Class factors, household politics have a profound and distinctive impact on a young woman. She is simultaneously a worker, a bearer of male heirs for the continuity of the husband's family line and of future workers for the nation's economy. It is thus inappropriate to analyze domestic organisation separately from the sphere of production. Biological reproduction may seem 'natural', but its social construction must still be analyzed from women's perspective.

There is an urgent need to develop alternative policies and programs that will correct the disparities that prevail and reverse the human and environmental degradation accentuated by the new policies. Actions in this direction are needed for human development.

Observations show that women may not continuously lose weight, but they are definitely lighter than their desired weights. Women have no energy reserves for emergencies their mortality rates are higher in the event of an epidemic compared to well-fed women. Women try to conserve as much energy as possible by cutting out on the quality of life; because they do not have surplus energy possible that their cells are converting food into usable energy more efficiently.

Thrust towards organizing and animating the women towards the movement of human rights and gender equality. For women inequity comes from the society's refusal to acknowledge and reward the services that women render to the society. These activities take place mainly at the household level; women's contributions go unrecorded. Women's work that is crucial to survival becomes marginal and they are believed to be dependent.

In agricultural countries such as India, the participation rates for women are influenced by their participation in the agriculture. The role of women in agriculture is crucial not only because of their number engaged in it but also because of the variety of activities, which they perform. Except for ploughing, women are involved in all the operations required for growing food-grains and vegetables and rearing livestock.

Their involvement in the agriculture can be observed in compost preparation and application, land preparation, specially clod breaking and land leveling, sowing and transplanting, weeding, harvesting, cleaning, drying and market-produce selling. In livestock keeping they collect fodder, clean animal shed, milk mulch animals and process dairy products. All this in addition to their regular household duties such grinding and de-husking grain, fetching drinking water, collecting firewood, preparing family meals and looking after children and the old. In reality women work harder than men and get little economic credit for doing so. Women are also seen carrying basketsful of vegetables, fruits and other agricultural produce on head or back for marketing or for door-to-door selling.

Technological developments have also harmed the interests of women. Because of rapid industrialization have destroyed traditional crafts, difficulties women face is illiteracy, low technical skill, lack of opportunities into the more structured units.

Over and above these, women's mobility is restricted due to family obligation as well as attitudes regarding what is permissible work for them. 'The major problem for women seems to be not so much being pushed out, which is true in some sectors, as staying where they are. While men move up through education to higher jobs, women continue to hold traditional occupations that ensure bare survival for the family, but do not assure adequate economic returns. They face lot of restrictions, taboos and do and don'ts. They are told to take up or not to take up particular job if the man of the house thinks for her what is good and what is not and she as a submission says Amen to it because the family priorities and concerns are more important to her, so she let go such opportunities that sometimes come on her way. She is the slaughter lamp who has to sacrifice her ambitions and dreams every time.

What does international women's day mean? Women most adored, but most neglected. Give me good mother, and I will give you good nation, commented Napoleon. From time immemorial, fascinating person and man has struggled to find adjectives to describe her. She is a woman dearer to the creator.

EMPOWERING WOMEN FOR CAPACITY BUILDING

Who live in hostile, endless saga of sufferings and challenges, unhygienic conditions for decades, night and day, they moan from their dignity world, and there are too few who would even dare take note of them. Deprived of the basic necessities of life, they exist only to fulfill the routine exercise of going through existence, with no real jest for life. There is no end to the problems these women with her grown up girls around has a lot to say about her pathetic condition. She is torn apart fulfilling the needs of the family, with limited resources. She has to quench the hunger of all empty stomachs lack of privacy, no security, no respect for her womanhood, in such a condition how are we to empower them and put an order so as to help her live a meaningful life in the midst of difficulties and challenges and elevate her from mist of inhuman condition to give them the ray of hope, stand on their own feet, to redeem. The women have long way to go in talking stock of their own lives, education is one of the way how they will be able to rise up in life.

Entrusted with the burden of housework, sibling care, and work outside the home at a tender age, does she even have a childhood? On her fragile shoulders rest so many responsibilities. She is eventually denied her own freedom and innocence. This sort of discrimination takes place, perhaps, because in the Indian society parents tend to prefer a son for vague reasons like entry into heaven being assured by the birth of a son. Sons are considered to be an asset whereas daughters a liability. The woman has to struggle against all odds.

Against religious and cultural prejudices, economic and political factors, and above all patriarchal forces which has neglected girls and women to secondary citizenship. Education the key to human development, in the case of girl child is considered to be expensive option and her low social status is reflected in her lesser entitlement to food, health services, care and affection. Violence against women is the gravest and most pervasive form of violation of human rights. Violence against women violates and impairs the women from enjoying human rights and fundamental freedom. Violence against woman has to focus on the face, a fatal blow of rifle but on the chest or the lighting of a kerosene soaked body that constitute violence. Rape, eve teasing, sexual harassment, kidnapped, torture women's endless struggle continues. Their living conditions most deplorable, a whole family is often accommodated on a single bed and some times a heap of filthy straw and a covering old sacking hide them as one undistinguished heap, debased alike by penury. Often more than one family lived in damp one-room cellars in the pestilential atmosphere from 12-16 persons crowded together.

These were the sources of diseases and premature deaths. Therefore, we find that in spite of overall development women are not empowered. She is not able to choose and has not enabled herself to stand by the choices. Come let us give a joining hand to march with them on every walks of their journey towards gender equality and towards a better society.

An old Tamil proverb says no peacock will shed feathers if you ask it to shed; you need to pluck them by yourself. This makes sense today, when we need to force our way through if we are serious about what we want. One of the best ways in order to get their way in is by creating ripples and disturbs the set order in society; so that the core of humanity could be visible from the shore. It is the time that they come forward to challenge some of the established social taboos and stereotypes. Once these taboos are broken, and then new social expressions based on equality of sexes, when there is respect and dignity for all could be evolved.

They are denied opportunities for personal growth and social development, in education, employment, marriage and family, professional and political life they are rated second to men. Solidarity of the suffering women; abortion of female fetus, female infanticide, dowry deaths, bride burning, rape, declining sex ratio, illiteracy, we can see the women are still in oppressed state. Marriage is the occasion when parents feel relieved of the tensions caused by the birth of the girl child. Child marriage, early pregnancy and an extra workload make a woman reach her senility, even in her youth. Even when she is sexually abused, she is forced into silence given the culture of privacy, female prestige and social fabric.

Education is the need of the hour, which will empower her with courage and confidence to speak. Women are worth listening. Therefore, speak your words of wisdom from the book of life experience to make life worth living. Speak out those emotions and sentiments that had robbed you of your dignity and honour, pour out those silent screams hushed into your frozen feminine that your is a saga that is turning a new leaf. Once your story takes a new birth, your life will not be the same again.

In agriculture, high yielding variety technology, along with irrigation led to increased use of labor time per unit area cultivated because of higher labor use in the application of new inputs, higher cropping intensity and higher yields. However, evidence from some village's surveys show that the demand for hired labor goes up with agricultural prosperity and irrigation, but such evidence shows only a shift from family labor to hired labor and not a increase in the overall rate of participation of the village population in the workforce.

"Being a woman means putting up with all this and not complains". The woman has always been the homemaker. If a woman is living below the poverty line, she will in all likelihood; go hungry in order to feed her husband and children, and put herself last always. Feel tired and stressed out playing her multiple roles of wife. Seldom talk out about what she thinks.

For women, a major area of inequity comes from society's refusal to acknowledge and reward the services that women render to the society. Women's contributions go unrecorded. Women work harder than men and get little economic credit for doing so. Women are socialized to being caretakers, and they almost automatically take on responsibilities that men might not even consider.

We have just left a century of remarkable human progress. The health gains of the 20th century count as one of the biggest social transformations of our times. Living conditions have dramatically improved for the large majority of people. Health needs trigger economies to grow.

Yet, denial of adequate food to girls, partly due to non-availability and partly due to discrimination, continues to be a major problem. An inadequate diet has life-long consequences for girls, as their growth and development is jeopardizes. Early marriage and early pregnancy further deplete their inadequate reserves.

Girls start working earlier than boys, work longer and harder throughout their lives. This results in a negative nutritional balances and calories deficit. The situation worsens when women also have to perform hard labor for wages: walk long distances to fetch water and fuel in environmentally degraded regions, especially in hilly areas; take care of large extended families, in which the caring of children, elderly, sick, husband and animals are done by women alone – with little or no help.

Even when women work outside the home, they do not get equal wages for equal work and are made to perform unskilled jobs, which are poorly paid, more hazardous and demanding.

IMPACT OF WOMEN'S LACK OF EDUCATION AND MISCONCEPTIONS

Society embedded in superstitious beliefs those that are good those which affect people's health needs to be challenged through women's education.

Rural woman believes that, certain people have an evil eye and they harm the family it is not because the evil eye that brought some misfortune but its strong belief they can do. As she is convinced with it, it becomes difficult for her to understand it. Today even educated people too have so many such beliefs deeply rooted into their system and they pass this fear to the next generation. While community works came across that people say that so and so has the power to make you ill. Now other people who know it is not true take the advantage of such feeble-minded peoples fear to deepen what they believe their own profit to earn money; therefore, where the problem does lie in our mind.

Years before we were living in bullock card age, people were living in close boundaries of their village and could not think beyond the limited world of theirs and also scientific knowledge had not advanced so much as today that time certain such beliefs were tolerable but not at this 21st century, things are not the same. Those years were not many doctors and medicines not easily available they would take home and herbal medicines go to witch doctors. Today times are no more the same, it is the time to eliminate harmful beliefs and adapt the useful and helpful one.

In the rural areas if some magicians make a hen turn into cat, such things excite innocent people and the other clever ulterior motive people start there business shop of cheating on the cost of the poor illiterate people, and take advantage of their ignorance. Which now and then we read in newspaper and in televisions that such people were at the end were bluffers. You show a note and they give you solutions for anything under the earth problems such as unemployment, loss in business, and failure in marriage, have no child; there is no curative medicines for such beliefs, and education is only solution to know what is good and what is harmful.

Due to such blindfold practices, advantage is taken by malpractitioners when the people are ill, they first go to such places and come back worse ill when no hope and situations are out of hands. This is a serious health problem even today in certain remote communities. If we are going for some good work and if any widow happen to see or any cat crosses the road, drop the milk, you already feel things are not going to turn good for you. If any crow cruces believe visitors will come, if night dogs cry you say something bad Oman some wicket is going to fall, that is someone going to die, as dog sense death. Door and vehicles put lime and chilies, child to put a black sport to save from evil eye, without knowing the meaning of certain things being passed on and carried forward from generation to generation. Some of these things believed is not life threatening yet it needs to be changed as education comes in.

In interior villages when any unfortunate things happen, such as a standing crop gets spoiled; or all of a sudden few animals die, or more than one person becomes ill, such as conjunctivitis, mumps, cholera, chickenpox; people try to find the solution for it, by trying to put the blame on an innocent defendless widow, or single woman. From here begins the plight of ill treatment for these women; all village community comes and gathers together and name the woman "witch" (usually they are women witch no male witch, why they cannot have male witch) who is possessed by devil and the one who drinks their blood, or harms them and the animals or crops; they mercilessly bit her, some time they throw her into well, tie her on a tree, make her walk on burning coal, make her eat cow dug, or human excreta, put her hand in hot oil, make her naked and parade her, put chilly powder into her eyes or make life miserable and unbearable to live and drive her from the village; or make her say what they say is true. Just few days back a man cuts the head of such woman and putting on his shoulder openly walked to the police station. All these kind of things are not revealed or officially notified unless if you work closely with them you come to know. In this computer satellite age such things still exist though it is lessened as people are getting educated. Education is the only things will change the face of the society.

Education is an essential powerful tool to bring the change in the attitudes. It is an effective drug in the treatment of illness. It is as an effective as an immunization, if it is carried out meaningfully. A mother should know the cause of her child's malnutrition and its effect on the child than only she can prevent it; will give frequent feed to the child, that contains the rice, fruits, vegetables, milk, eggs, essential nutrients. To have good health is an asset, which helps people to solve their own problem in their own way.

Education creates awareness to take away the misconceptions, bad habits, doubts, and ignorance. It motivates and helps in changing beliefs that are harmful. It helps in learning new skills, increase and improves knowledge, and builds self-confidence.

Teaching is the cheapest and most effective way and is a core of health work, which helps to persuade people to discard certain habits that are known to be harmful to self and others; learning and teachings, is a continuous process. Education brings about a transformation of behavior, and helps to take up responsibilities. It moulds our character and morals. Thus, making life dynamic and progressive, it leads to integrated growth, new powers and values become part of life.

Education directs the capacities, attitudes, and interest to desirable channels. It liberates and frees us from ignorance and superstition, prejudices, blind belief and customs and thus leads to the light of knowledge, freedom and self-realization. It develops personality and modifies the behavior. It helps to improve the quality of life. Helps to discover talents and provides the opportunities, self-expression, creative thinking and creative awareness, enables to make correct choices. It is a life long process. From womb to the tomb, cradle to the grave. It develops person, family, community, thus it develops nation.

Awareness comes, as health is a vicious circle. If the mother has good food during antenatal period, she has less risk of health, more strength and stamina, better blood hemoglobin, healthy baby, good lactation, more vitality to work and fewer infections, better quality of life and more chances of survival. Women continue hard physical labor till last stage of pregnancy. In addition to their household works, working beyond the limits of physical tolerance, their babies are depleted of essential resources thus resulting in low self and baby weight.

With education many women have secured jobs, there is greater awareness of the world around. They are more self-reliant and independent, foster habit of saving being learnt with that improved life-style, got better facilities at home, better food, clothing, medical facilities, are more confident, alert and motivated, learnt with the education to live fruitful life. Educational, economic and social life has improved, talking personal responsibility and moving ahead.

Impact of education of women there is a marked difference in the attitude, they want to live better life and face their future courageously. Education and health has done many good is being done to the women – medical facilities have reached to the remotest villages and are made available for the people at minimum cost. The women and children have received special attention and care. Health status of the families and villages are better organized, thus increased personal responsibility. Now these women enjoy a certain amount of dignity as a human being.

Common vision, which would act as a guiding mandates to build peoples lives. The need to build a competent and credible body that would foster, support the vision as well as dialogue with them, so that better planning and coordination could render them more effective benefit.

A radical attitude to be more centered in the building of a preferential priority to work with women and children; to interact with other secular NGOs who have similar aims in terms of human rights and democratic values. Work and labor: However, as time passed, new ideas of production, new technologies, led to determine the type of society man creates with all its advantages and pitfalls.

To improve the standard of education of the pre-school going and primary school going children; to improve the food security situation by an increase in the food production through education, land leveling, seeds and fertilizers distribution, milk cooperatives; and through various income generating activities through the Mahila mandal.

To release human potentials through organizing the women at grass root level into various people organizations and providing them necessary trainings and exposures to meet their challenges; promoting solidarity among the people through network organization.

Education is knowledge, and knowledge is third eye. Education opens man's inner eye, flooding him with divine light and protects him like a mother to follow the path of good conduct. It forms character, develops personality, provides for earning a livelihood, trains for leadership, trains in art of living, supplies professional skills.

Government is investing a lot on developing infrastructure facilities such as promotion of housing, safe drinking water, sanitation, roads. which helps to improve infrastructure facilities of rural areas; giving lot of scope for people to take part in development giving priory to women in development process through channelizing programs through self help groups.

Women are no way intellectually inferior to man, she possesses excellent memory, intelligence and other mental powers and she has the capacity to obtain any kind of education. It is aimed at equipping the person for the struggles for existence. It reduces poverty and exploitation of man to man, they grow into their full stature; there is scope for self-expression.

According to the potentialities, education is the weapon of democracy and without good education democracy will not be successful. The purpose is to ensure behavior reforms to the value and ideals of democracy and must build the democracy. Thus, it is clear that democracy can be successful only if all the members of the community especially women are educated up to a certain minimum slandered. Creative qualities of every person are encouraged by education.

Awareness is created among the people as personal responsibility of each one for their own health and the health of the community. Superstitious beliefs on health and sickness have been removed. The problem of tuberculosis is being tackled concretely. They enjoy a certain amount of dignity and well being as they step into the new millennium.

During Vedic and ancient days, women education was encouraged and number of women Vedic, Upanishads created great women in different walks of life like science, literature, various disciplines of studies in the universities and in the political life of a country, so still we have to make effort to expand women's education. Women have special inclination towards teaching line; they are also attracted towards various professions such as medical, engineering.

Today due to television network, Internet, web brings the educational conferences to every living room or work place which can be downloaded and later printed for future use; it is one of the significant developments that the new technology of education have made possible and opened the wide horizons and sky is not the limit today. With it all barriers of remoteness, isolation, deprivation and distances are thus countered and conquered.

Female feticide: The inhuman and uncivilized practice of female feticide. No nation, society or community could hold its head high and claim to be part of a civilized world it condoned the practice of discriminating against women growing economic prosperity and education levels had not led to a corresponding mitigation as far as reducing female feticide was concerned. Every citizen to step forward and help in empowering the girl child. The action must begin at home, in our families. A longer jail sentence along with a higher financial penalty and a 24-hour toll free number to record complains against doctors conducting sex determination tests is health minister to tackled female feticide in India planning many a slew measures. As every girl has right to life, liberty, security, and protecting the unborn child in the womb with a mother.

To make the illiterate women literate which will change the face of our nation? Society is a web of social relationship, time and world does not wait or stand still for anyone to get up and rise, ever organism grows, every life flows, social changes reflect the dynamic nature of society, everyday women are faced with new situation, no society remains stake but the speed and direction of social change differs from society to society and with this signs of the times women too have to grow and bloom. These are, in brief, some of the significant areas of the process of organizing and building an effective women's society where they live with human dignity, self-esteem and wholesome person for which God has created her for, one hopes it will gather more momentum as time passes.

Today we see modern woman working in post office, school and colleges, nurses, research centers, doctor, engineer, every field she is taking part and coming ahead. Times have changed women needs strong determination and will power to overcome any obstacles and March ahead in believing in herself that she can do and no way is she less.

To uphold the dignity of women; though Indian women are granted equality of status as well as freedom to enter diverse occupations, the realization of these constitutional and legal rights and opportunities is yet to be achieved.

Woman was made from the rib of man. She was not made from his head to rule over him, nor from his feet to be trodden on. She was made from his shoulder to be equal to him. From beneath his arm to be protected by him. From near his heart to be loved by him.

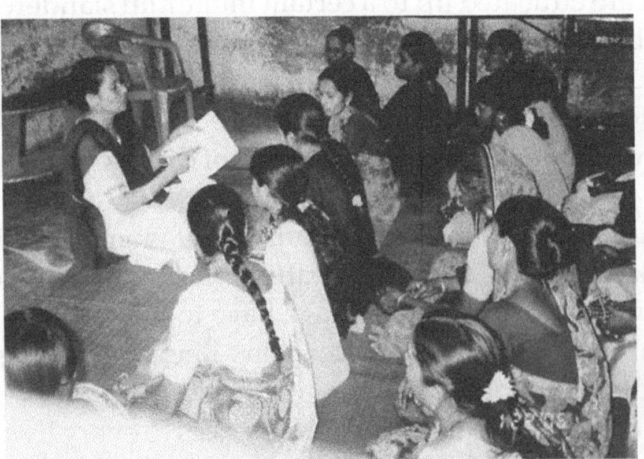

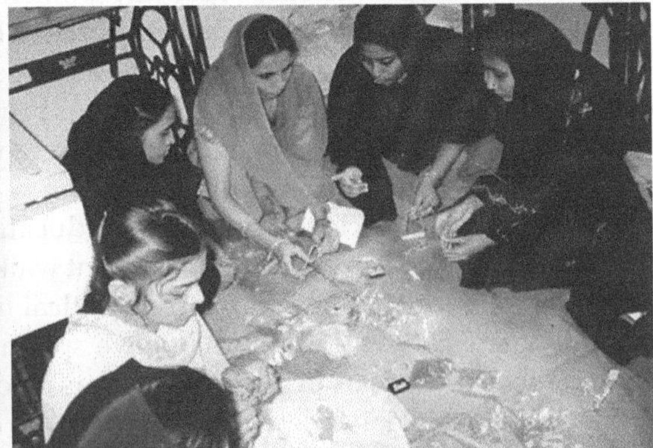

Figs 10.1 and 10.2: Skill development and training programs. Income generating and community development activities

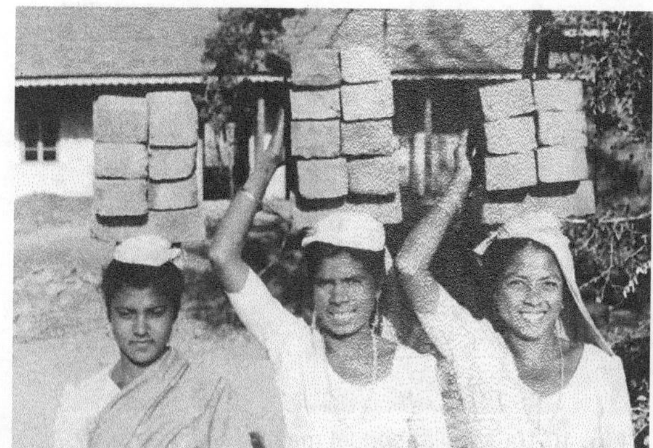

Fig. 10.3: Other trades such as brick/block making for rural housing

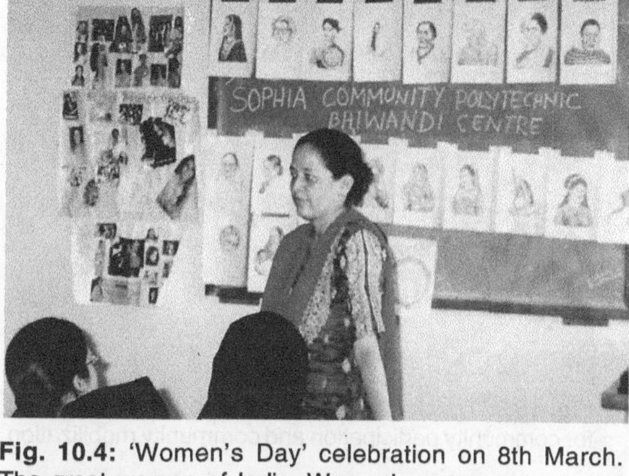

Fig. 10.4: 'Women's Day' celebration on 8th March. The great women of India. Women's empowerment and health awakening program

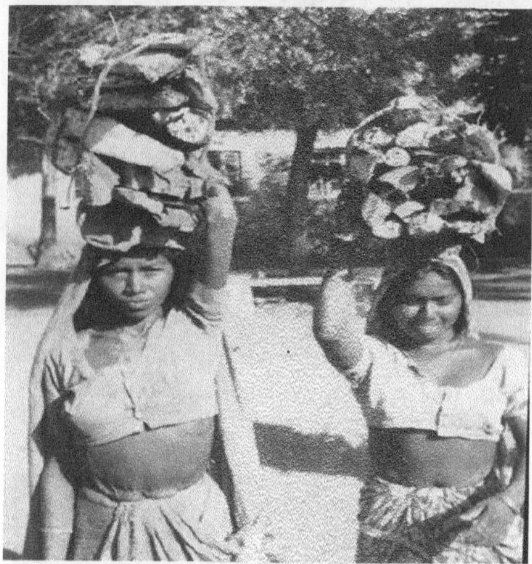

Fig. 10.5: Daily labor; daily wages: Health and socioeconomic status, environmental sanitation, which affect health

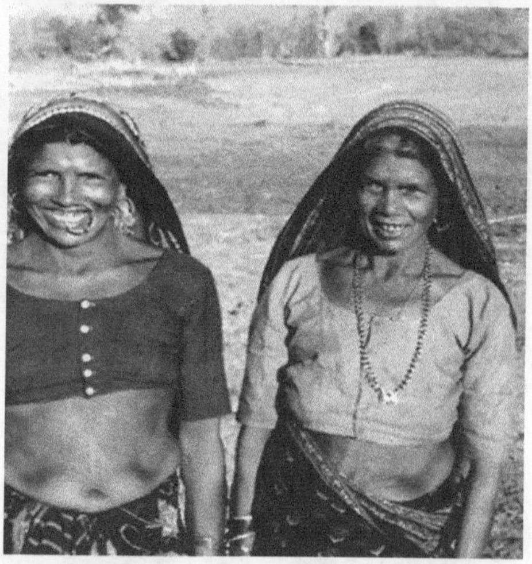

Fig. 10.6: Women with wisdom and smile cultural values, beliefs, attitudes and practices, inadequate food, housing condition which have a basic bearing on health

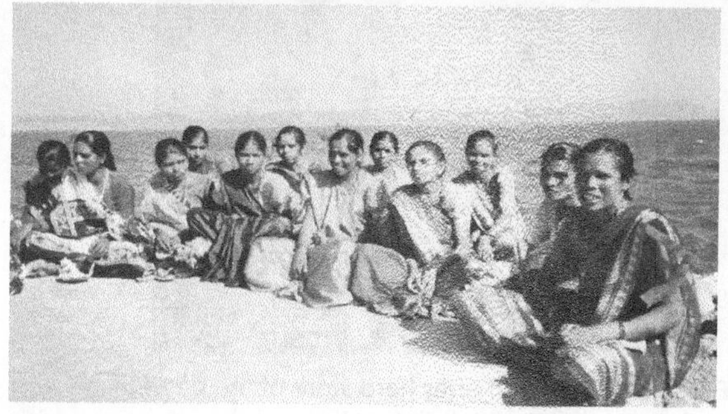

Fig. 10.7: Rural exposure program for women to show the world that is beyond village boundaries around which is so different then their own

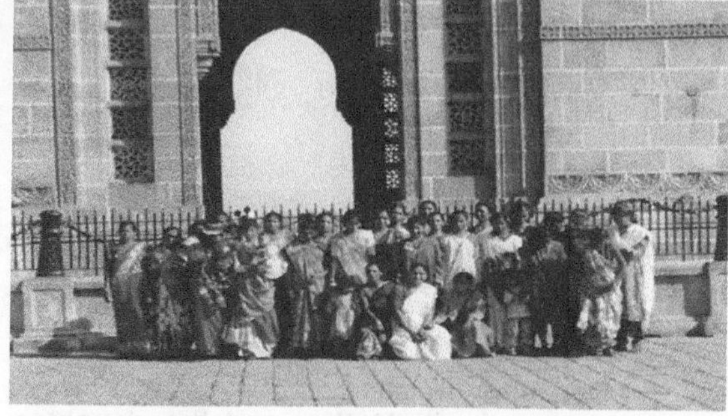

Fig. 10.8: Women do not get chance to get out of the house, hence remain unaware of the world that is somehow affects their life

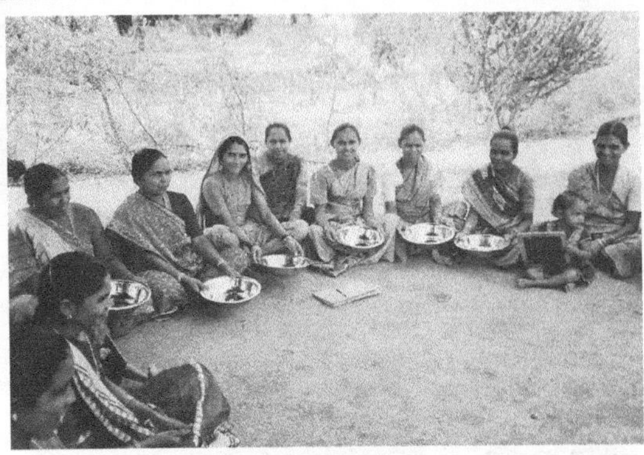

Fig. 10.9: Training through the demonstration. Scope for community participation and community mobilization

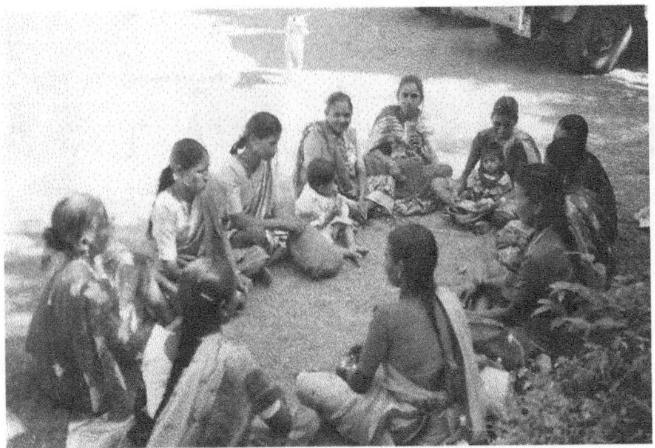

Fig. 10.10: Mahila mandal meetings and saving schemes

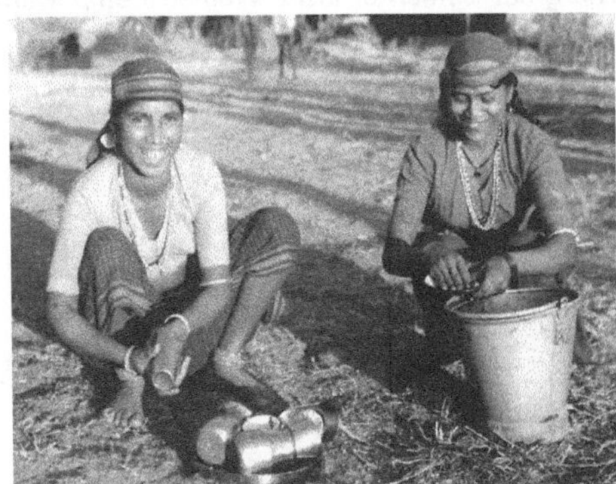

Fig.10.11: Women with household work. Improving family income and standard of living

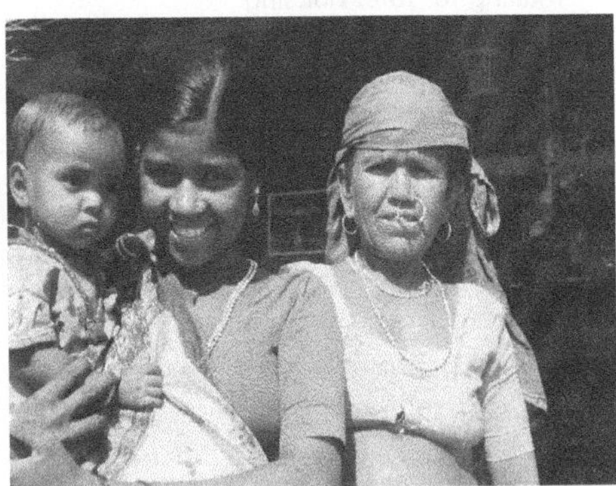

Fig. 10.12: Happy relationship in the family

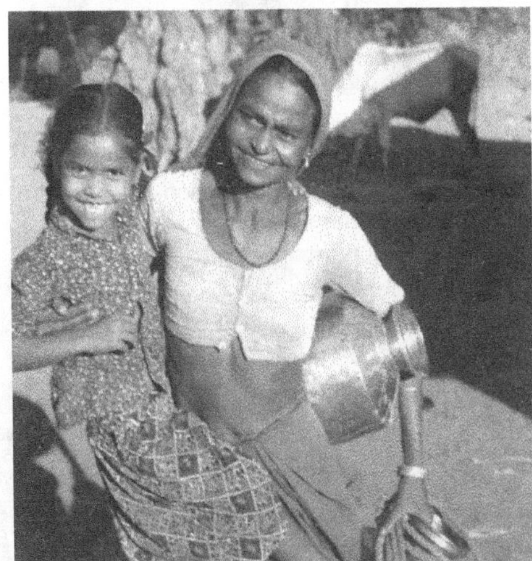

Fig. 10.13: Allotment of social welfare scheme water scarcity:Mother and the daughter relationship. They love their children very much

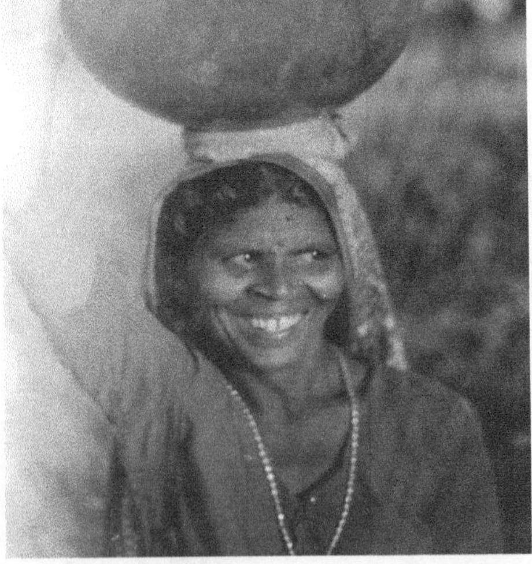

Fig. 10.14: Women after hard work of the day, go far distance to fetch the water

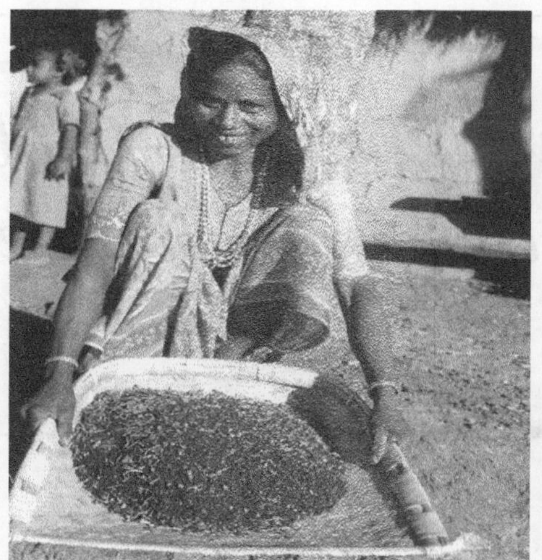

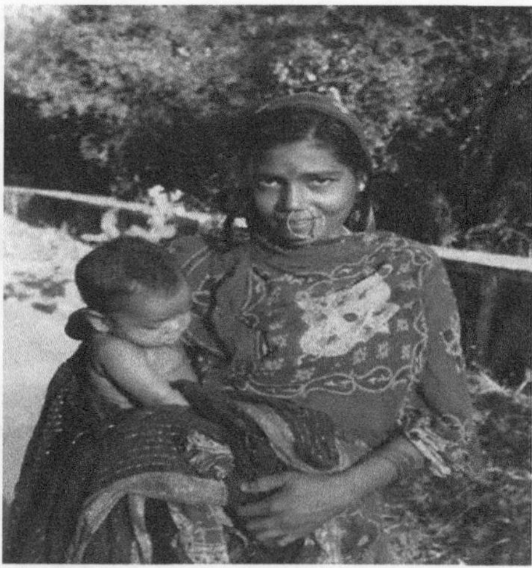

Figs 10.15 and 10.16: Socioeconomic condition of rural women

11 Our Environment—Global Warming and Climate Change

God gave us a land of ours with all its richness. However, it has been used and even abused by a few powerful rich. In order to improve our motherland we have to be a shine light. Appreciate and protect the tremendous natural wealth of our country and to make our mother land a better and more beautiful place to live.

To enjoy the beauty of nature by listening to the chirping of birds, the sound of the breeze, movements of trees and plants. What are we doing with our natural resources, and wealth? Is it possible to give plants as gifts or adopt a tree when we have special occasions and celebrations?

The environment protection Act 1986 is a fundamental duty of every citizen to protect national environment; including forest, lakes, rivers and wild life and to have compassion for living creatures. Awakening environmental consciousness demands that issues like garbage dumping, recycling waste, preventing pollution are raised. Efforts at keeping the environment clean, planting trees; encouraging use of organic fertilizers to replace chemical fertilizers is encouraged.

The world is our home. It is not a toy that we can use merely to entertain ourselves. Everything in the world, the air, water, plants and animals are also part of our existence and we are related to them. Only when there is a harmony among all these elements that constitute the earth, can we have a real home to live in and experience the joy of a genuine family life.

Climate change is one of the emerging threats to human health. Protecting health from climate change is urgent need of the hour as we look at the signs of the time. Environmental problems have become serious in many parts of the country. The main environmental problems in India relate to air pollution, and water pollution, particularly in the metropolitan and industrial zones.

The degradation of common property resources affects the poor adversely due to degeneration of their life support system. Even the rural population is not free from the ill effects of air pollution. Rural population uses substantial quantity of non-commercial fuel, i.e. crop residues, animal dung or wood. Air pollution due to biofuels largely released directly where the people are, inside or near homes at mealtime everyday.

Today Asia is melting, areas sinking in the sea, forest drying, animals fitting for survival. It has good and bad effect as coal, **petrol and diesel** gives us energy but too much of it pollutes the air with carbon dioxide and all living being need oxygen and therefore excessive carbon dioxide in the air have an imbalanced effect that disturbs the ecological system.

Sea water warming has increased, heat waves, drought or floods, cyclones and typhoons have given way much more than in the past such as in USA yearly it is to be said seven typhoons maximum now last year they had twenty two of it recorded.

Due to this climatic change we in India trying already to do some concert steps such as, we have begun using as a prevention ONGC vehicles, constructing building towers earthquake proof, renewable energy used, replacement of coal and gas by electricity. Lot of trees being advised to plant, growing more vegetables, and trying to move ecofriendly vehicles. Whole world join hands in fighting this global warming as a common goal as earth matters and we are part of it; let us united fight to create green earth. Scientist develops way to create biodiesel fuel for cars from coffee waste. Therefore, lot of research being experimented world over to balance the imbalance.

Need to act and take steps for prevention—Industries need to be warned to keep under control the causative agent of pollution. Control of population growth to reduce congestion of air and space and thus lessen the crowded areas, the air needs to be constantly circulated and replaced by fresh air more tree plantations between residential zones and industrial zones; and call this areas as green belt, green zone. Have more ventilated windows with inlets and outlets.

No living organism in nature is independent and can live by itself without environment. We can make a long list of plant life that we human beings depend on. We can make a list of animals that man depends on. More and more forests are being destroyed to make place for new homes, for factories, roads, farms, holiday resorts, entertainment parks etc. When will man realize that if he does not put a stop to his own population explosion then because of his ever-growing numbers all life on earth will slowly die out?

The needs of a family keep increasing with the increase in the number of members in the family. Where would more space come from except by clearing up any and every piece of forested areas; if such a trend continues with the population doubling in every twenty years?

When man first set foot on the earth as a cave man, he was very much part of nature and nature pampered him with an abundance of his only two needs food and shelter as clean air and pure water was in plenty. But, as time went by, man gained knowledge and used it to improve his standard of living. Better living conditions increased the life span and lowered the death rate leading to increase in human population. Everything in nature that man makes use of to sustain or improve his life is termed as natural resources.

Sometimes it happens when the Municipality people inform a whole locality of people that there would be no water supply for a day or two because of some pipe breakage or other. What do we do at such times?

Natural resources are sunlight; wind, tides, and flowing water, renewable resources air, fresh water, soil, plants and animals, non-renewable resources are coal, oil, natural gas, metallic minerals and nonmetallic minerals.

How serious is this problem of climatic change? Due to either excessive heat waves or floods affect the crop pattern and harms the production in both cases. It is evident today with scarcity of food grains all over the world, high food prices and shortage of essential commodities. Solution is Agro industries to make the food available and to create jobs within the system. The problem is big yet manageable.

There are so many questions we can ask such as, what do you understand by the term environment? A lot is heard about environment these days, why? What steps do you think should be taken to make up for the negative effect? Why is Mother Nature not able to control human population? What comes to your mind is the single most important factor responsible for life on the earth? Why should we conserve natural resources? Where does all the energy required on our Earth come from? Imagine you found yourself in a very crowded place what difficulties you faced. What do you think should be done to prevent people from cutting down trees? What is environmental pollution? Why was pollution not a problem during the earlier part of human history? How does air pollution affect human beings? What is one of the main causes of air pollution today? What is global warming and climatic change?

Has your mother ever punished you for some mischief you did, by depriving you of a meal? If so then you must have felt quite hungry and as the time for the next meal approached slowly, you felt more and more hungry. What else did you feel with the hunger? You most certainly felt yourself feeling weak with the energy in you becoming less and less. Yes, it is food that gives us energy to live. If food is our source of energy, then where does food come from?

All our food directly or indirectly comes from the plant world. Yes, our mother earth. And where can you tell do plants get energy? Plants are our Earth's powerhouses. They trap sun's energy in the form of sunlight and prepare their own food using carbon dioxide, water and mineral salts through the process of photosynthesis. The food that plants manufacture, store and share with us is in the form of chemical energy converted from solar energy. Air pollution can affect the lives of plants and animals and can damage the building constructions too.

Impact of air pollution can cause respiratory illness, bronchitis, asthma, respiratory death due to suffocation. Several health effects are suspected, like respiratory infection in children, chronic lung disease and lung cancer in adults, adverse pregnancy, such as low birth weight and stillbirth.

Much of the air we breathe is polluted. Due to domestic reasons such as burning of coal using coal gives away smoke,, wool, oil, industrial factors such as mills, automobiles, motor vehicles running on the road, railways and other causes such as nuclear explosion, over population affects the air. Bad fumes and gases needs to be changed for alternative fuel gas, chemicals, dye etc create grave danger to health. Air carries oxygen, the essential gas, for human survival, it keeps the body temperature cool; and constant change talking place in the environment affects the health as only pure air can help to prevent diseases and promote health and remove impurities in the air or this pollution can cause irritation of the nose and throat. Cigarette smoke can pollute air at home and at work. How fresh is the air where you live?

We need air to breathe to live. Fresh air contains oxygen. Where there are lots of factories and industries, the air contains many impurities and other substances, which can harm us. The problem of air pollution has become acute today. Condition of hot layer of air pressing over coal layer of air helps the impurities to be trapped in lower zone making the environment dangerous. Air pollution is more intense in towns and cities then rural areas.

The sunlight kills the harmful organism by heating, wind carries away concentrated impurities, rain washes away dust and gives us clean atmosphere, and the green plants utilizes the carbon dioxide and gives in return oxygen this helps to maintain the balance between both gases.

Due to over population and congested living in small room with more people the atmosphere there becomes warmer, due to talking, coughing, the room becomes stuffy and can cause headaches, breathlessness, tuberculosis, and lethargy. As the organism circulates in limited area and all breath the same air repeatedly.

There is an imbalance in body temperature due to extremely hot, intolerably hot, uncomfortable feeling is experienced. Ill health is the cause of environmental factors, high death rate, epidemic diseases, poor standards of health, to maintain good health surrounding needs to be clean from pollution.

Safe wholesome **water** is essential which has to be free from organism, harmful chemicals. We pollute our precious water. Pollution of water is another growing problem. The major sources of water pollution are domestic wastewater, industrial wastewater and effluents, and agricultural run off. Water pollution from domestic and human wastewater causes many severe water-born diseases. The major water pollution industries are leather, pulp and paper, textiles, and chemicals. Water also gets polluted due to bad sewage which contains organic matter which carries bacteria gives rise to disease. The production of many such industries, which poses high risk to human health and environmental quality due to the disposal methods used for wastes, has multiplied. Household purification of water by boiling and by other means as chlorination and regular checking for impurities will help to prevent diseases.

Impact of water pollution and poor sanitation, diseases commonly causes diarrhea, trachoma, intestinal worms, hepatitis, etc. Health hazard such as malaria, filariasis and even epidemics such as cholera can spread. The children in villages suffer from parasitic helminthic diseases caused through mixing of human waste in open water sources; deterioration of village by deforestation and soil degradation or other major environmental problems that affect a large part of the population directly.

Water is used for various purposes. We brush our teeth and rinse our mouths with water as we wake up in the morning, we bathe, we wash our clothes, and we wash utensils, wash and clean our house floors; in the end of each activity, wastewater is produced. In cities, dirty water or sewage water is drained into rivers and lakes. Many people use water from the same rivers or lakes in raw form.

In many places, people wash their clothes and vessels on the banks of the rivers or ponds. They also wash their animals in the same places. They sometimes defecate in or near the water sources. This water thus is much polluted and can cause serious diseases and yet further down the river at the next village the same water is used as drinking water and for all other purposes that the earlier village needed it. The water that leaves the shores of this village is that much more contaminated.

Some rivers are considered holy, and are used to have a dip, also certain places where they have ceremonies and cremation at the banks of the river and they throw bodies not burnt sufficiently put into to river according to their sentiments at the same time others drink water rawform from the same river which is considered sacred .

Cultural practices: Some are good some harmful like unless they do puja in the morning and have bath will not have food, clean house and do regular white wash. Due to religious ground, some do not take onions, garlic. Some deep-rooted beliefs, men eat first and women eat last, poorly, and left over; some foods that are forbidden during pregnancy, branding the skin with iron rod, chewing tobaccos, pan, and wear chappals. Sociocultural practices too affect the environment.

As it is the **responsibility** of community health nurse needs to incorporate these cultural good habits in promoting and integrating while determining the priorities of health care. Fairs and festivals expose the people to the risk of infectious diseases. Going on pilgrimage is part of people's customs; it is an important event of life of people to visit holy places. Community health nurse has to see that sanitary arrangements recommended safeguarding public health.

Food handlers are **ignorant** and do not know hygienic ways to deal with food and they can spread disease, with education community health nurse can prevent many health problems. The health workers make a large chunk of health care delivery of the people, public relations are essential to understand the tactics of handling human beings, health is an organized effort and its common purpose is to raise the stands of care.

Each one of us contaminates the environment around us. How lack of personal cleanliness can contaminate the food, what we eat can lead to food-born diseases. Food is a basic need for survival, so it is vital what we consume is pure and nourishing. Need to prevent food adulteration, eat food hot and well cooked, specially certain meats, and non-vegetarians, keep kitchen clean, store food carefully, be conscious when you buy food items, food safety is an essential, eat quality diet that is wholesome and balance.

The battle against climate change is all set to go down to every village in the country. In bid to create awareness about global warming, the government has decided to train and appoint climate manager in villages whose main task steps for sustainable development at the grassroots level. Besides they will be trained to handle natural disaster and prepare them areas to face the crisis. People at the grass roots will be the first to bear the burden of climate change. The 11th plan has set aside allocations for capacity building and skill training under the minister of HRD and Panchayati Raj, which will be trapped for this project. The task of managing climate change a man and a woman climate manager from each Gram Sabha will be trained in the science and of managing climate change and enhance their capacity to cope with natural calamities.

Heat pattern is changed in globally is a dark side as regional weather changed, extreme weather conditions, rising sea level, extreme cold which never experience before, and so positive attitudes towards this weather climatic change need individual effort and attention, community education, counselling, as it is an multidimensional factor needs multidisciplinary action. Danger of technology mobiles, electronics increased with in radiation have increased which are harmful to health, over population crowed cities, traffic jams, noise pollution, air pollution with increase of carbon dioxide, over uses of gases and exhausting earths resources. The situation is not yet out of hand if and only if we start acting and making the people aware of the gravity. Sometimes without a real need, water just runs, gas just burns, batteries just charges, plastics just thrown away causes clogging, building the towers on salt pans and not keeping the outlets, let all work in cooperation as a team.

Environmental pollution is one of the most serious problems facing humanity today. Polluted water kills fish and other marine life. Pollution of soil reduces the amount of land available for growing food.

With **soil degradation** million hectare of land is affected by serious soil erosion through ravine and gully, shifting cultivation, cultivated wastelands, sandy areas, deserts and waterlogging.

Soil is used for cultivation, forest, solid waste in the form of tins, glass pieces, rags, plastic, human excreta at road side give rise to health hazards.

Have you ever traveled in an **overcrowded** train especially during the monsoon season with all the doors and windows shut? If you have then you would have experienced the atmosphere as being very stuffy humid sticky almost suffocating. You may find it quite difficult to breathe and you must have longed for the station to arrive so that you could get out and breathe in fresh air.

Can you imagine our earth to be like a closed train compartment? If you can, you will appreciate the fact that we are constantly adding to the number of people on our planet, we are constantly and increasingly polluting our air filled envelop that surrounds our earth. We each have to spend our whole life therein. if such is the hard reality then why is it that we cut down trees that supply us with oxygen to breathe? Why? Why are we murdering our earth by suffocation and strangulation? In addition, increasing to global warming and climatic changes?

Prompting , protecting and preserving earth how will you do it? Our **atmosphere** is like a protective blanket around the Earth. This blanket holds the air close to the earth so that we can breathe and live. If the blanket were removed or destroyed then all life on earth not only man but all plants and animals also would die out. More and more trees should be planted wherever and whenever possible. Every man on earth should become nature friendly. Each human being must make the surroundings green. Because this issue is not a distant reality but we have already have started to sip the bitter cup of its effect on the earth and on each of us.

So many calamities which were never heard with this frequency have started hitting the earth and slowly destroying the human race bit by bit ; in this rate things continue, the humanity will be vanished from the face of this earth. Therefore, we have to take these issues seriously, and try a bit of our effort to motivate and awaken self and others towards its cause. In unity, there is strength and all together we will march towards tomorrow together; and make the earth green and ecofriendly paradise; truly heaven on earth in every sense as God had destined and created from the beginning of the world originally from the start.

Chemical fertilizers pollute land, water, air and the food we eat. Organic manure is ideal but difficult to produce according to demand. All the trees have been cut down. There is no fodder available. His bullocks starve in summer. To protect the crops in which he has invested so much money, he applies banned pesticides at very high levels. If his animals die or become sick from eating crop residues with so much pesticide in them, his available organic fertilizer will decline even further. He and his family are prone to jaundice from pesticide exposure. What is happening to that farmer is happening to other farmers as well all over the country. The nation's money meant for fertilizers is spent only on chemical fertilizers.

The **green revolution** model is reducing this country's economy and rural societies to beggary. The harder we work, the more chemical fertilizers and pesticides we produce and use, the poorer we become and the more people will starve and be malnourished.

When man appeared on the earth he found himself in a wonderful world thickly inhabited by plants animals living. When man first appeared on our planet earth the entire globe was living with nature in complete harmony and earth was beautiful. Man being a superior, being started challenging the laws of nature. He was then a primitive man, he is now modern and well educated and yet he continues to bleed his environment for the sake of his own personal pleasure, thus creating unwanted environmental problem. From his earliest days he has been dependent on his environmental for all his needs namely, food, clothing, shelter and raw materials to feed industries.

With time **human population** grew increasingly, the use of natural resources went beyond a certain limit and harmful side effects began to become evident. Man was far more intelligent as well he lost no time to challenge mother nature of which he was an offspring. He considered himself as the dominant master of nature and ruthlessly began to use and destroy natural resources for his own comfort. Intelligent as man still is, it is time that he realizes that excessive pollution will eventually suffocate life on earth and so it is about time that serious steps are taken to undo the harm done through pollution and to stop further pollution. More and more trees should be planted wherever and whenever possible. Every man on earth should become nature friendly, and make every effort to make our surrounding green.

Biomedical waste management: It is a challenging task in the prevention of infection as well as achieving clean atmosphere. Segregation, collection and proper transportation with decided colored bags and codes.

Effect of pollution is both immediate and delayed. Household waste can be best used as manure such as 3 feet pits are dug and alternate layers of refuse and night soil are spread proportion 6 inches when the content reach above the ground level, the pits are covered with earth and compacted. Because of bacterial action, intense heat is generated with the composite pits. At this temperature, the pathogenic and other organism will be killed. At the end of 4-6 months decomposition is complete and manure is formed.

Ecological protection of the environment is for the good of humanity. Respect the earth as God's creation and preserving the humans as its caretaker. If we scan the regions of our planet, we immediately see that humanity has disappointed God's expectations, man, especially in our time, has without hesitation divested wooded plains and valleys, polluted waters, disfigured the earths habitat, made the air unbreathable, disturbed the hydrogeological and atmospheric systems, turned luxuriant areas into deserts and undertaken the forms of unrestrained industrialization, degrading of earth our dwelling place.

We live in a broken world. Healing our broken world, human beings role in the cosmos, human beings are embedded in nature, responsible use of natural resources. Preventing factor **ozone destructions** from supersonic jets, acid rain, cloning, animal clothing, human cloning, and ethical issues of cloning, abiding presence God of creation, feeling one with nature, preserving and admiring the universe, glorifying God through nature. Major issues challenges before us. We live, move and develop our being in and through this environment. Therefore, it is essential to understand it.

Problems of health in the broken world—big factories, excess **motor vehicles,** overcrowded cities and nuclear plants are among the major sources of environmental degradation, cough, bronchitis, TB, asthma, allergies, cancer, diarrhea, cholera, hepatitis, typhoid, skin diseases are among the more common ailments.

The root cause of environmental degradation is greed-based on the existing developmental model. It has to be community oriented fulfilling basic needs. To be actively involved in environmental protection programs. Today people have tall buildings, buying more, spend more, fancier houses.

Due to **deforestation** merchant invasions, land-grabbing businesspersons the trees are cut down; a new mind-set and a new attitude towards developing humane relationship with environment. We, the modern-day humans, have the obligation to protect the earth and its closely inter-linked eco-systems. We have no right to poison the earth or damage its environment for our immediate benefits.

Training sanitary workers: This is aimed to improve the village level sanitary conditions near water sources and also around the houses. Sanitary workers are trained on water-borne diseases, communicable diseases, etc. and also its prevention measures. These paraworkers motivate the self-help-groups to take up sustainable sanitation measures. At village level as well as at household level. These workers are also going to be trained in restoration of hand pumps and provided with centralized tool kits. These people will take care of hand pump, which assures safe drinking water to the community without any break. Cost latrines with the support of government to reduce open defecation practices by that addressing the issue of facial and communicable disorders. Improved consumption of consumable forest produces. Increased income levels, increased transparency and accountability.

Germs are all around us, in the air we breathe, and often in the water we drink, they find their way into our food, usually because of poor methods of handling. Rain and snow are the original source of all our drinking water. Water is truly liquid of life. Nothing else can ever take its place. 2008 international year of environment is declared. As Environment includes water, air, housing, soil waste, radiation and also social customs, culture, habits, and economic income, occupation, religion, bacteria, viruses, insects, rodents, animals, etc. conditions under which we live.

The key to man's health lies largely in his environment. If clean water is not provided we can get water related diseases; ill health can be due to water pollution, soil pollution, air pollution, poor housing conditions, presence of animal reservoirs and insect vectors which pose constant threat to human health.

Often man is responsible for it by urbanization, industrialization and other human activities. As we can see from the past that old problems solved, new come up like air pollution, radioactive pollution is growing problem faced by the society. "Sanitation is the way of life". It is a quality of living that is expressed in the clean home, the clean farm, the clean business, the clean neighborhood and the clean community. As it is being way of life it must come from within people, WHO – "the control of all those factors in man's physical environment which expresses in man's physical development, health and survival".

Adequate **food**, safe water, clean environmental sanitation, good hygiene and health habits are the pillars of health. These are dependent on people individuals, families, and communities. Therefore, 'Health for All' cannot be achieved unless people are empowered enough to participate fully in health programs.

To improve the quality of life and to have a good standard of living we have to focus our attention on to the healthy lifestyle which includes not to deposit feces near homes, diseases carried from excreta, human excreta is the source of infection; it contains pathogenic bacteria, protozoa, it can contaminate drinking water. Therefore, it must be disposed of in a hygienic manner. Self-care has to be taken.

Hygiene: It is important for washing hands after defecation and before preparing food. Inadequate water supply increases health hazards like skin infections, eye infections, and guinea worm. Without abundance water around home personal hygiene becomes difficult. Water has to be free from pathogenic agents, and also from harmful chemical without ample and safe drinking water, we cannot provide health care to the community, water requirement in sufficient amount is necessary.

There is a need of sufficient **water** for domestic use that is for drinking, cooking, washing, bathing, flushing of toilets, gardening; water for public purpose such as cleaning, swimming pools, public parks. Industrial purpose water needed for processing and cooling; agriculture purpose such as irrigation. Therefore, water is essential for economic, social and cultural development of a community. We can get water from rain, rivers, streams, tanks, ponds, lakes, ground, wells, springs, tubewells.

It is another environmental issue is to get **pure air.** Due to pollution in the air there is a transmission of stimuli by dust, smoke, toxic gases, chemical vapors has resulted in sickness and death. Air can get impure by so many ways such as respiration of men and animals, combustion of coal, gas, and oil. Also decomposition of organic matter, trade, traffic and manufacturing processes, which give off dust, fumes, vapors, gases. When there is an air pollution people will have adverse effects on their health such as exhaust, respiratory tract irritation, bronchial hyperactivity, lung cancer, cough, discomfort, asthma, death may occur in severe exposure. Though the wind sweeps away the impurities, sunlight, rain, plant life cleanses air. Air disinfections is still in the experimental stage.

Whatever be the beneficial **effects pesticides** have in crop protection, vector control, etc. they should not be at the cost of human life and environment. The Bhopal tragedy of 1984 is a classic example of pesticide hazard in our country. Thousands of people died due to the leakage of the gas. Pesticides can reach the human beings through the food chain. Much of the spray will remain on the plant/tree parts and get washed into the soil and then to the nearby water bodies. The pesticide can enter the body of the fish, which is a staple food of the humans.

Sanitation is a way of life, which comes from within people expressed in cleanliness. Fairs and festivals expose people to risk of diseases. People need to be protected. It is vital to take measures during the festivals and fairs and community nurse cannot avoid it. Educating people on proper cooking methods adopting hygiene habits close association of animals to be avoided, which are hazardous therefore continuous efforts to see people do not get affected, therefore environmental sanitation is a great challenge.

Today ultramodern fast forward **technological advancement** called jet age life has its effects on human. Noise exposure, such as unwanted sounds, or wrong sound, in wrong place, at wrong time it could increase stress factors. With its loudness, intensity, frequency, will result in auditory effects. Deafness, interference with speech, annoyance, rise in blood pressure, increase heart rate, breathing, sweating, giddiness, nausea, fatigue, visual disturbances, interference with speech and communication. To control this noise, the apt planning cities, separation of residential areas, and control of vehicles, blowing of horns prohibited, soundproof building, and silence zones needs to be created more and more.

Radiation exposure is also harmful such as medical, dental, X-rays, radioisotopes, there are also other occupational exposure, TV sets, radioactive dial, watches all these radiation where we can get affected with radiation sicknesses such as acute radiation syndrome, Leukemia, carcinogens, fetal development abnormalities, shortening of life, chromosome mutations, sterility etc.

"**Home** gives experience of heaven on earth". Good well lighten, well ventilated and proper site of house also is an important part of man's environment. The 'Physical structure of the home also providing shelter' facilities, equipment, devices, social well-being sanitary shelter, preparation and storage of food, meeting, sleeping, basic activities, access to community facilities, school, shopping area, places of worship, help in times of need, physical protection, provides adequately for cooking, eating, washing, and excretory functions is designed, constructed, maintained and used in a manner such as to prevent the spread of communicable diseases, provides protection from hazards of exposure to noise and pollution, free from toxic harmful materials, encourages personal and community development, promotes social relationship, promotes mental health. If we see the urban slums they live in over crowed areas.

More people living in single **dwelling space**, their movements are restricted, they have no privacy, there is lack of hygiene, they find it difficult to rest and sleep, there is constant feeling of irritability, frustration, anxiety, violence, mental disorders, unhappiness, psychosomatic effects, prevalence of communicable diseases. They dispose the wastes garbage, such as food, rubbish, paper, plastics, wood, metal, glass, etc. anywhere just throws away. Even the dead animals, heaps are nuisance with bad odors, which later decomposes and favors fly breeding, attracts rodents.

We have to educate the public for health protection. The control of all these factors is important component of community health, because much of the ill health is due to these factors. It is the responsibility of community health nurse to educate people about hygiene and improvement of sanitation to prevent disease. To educate the people and get their cooperation in order to maintain good health, the physical and mental health care is not sufficient; it is necessary to take care of surrounding hygiene.

Create an awareness attitude to help each individual to develop a healthy and positive attitude impart knowledge and inculcate skills of understanding to be sensitive in minimizing the problem. So that man lives on this planet with complete harmony in this wonderful world by stopping further pollution. Trying to reduce the threat by spreading the message and planting more trees, recycling and proper garbage disposal, sweeping, educating and motivating people, keeping the surrounding green and avoiding any act that pollute the mother earth. In addition, talking the care of nature gifted by God freely to humankind.

Awareness and sensitization of the public on the science of safeguarding health through clean environment; to create awareness in every individual and in the society about the environment and environment-related problem; to help each individual to develop a healthy and positive attitude towards the environment; to impart knowledge about the essential environment and its cause; to inculcate in the students the skills of understanding the need of a healthy environment and also help develop skills to be sensitive to environmental problem and to solve them. Let us ask ourselves these questions— How are we to conserve natural resources? Here is one concert example stated below will explain the gravity and urgency of the collective responsibilities and action.

Mercury, mars can destroy earth. Before sun eats us up, earth could collide with either planet, predict scientists. No one knows exactly how life on earth will end.

In another 100 years, the hungry tide will swallow sunderbans. Global warming has become a major cause of concern for the mangroves; rising sea levels and melting glaciers will submerge the world's largest tiger reserve. Scientists say Sundarbans islands would be completely submerged under water in Bengal would be wiped away. It is a slow disaster. The destruction of the mangrove covers, rising sea levels and melting of Himalayan glaciers are the main causes behind the changing geographical conditions. The region has been witness to an abnormal rise in the sea level in the last four decades. This has led to massive erosion. Lohachara Island was the first inhibited island to disappear. Now, even the animal kingdom is feeling threatened. Geologists say the people of Sundarbans are the first global warming refugees. Four million people, who inhabit the Indian side, are dreadfully vulnerable. To stop erosion massive plantation campaign the problem can be tackled help to ward off natural disasters and maintain ecological balance. Says environmental scientist.

A letter from soil to man—Dear people, I am the soil. I am the "top-covering" of the Earth and under every step, you take. Will you please listen to my story, before I completely disappear? My body is like a big warm blanket wrapped around the Earth. I have many different textures from hard to silken soft. Imagine all the different shades of brown, yellow, red and black and you will know a part of me. I am a "home" for seeds and plants. Plants get their water and nutrients through me. In my layers, there are tiny organisms that are necessary for my fertility, breaking down humus and making pathways for air and water. I filter the rain that falls to the ground, slowing its flow to rivers and the sea. In this way, I help to keep my friend – the water, clear and clean. You need me. I need you to look after me. I take lots of time to make, and you can destroy me in a minute. Please help me. There are many people on the earth and the population is growing. Much of me have been lost by erosion. Yet there is still time to secure me, before I get swept away completely. You could cover areas of me with grasses and trees. You could see different techniques of farming which strengthen me slowly and surely. With warm regards, yours sincerely, the soil.

Living a simple lifestyle: A simple lifestyle that respects the earth as God's creation, and perceiving the humans as nature's caretakers. In the fast changing health scenario of the country, collective vision and efforts would take the country to greater heights in health achievements. We have no right to poison the earth or damage its environment for our immediate benefits. Protection of the environment is for the good of humanity. We, the modern-day humans, have the obligation to protect the earth and its closely inter-linked eco-systems. The Bible tells us, "God created man and woman in His own image and likeness". What a profound revelation! We are not just chance products of physical and biological processes. Nevertheless, we are precious beings having divine dimensions. Being His image, we are also co-creators of this ever-changing, ever-expanding and ever-developing universe. Persons created in God's image invite relationship, response and respect our mother earth.

CONCLUSIONS

Climate change is one of the greatest changes of our time. Protecting health from climate change the theme of WHO 2008 puts health at the center of the global dialogue about climate change, which is posing global threat to public health security. Through increased collaboration, the global community will be better prepared to cope with climate related health changes worldwide action- strengthening surveillance and control of infectious diseases and coordinating health action in emergencies. There are many factors explained above contribute to the upsetting the delicate balance with the earth and its inhabitations have shared ever since earth came into existence.

WHO aims to put public health at the center of the UN agenda on climate change.

Create advocacy campaigns for generating momentum that compels governments the international community, civil society and individuals to take action to anchor health at the heart of the climate change agenda.

Goal is to raise awareness, advocate for interdisciplinary and intersectorial partnership generates effective actions, demonstrate the healthy communities' role, and spark commitment and action.

Health is one of the areas most affected by climate change. The science is clear; the earth is warming for which human actions are responsible. If the same tread remains, uncontrolled humanity will face health problems. As glaciers, melt the hydrological cycle shifts and the productivity of arable land changes. Human activities are a prime cause and human can be a solution. We must act now; together find solution to find ways to stabilize the imbalance. Action must begin now before catastrophic climate changes destabilizes beyond control. Awake.

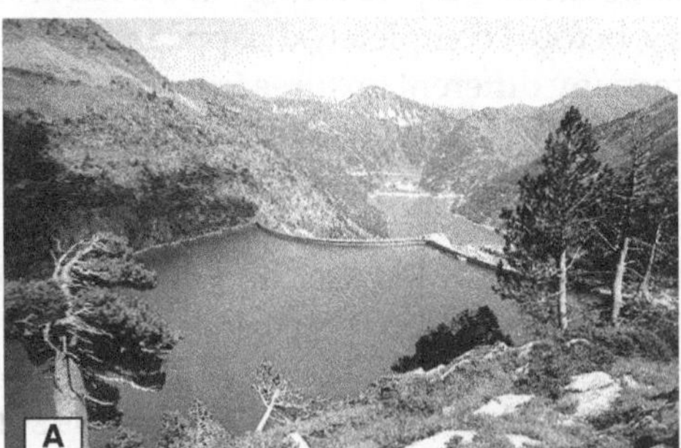

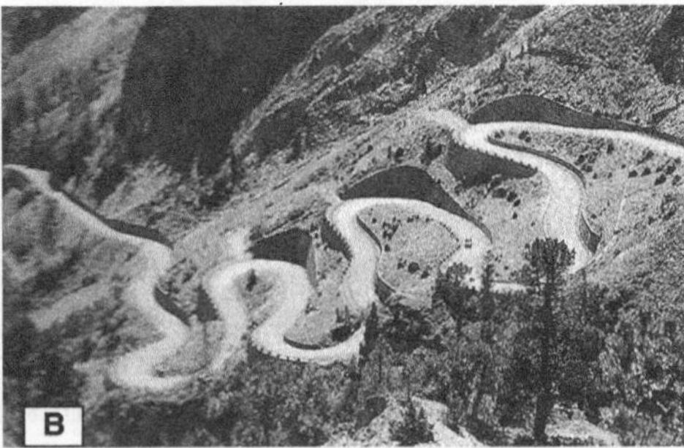

Figs 11.1A and B: God's wonderful creation of the planet earth. The beauty and the awesome sight of the nature. The peace and the serenity, purity that blends together harmoniously which pleasing to the eyes

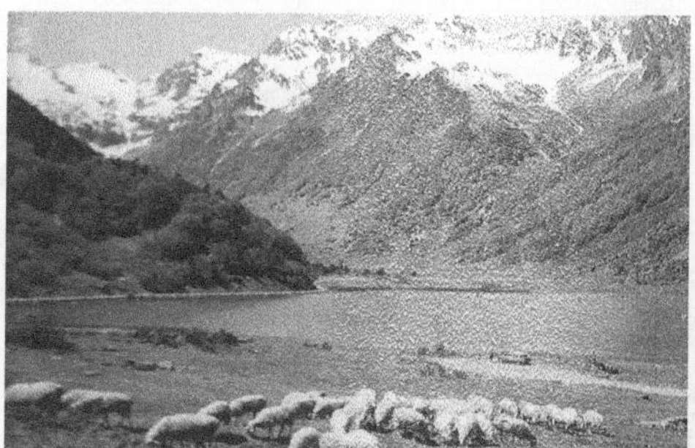

Fig. 11.2: Clean air and safe environment. Free from pollution

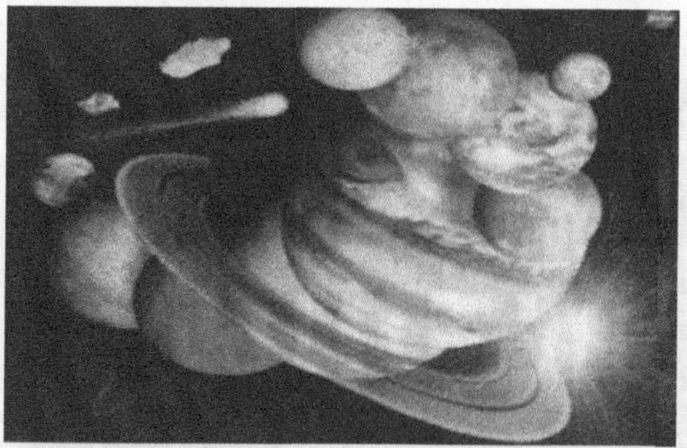

Fig. 11.6: Climatic change due to global warming. Changes in the galaxy

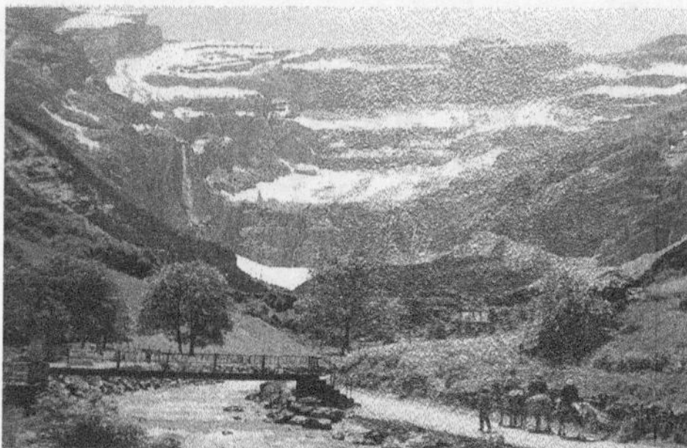

Fig. 11.3: Water, the liquid of life. Sources of pure water

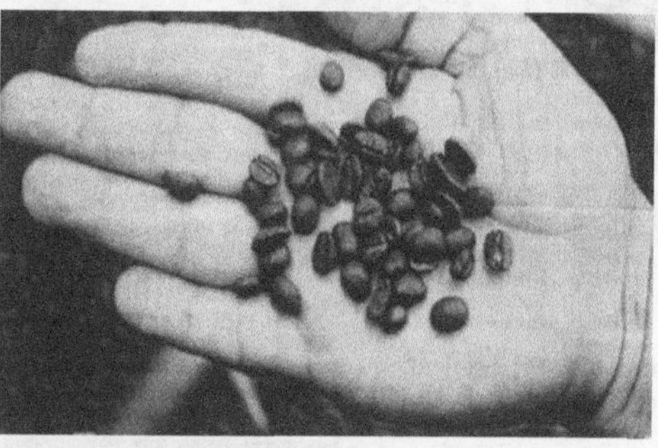

Fig.11.7: Scientist develops way to create biodiesel fuel for cars from coffee waste, which is ecofriendly and can prevent pollution

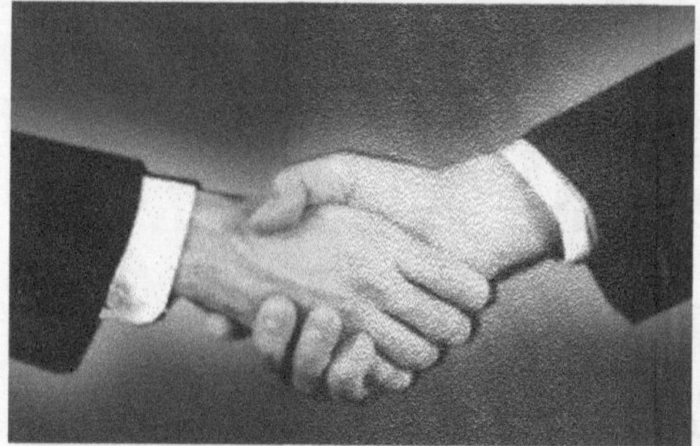

Fig. 11.4: Let us join hands in common effort to save our earth

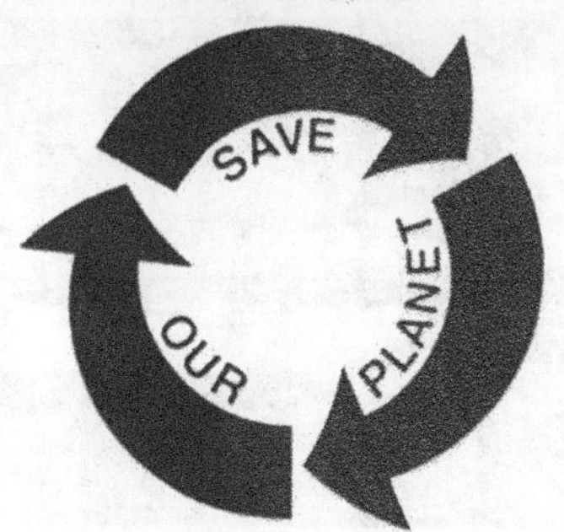

Fig. 11.5: Recycle

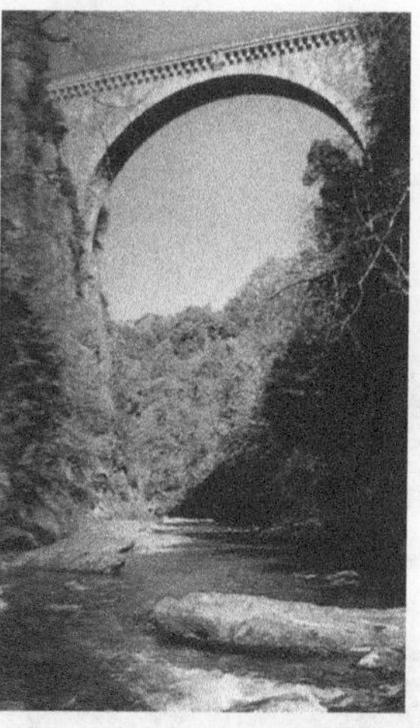

Fig. 11.8: Green belt and flowing water. Deep forest with plenty of trees with natural habitat

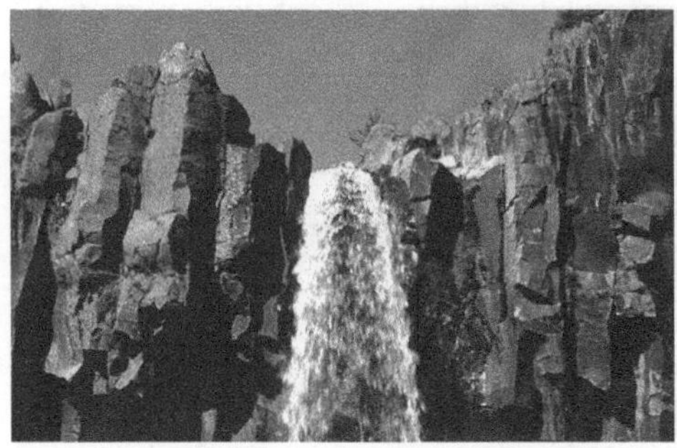

Fig.11.9: Environmental preservation

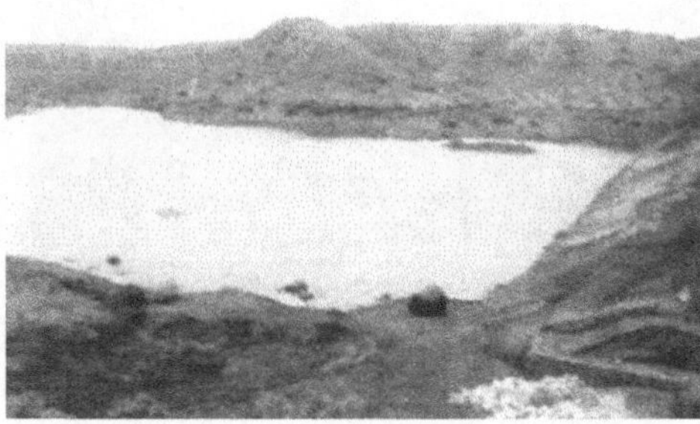

Fig. 11.10: Rural water resources. Used for common purpose

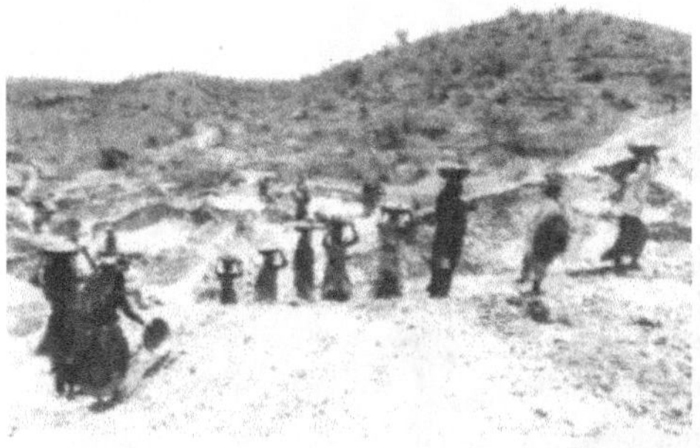

Fig. 11.11: Lack of monsoon, due to climatic change, people working in hot scorching sun

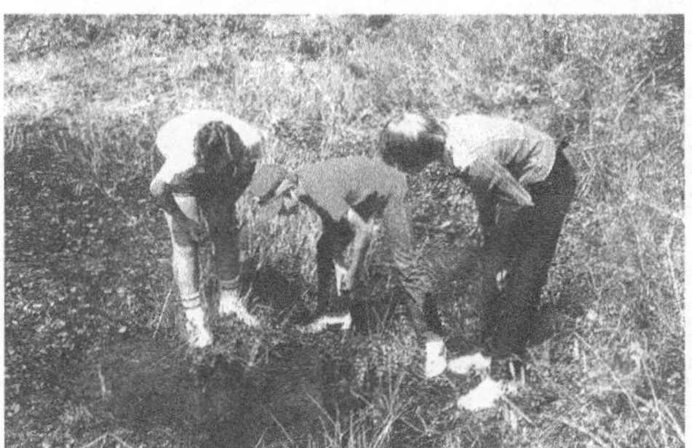

Fig. 11.12: Environmental sanitation

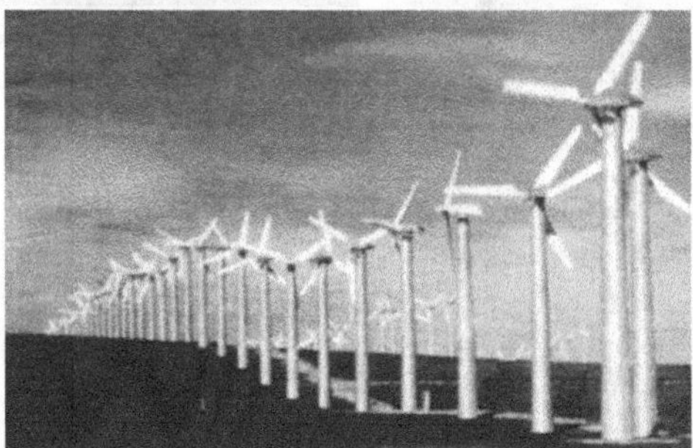

Fig. 11.13: Wind farm, producing electricity

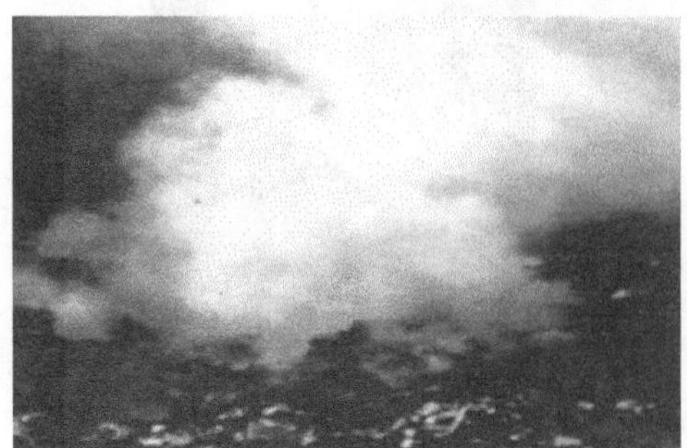

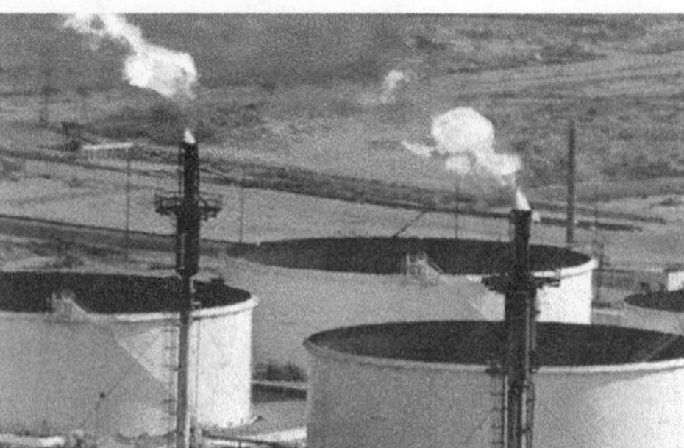

Figs 11.14 and 11.15: WHO theme for 2008 environment and climatic change. Environmental air pollution which give rise to ill health

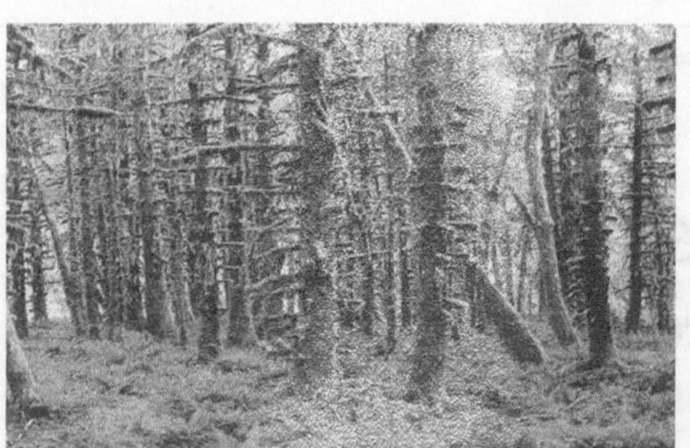

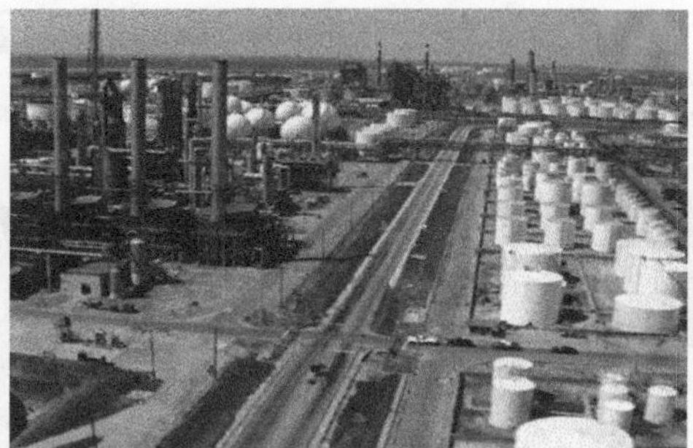

Figs 11.16 and 11.17: The green house. The forest with tree plantations. Preservation of soil erosion

12 Disaster Management: The New Challenge

The famines, droughts, floods, devastating earthquake; and many other natural calamities, that takes place on and off in different parts has called attention of the whole world. On this destructive day thousands of people lose their lives, many lose their parents, brothers, sisters and relatives, many became homeless, people became jobless and many who lose their property and all the earnings of life. People lose confidence. This shocking moment lift people in trauma and terror. In short, people lose life and community.

It is now the **responsibility** of the world community to build human community and give dignity to the victims of earthquake and other such disasters that strike on and off in different parts. It is now our responsibility to give them confidence and support to face the life and to build up community especially in the poor village community. We have to form village committees who will be responsible for the development of the village. Together with community organization, we have to propose 'Livelihood Program' to promote life and dignity to the victims of disasters. Learns to cope with the loss of life, shelter and livelihood that causes by the disasters such as earthquake, where the survivors have to 'pick up the pieces' and resume their lives which can bear testimony to the indomitable spirit of humankind; as nature is not entirely unkind if we live ecofriendly life.

Since the beginning of time, disasters have been a part of life. Disaster can violently disrupt our day-to-day lives and change the history forever. There are times calamities and the disaster has wiped off places from the map of the world. People and the places are no more the same after the disaster. Large number of people are displaced, killed or injured. Disaster is an occurrence that causes damage, economic disruption, and loss of human life. In primary prevention awareness and educating public of risk factors, individual and community safety practices. Secondary includes interventions like immediate rescue, preventing additional injury or death, first aid, organized community responses, medical care, shelter; various actions to be taken for rehabilitation and disability.

American Red Cross defines disaster as the occurrence either natural or man-made that causes human needs that the victim cannot elevate or solve without the assistance (1975).

There are different types of disasters such as earthquakes, floods volcanic eruptions, hurricanes, tornadoes, landslides, tidal waves, epidemics etc, in each of this calamities the casualties are very high, for example, in 1985 Columbia there was volcanic eruption and 23000 deaths were reported that is the mortality was very high.

There are also **man-made tragedies,** which also cause the disaster that can be worse too. Such as for example, Bhopal gas tragedy in India on third of December 1984; in which a leakage in the storage tank of union carbide pesticide plant released tons of methyl gas; which was pumped into the air, about 2 million people were exposed to this tragedy living 2000 people dead, and people are still suffering of the adverse effect of it which will go on for few generation.

In this fast growing technology ultramodern electronic media; there are insidious disaster of chemicals exposure, radiation exposure specially in nuclear weapons producing factories, in research of lab, results in radioactive substances into the air, soil, underground waters where chemical plants release toxic substances, adding to global warming**, wars and civil conflicts,** for example, where we had the attack on the twin tower of the world trade center in New York in which 6000 people lost their life. These are man-made international disaster including the atomic bombing.

Principles of disaster management—Sanford in 1984 listed eight principles—prevention of occurrence of a disaster whenever possible by observing warning signs and predictions done by weather for cast through radio and televisions, minimizing causality number, preventing further casualities, rescuing the injured, providing first aid, evacuating the injured, providing definitive care and facilitating reconstruction-recovery; preventing migration. The community health nurse who will be assisting in disaster relief efforts must be as healthy as possible, professional preparedness. Community preparedness—for emergencies can rescue people rapidly and provide life saving first aid. A vigilant, attunes, alert and focused to act promptly to take decisions to save life that is timely intervention.

Rescue emergency medical care by locating the trapped victims and transferring them to safe places, to save maximum lives categorizing the treatable victims from untreatable ones and color code could be given to them such as color Red fist priority those having life-threatening injury and those who experience hypoxia, unconscious, shock, chest wounds ect. Yellow the second color for those mostly with multiple fractures, spinal injury, and large laceration sect. In addition, the Green colors the third category for minor burns, closed fractures and the last category in Black color for the ones who are already dead.

All the different agencies pull together to restore the economic and civic life of the community. Keeping in mind the rebuilding effort. Provide disaster education; seek to keep a safe environment, on going assessment or surveillance reports, which includes statues of affected population, observation, physical examination, interview, health and illness screening, surveys and records. Vigilant in teaching proper hygiene and making sure immunization records are up-to-date. Remain alert for environmental hazards during the recovery phase of the disaster.

Home visits may lead her to uncover situation such as faulty housing structure, lack of water supply or lack of electricity; Danger of dead animals and rodents; psychosocial intervention in the aftermath of disaster. Keep the people in their natural groups if they must be relocated. Provide social activity for new community, encourage families to talk to gather about their experiences, losses and feelings encourage families to resume normal activities to the extent possible, and help families handle conflicts appropriately so as to minimize negative encounters caused by the strain, fatigue, and irritability that often follow trauma.

To rebuild villages, and rehabilitate the lives of the people affected by the disasters of earthquake and other calamities. To enable the villagers overcome the trauma through counseling by the animators, to help rebuild the social life of the village. To identify the people most requiring assistance to restart their livelihoods and provide appropriate materials.

The result of devastating and destructive earthquake and calamities has loss of life, property, infrastructure; terror, fear and depression, lack of confidence created in high intensity. In short, the life and community are destroyed if you glance through the serious of recent disasters that took place.

This kind of different livelihood project helps the poor to up grade their social, economic, physical and educational status in the society. Due to this project family assets will increase. After two years family get more profit. The life standard of the family will come up. With milk and the product of the milk and cow dung that is obtained everyday, the economic status of the family will improve in the society. For that we need to create a disaster management cell. Disaster of all types, natural and man-made has been experienced all the times. They always have serous effects on human and other living species in varying degree and kind. They have human, social, psychological and economic effects on mankind.

Planning: The well planned and prepared health delivery system would reduce loss of lives, prevent epidemic spread and ensure essential services like water supply, food stocks, sanitation and sewage facilities; grass-root level vocational training institutions designed for bringing the gap between the available technologies at one end and their application for increased production at the other. Identification of training areas, target group, effective program, technical and training needs of villagers. They may also be approached for rapport building and for creating awareness among the community regarding the scheme; as the success of the program depends largely on the local collaboration.

Emotional shifts in disaster sufferers: Disaster, weather natural or human made, is a life-twisting event for any person. Emotional changes, responses and traumas, the affected people go through would enable the caregiver and volunteers to act accordingly and effectively.

The very **first reaction** of a person hit by a disaster is denial, and a search for the causes of the happening. This cannot happen to me. My dear ones cannot die. My home cannot get dismantled. They become excessive active or passive, move around like hysteric.

Human tendencies: As we are, we would like to find a reason for such a happening in life. Why me and not the other? Where did I go wrong? Why has God punished me? Once the people are able to recognize that the inevitable has happened, they usually try to find solace in fate. Some others would see it as anger of God for the evils they have done all through their life. Then the person comes to know that not only they lost dear and near once and valuables but there are others too who share the same fate.

They lose everything that they had built up over the year. They know the future is bleak and they have to begin from scratch. Anger and frustration crisp in them. The loss of dear ones as well as belongings and properties brings in a feeling of lethargy and helplessness. There is no more enthusiasm to fight back, at this time many people come to their aid. After few months, the affected people try to accept the situation as it is; acceptance to live in spite of all eventualities that rocked their lives. There comes the new enthusiasm to live. There is a tremendous attitudinal change; and there is a mood to fight back in life. Try to rebuild their lives and communities. Give them psychological counseling and emotional support to help them to come with terms and return to normal life. Application of professional nursing skill to recognize and meet the physical and emotional needs; nursing part in primary prevention is to remain in disaster place until the situation subsides. During that time, assessment data is collected and analyzed so that it can help in nursing diagnosis, use crisis intervention technique based on assessment and then set goal to be established.

Throughout the history, the violent side of nature has manifested itself in destructive phenomena such as folds, volcanic eruptions, severe storms, earthquakes and so on. Disasters will continue to threaten, kill and destroy. It is virtually impossible to prevent most disaster. Nevertheless, we can forestall or alleviate many of the effects by anticipating them and by being adequately prepared.

India is considered one of the places most vulnerable to earthquakes and other natural disasters. Human-made disasters are on the rise in our country, which adds to the already-existing precarious situation. One of the crucial aspects during disaster response is finance. Identifying credible donor agencies that would support the work financially and logistically is important. Their assurance of support needs to be ensured.

A disaster situation may need many **volunteers**. They should be adequately trained in dealing with the disaster situation. They should prove themselves sources of strength and instill confidence and courage in the victims. They are to be skilled in listening to the victims, not to offer any solution but just to allow them to ventilate their feelings. It is crucial for the agency to place right people at the right time.

There are many things that **NGOs** can do more effectively than their partners because of their community level activities, their capacity to be innovative, their focus on vulnerable communities the trust and credibility that they have built up over the years and their capacity to listen to and involve people.

Teamwork is the most efficient way of dealing with the aftermath of a disaster. Networking among the various agencies before the actual disaster is important. Each of them could complement the work instead of duplicating the work. A flood will be different from an earthquake or a communal violence. A core-team is a must. This means there are to be leaders who are able to make decisions and guide the volunteers and others in the relief operations.

Human energy is precious and it cannot be wasted, especially during a disaster situation, and hence sending the minimum number of people with necessary expertise and proper attitude is very important. Apart from the material facilities (food, water, shelter, and clothing and medical care) one of the crucial factors we need to take care of is trauma management of the victims. The volunteers are to be trained in handling a trauma situation. In a disaster situation, where all are affected and the people who can offer solace to the victims are the outsiders. The most important aspect is listening; listening to people individually and in groups.

"**The most vulnerable victims** are the poor and the marginalized, most of whom live in low-quality housing in flood-prone or drought-prone regions." "In periods of drought, their desperate search for water leads them to drink contaminated water and fail to exercise personal hygiene. And those fleeing floods often drink unclean water too." "If the drinking water supply and the sanitation systems are already inadequate, flooding poses a major health threat. Inundated industrial waste such as used engine oil and refuse dumps add to health risks. People who have lost everything in the flood – their homes, their food, their livelihood – are all the more vulnerable to disease."

Floods are the second most frequent cause of natural disaster after windstorms, but affect more regions and more people than any other phenomenon. Drought is the largest cause of death because it often leads to famine.

Receding flood waters provide an ideal breeding ground for mosquitoes, and create an increased risk of such diseases as malaria, dengue and rift valley fever. Flood water combined with effects of open sewage and reduced opportunities for good personal hygiene, lead to cholera, diarrhea and gastrointestinal viruses and displace rodent population, which can cause outbreaks of leptospirosis and Hantavirus infection. Flooding is visible to everyone, but drought is a great deal more difficult to recognize. Drought triggers or exacerbates malnutrition and famine. Deaths are mainly due to lack of food and the worsening of pre-existing malnutrition, but also to migration, homelessness, and damage to public health infrastructure, to water distribution and to health care. In hot countries or during heat waves, deaths may be caused by a combination of heat and shortage of water.

Disasters like drought, flood, tsunamis, natural calamities etc. aggravate these situations. When calamity strikes be it a natural or man-made it takes a form of disaster. For the people who die in the attack is also a disastrous. We need to extend our support for the survivors who remain in the relief camps. We have to help them to build up. Nothing can justify the killing of the innocent people. We have to take preventive measures to rescue people who are in great trouble. Disaster does not see the face of color or cast it affects all equally and humanitarian aid at such time is the only need of the hour where all join hands and help voluntarily. And that is a God experience and by which still the humanity has survived.

INITIAL FIRST AID FOR NATURAL CALAMITIES

The difference here is about the number of casualties, which may be more enormous. However, principles related to the single casualty type of emergency may be expanded to apply to mass casualty type of situation. Principles of initial first aid are considered to be:

Assess quickly the situation and the casualty and take measures indicated as life saving first aid. That is control hemorrhage, maintain respiration and take any action indicated in case of accidental poisoning.

Keep the casualty (client) in lying donor position and, if on the ground prevent loss of body heat by placing a coat, blanket or newspapers between the casualty (client) and the ground.

Avoid unnecessary handling or movement except to remove the victim from additional danger.

Assure the client that everything is all right.

Prevent shock, which may be anticipated with any major injury, loss of blood, fracture of large bone or crushing injury to a extremity.

Do not give fluids in the presence of any question of abdominal or if other injury is of sufficient complexity to indicate that a general anesthetic may be used within a short period of time.

Do not transport client except for a life saving measure until first aid has been completed, fractures are splinted properly, and the best means of transportation is obtained.

Appropriate case of the client is more important than speed is reaching a medical facility. Only a very few emergencies such as respiratory difficulty, uncontrolled bleeding and imminent delivery require movement as rapidly as possible to a medical facility.

As the number of casualties increases two additional principles become important.

1. Professional and nonprofessional personnel and supplies and equipment should be brought as close to the scene of the disaster as possible to permit the earliest possible initial treatment.
2. Treatment should be continued during the evacuation of patients from the disaster area to facilitate more definitive case.

Aspects of relief work in disaster when disaster strikes, how many people will be it's victim and whether they die or are crippled will depend to a great extent on how will the community and it's homes are prepared to meet such emergencies. Today thermonuclear warfare is considered to be ultimate type of disaster, but the local community stricken by storm, fire, earthquake or explosion may, will face almost as high casualty rates as would the nation in case of nuclear war. A village inundated by flood, with a loss of water over 4,000 lives is devastated as surely as if it were hit by a bomb.

WHEN THE CALAMITY STICKS

What happens to the average community or family in a disaster area? First of all, the electric power supply is impaired. Without electricity there will be no lights, radio, and television sets will no longer function. The telephone lines may well be out of operation, making it difficult to summon help from the fire or police department or to contact the family physician or local hospital. Even if they can be contacted, the condition of the roads and streets may make it impossible for them to reach you. If the grocery store survives the disaster, their contents may be so damaged to be unsafe to use. The water of many communities is pumped from a well, reservoir or lake by electric pumps. If the pumping station is damaged, the water supply will quickly be exhausted or the disaster may damage water mains so badly that contamination makes the water no longer safe. They will be cut off and will be in a place difficult to reach.

Disease thrives under disastrous conditions prevention of disease involves sanitation, isolation and immunization.

Sanitation involves the proper disposal of waste, especially human waste and the control of whatever may cause disease. Disease carries include rodents, house flies, mosquitoes and other insects.

Isolation refers to the process by which the individual with a communicable disease is kept separated from healthy individuals, as nearly as possible, to prevent the spread of these diseases. Isolation is always not easy under disaster conditions, but may always be carried out to a certain degree. The person who covers his mouth while coughing is practicing isolation.

Immunization is the best form of preventive medicine. It is, especially, a practical step in preparing for disastrous situations, because it can be taken in advance.

Every community should have a civil defense plan and organization. This can be used not only for nuclear attack but also for any other kind of disaster for effective and successful relief work in disaster, doctors, and nurses, paramedical personnel, police, military and other volunteers must participate.

RESPONSIBILITIES OF HEALTH WORKERS

To care for injured and sick persons during disaster, needs ingenuity and imagination to utilize things, which are available at hand. The temporary relief centers need constant medical and nursing care. During such times of stress, health workers have following responsibilities:

1. To look often injured and sick persons provide them medical and nursing care.
2. Prevent communicable diseases to spread.
3. Constant observation and treatment to seriously wounded person.
4. Maintain sanitation and cleanliness in and around relief centers.
5. Manage the temporary shelter place effectively.
6. Initial examination and health check up of all those coming to the relief centers.
7. To care for nutritional problems of infants.
8. Food and drinking water for all the residents of relief center.
9. Special care for pregnant mothers, infants, old people and persons with previous illnesses.

Rehabilitation is an integral part of service where community health nurse helps the client to attain social independence. If they are not guided and helped they pose severe disability- community based services can be provided such as physical medicines, physiotherapy, speech therapy, auditory and psychological support and counseling, vocational guidance, occupational guidance and placement service.

Building the lives of the people is very important after effect of disaster and calamities; as when fresh disaster sticks all rush at once to help and show solidarity and then people who are survived no follow-up done affects the development. What can be done to build there lives and brings them to cope up and look ahead with hope. According to the disaster and the types of region and damage, the ongoing projects could be implemented. Such as educating the group for income generating which will give them the regular income in the family, they will be able to educate their children. Give them something, which will take care of health and sociocultural background of work according to the region. For example, if you give them some goats, cows, buffaloes.

HEALTH

The milk of a goat is medicinal and is good for the children. Health status of the family will be improved; ghee, butter and buttermilk from milk, which is nutritious. Since the family gets nutritious food, the health of the family will improve. Social: the chain will continue of generating and regenerating of the income. Through schemes and project implemented, other families of the community too will come up. The value of community responsibility and concern for others will be practiced. Manure: the manure of a goat is good and expensive compare to other nature. This can be used in their fields and they can yield better crop. The activity is in tune with the culture of the village; regular cash flow from daily selling of the production of egg and fertilizer which will upgrade the economic, social, and health status of the beneficiaries? The group of people will manage the poultry and the profit will be shared equally in-group. The beneficiaries also will share the labor equally. Slowly they will build lives and try to overcome the trauma and the loss.

Community organization is a process of organizing the community towards value, purpose, goal, and activity. When the rich becomes richer and the exploitation of the poor increases we need to organize the poor to demand their rights and break the chain of exploitation. That is to empower the powerless. But this is possible when people are motivated. To motivate people we need motivation.

BUILD PEOPLE

To give life to the people who have lost their life due to many reasons due to devastating earthquake or any other afflictions like failure in crops, sickness. Life means not to be alive only. Even animals too live, that living is vegetation. But living means: living with a purpose that includes living with the values, goal and activities. Bringing self-confidence who has lost their self-confidence, bringing out the potentialities, that is in short giving dignity. People have lost their dignity because of the social system, which dehumanizes people. Bringing self-confidence through awareness of particular areas, issues, problems, social structure, social system etc. among target groups and marginalized. In addition, restoring the lost dignity to the people is an animation. The relationship of a human being also depends on the values. A human being is related to a supernatural environment, society, others and one self. Unless human being changes his or her behavior, attitude, norms and values, the system cannot be changed. Let us all together join hands to reduce man made disasters and redeem the affected lot. What so ever you do to the least of my people you do unto God, that is to clothe the naked, shelter the homeless, visit the affected, water for the thirsty and comfort the dying. Here you will see the face of God.

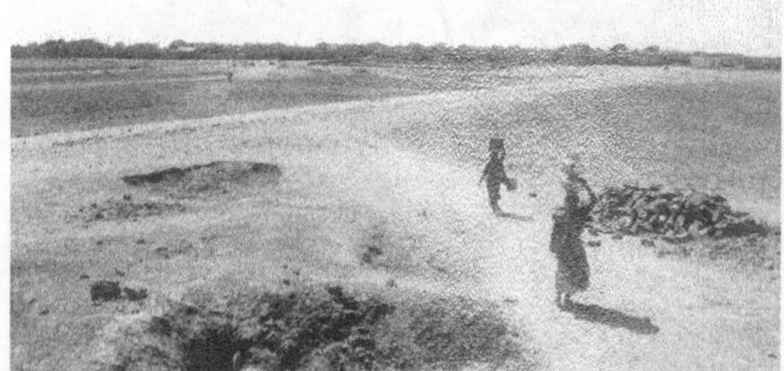

Fig. 12.1: Distance of water collection during drought and hot summer days

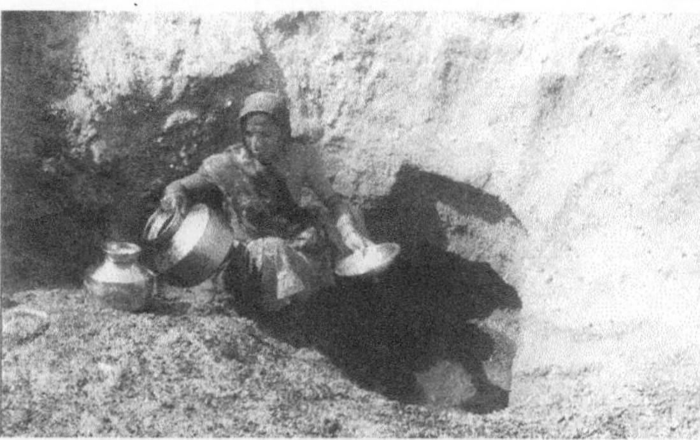

Fig. 12.2: Water scarcity: Water pollution leads to water born disease

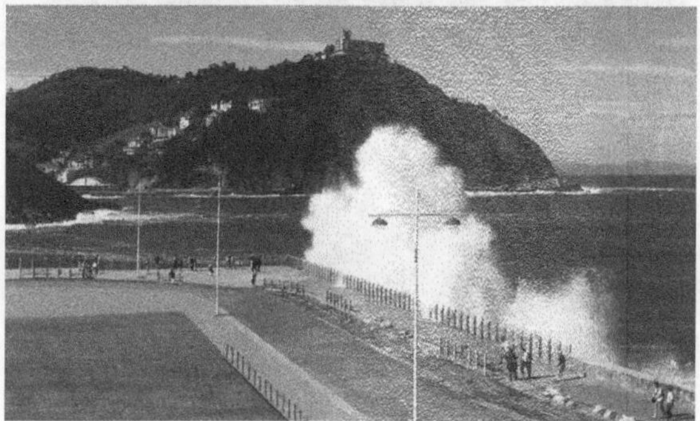

Fig. 12.3: Tidal waves

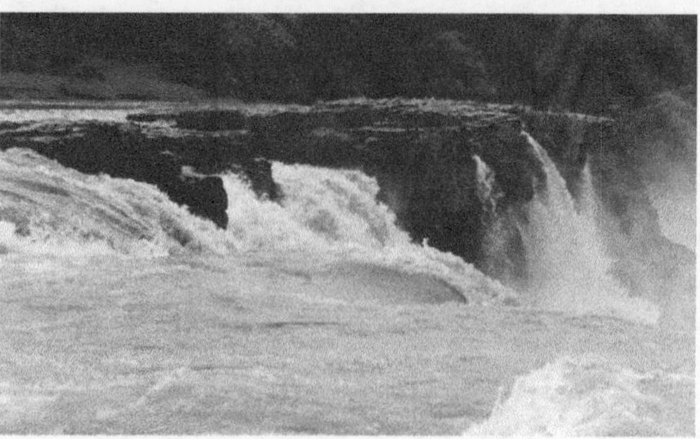

Fig. 12.4: Floods with excess water lives people helpless

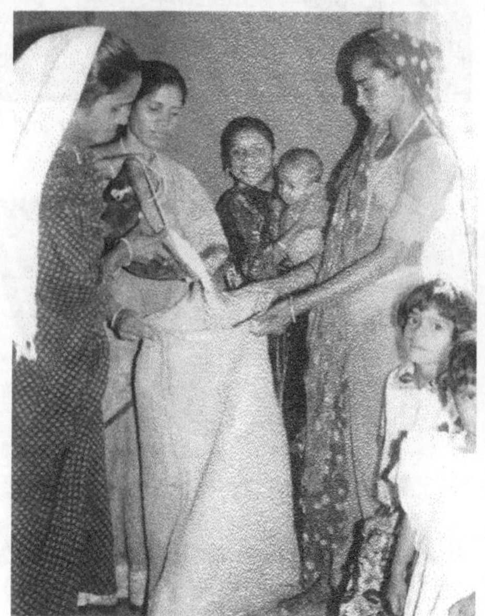

Fig. 12.5: Grain distribution

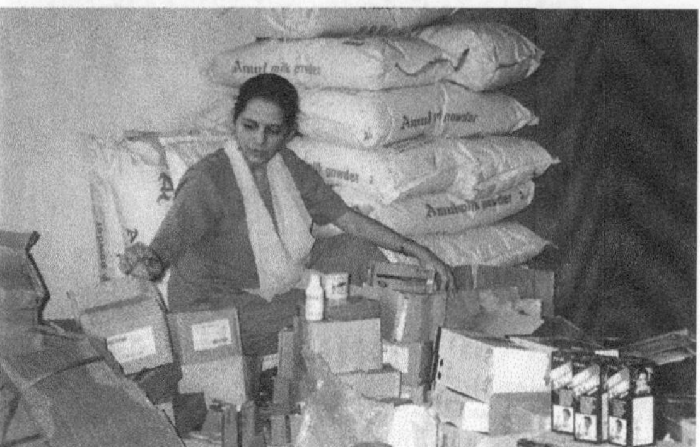

Fig. 12.6: Rescue, relief and emergency medical service

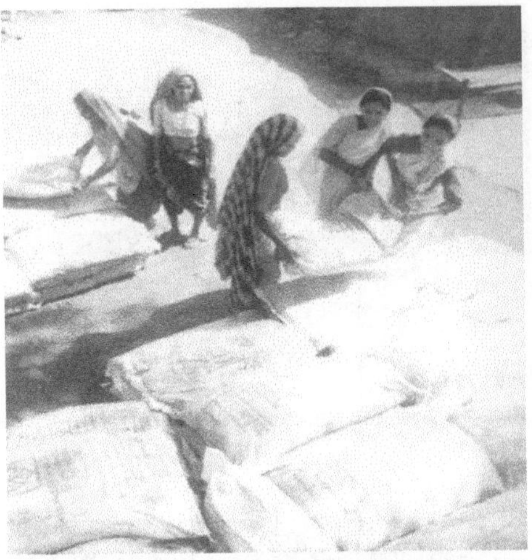

Fig. 12.7: Drought relief service

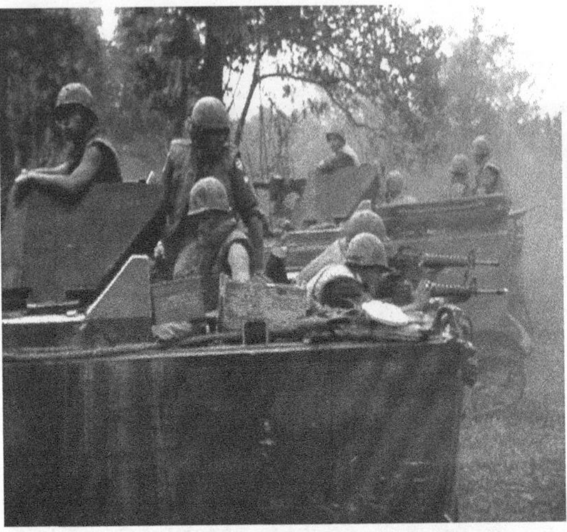

Fig. 12.8: Man made disaster and nuclear weapons—its ill effects

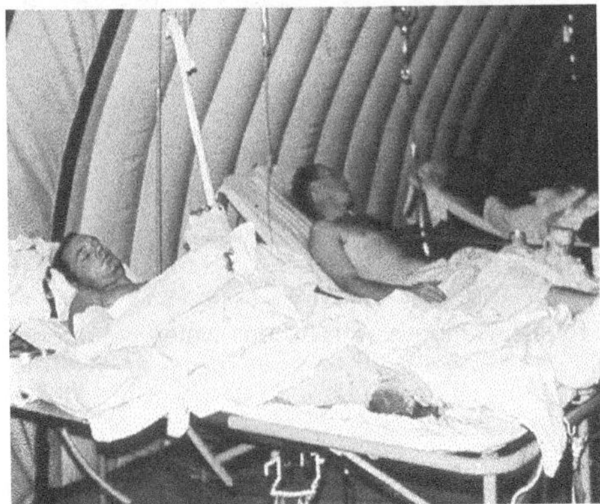

Fig.12.9: Calamity and disaster affected casuality victims

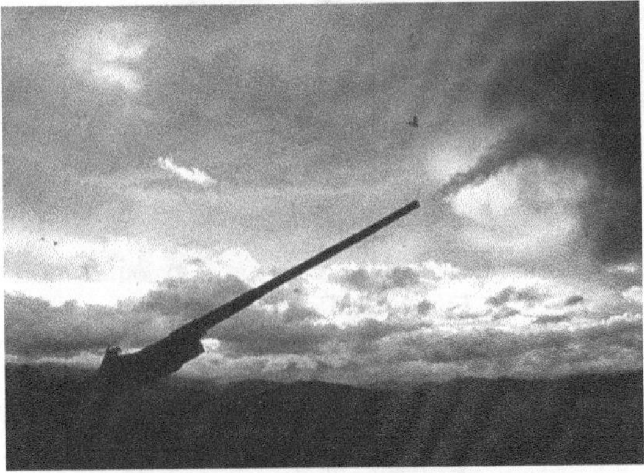

Fig. 12.10: Modern age technology and its good and bad effect

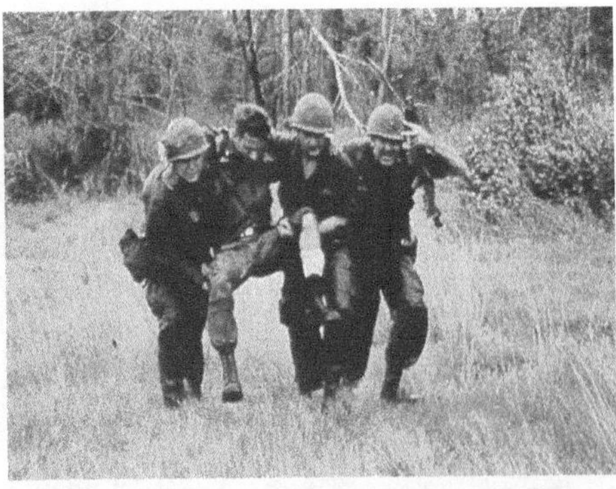

Fig. 12.11: Injured victims of the man-made disaster. Nursing management and first aids to be given

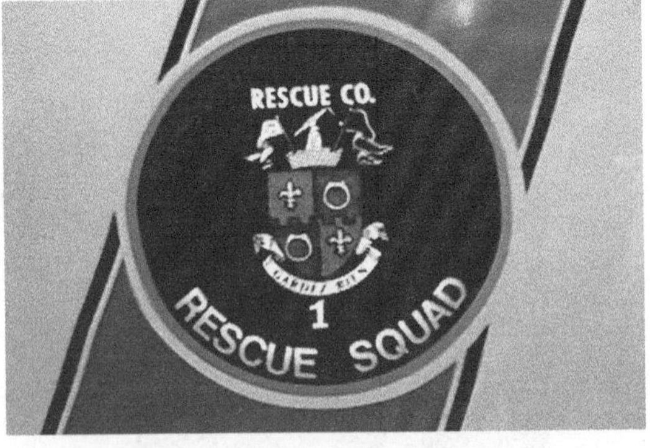

Fig. 12.12

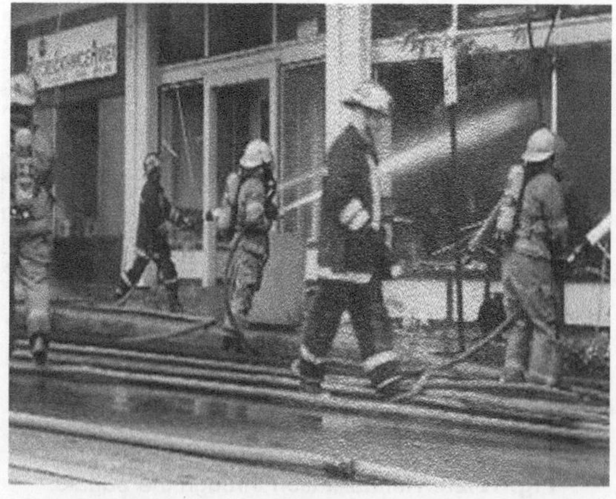

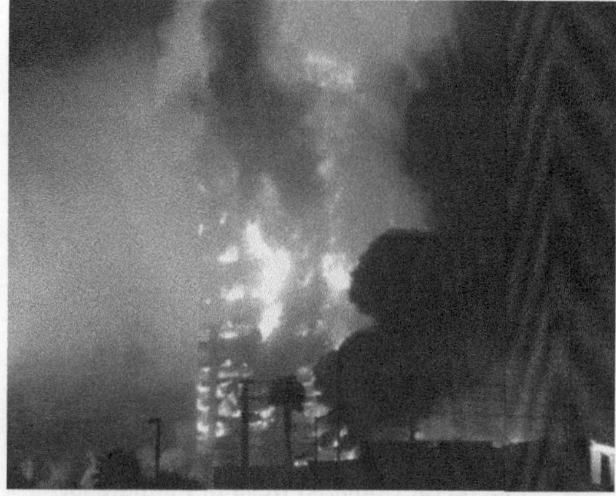

Figs 12.13 and 12.14: Building on fire and rescue operation. Environmental pollution and loss of human lives

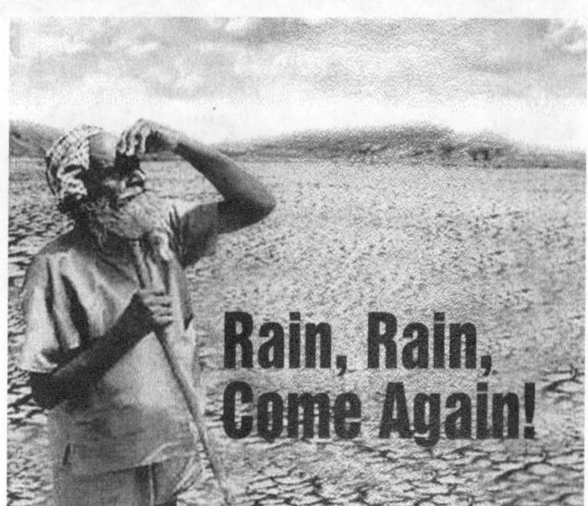

Fig. 12.15: Environment and effects of climate change

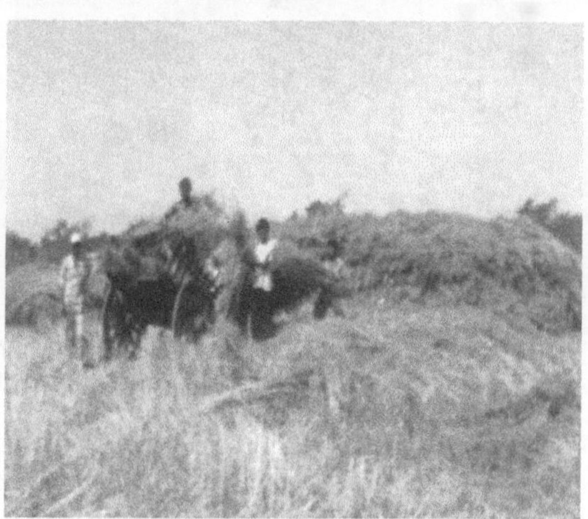

Fig. 12.16: Livelihood program after disaster

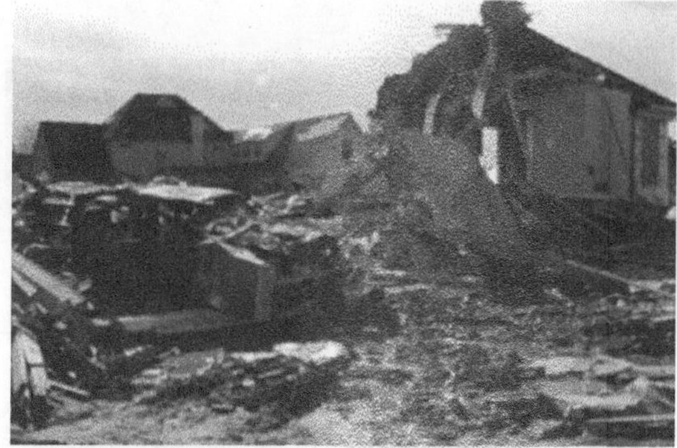

Fig. 12.17: Natural calamity of earthquake and its debris: In moment life changes drastically, never forgetful day

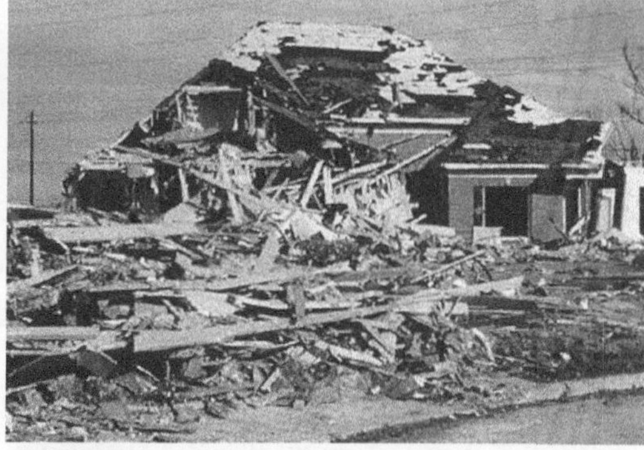

Fig. 12.18: Loss of life and property, the traumatic experience

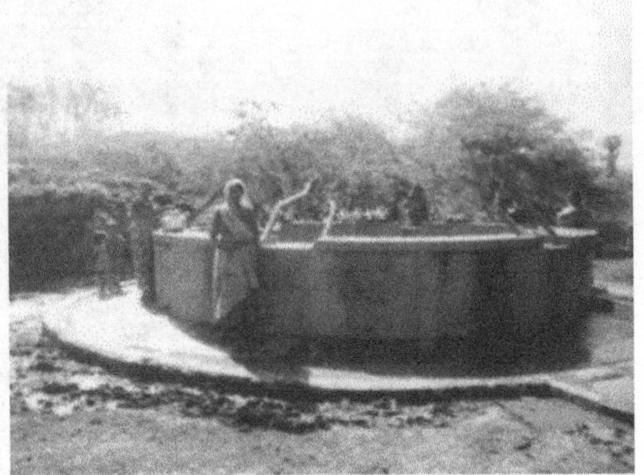

Fig.12.19: Common wells of rural areas. Chlorination and proper disinfections to be followed

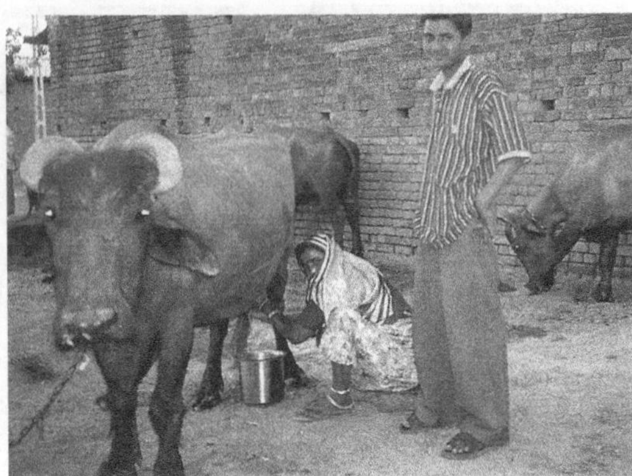

Fig. 12.20: Rehabilitation through the buffalo; financial security and income

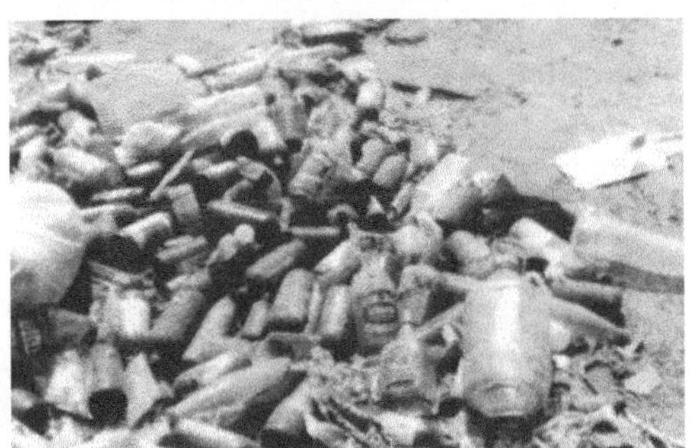

Figs 12.21 and 12.22: Loss of property and devastating effect. After effect of disaster, the remains and the broken situation

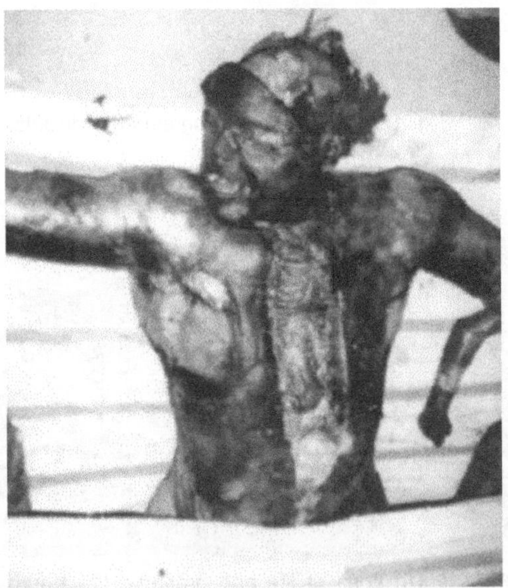

Fig. 12.23: Man-made disaster and its effect on innocent lives *(For color version see Plate 2)*

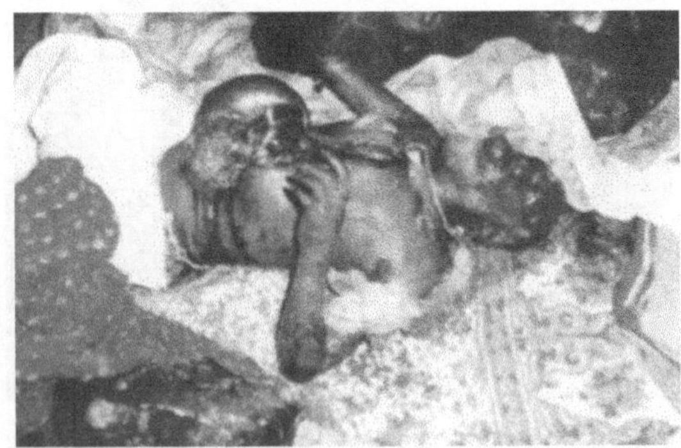

Fig. 12.24: Fundamental respect for human life. Loss of life, pain and suffering that is inconsolable *(For color version see Plate 2)*

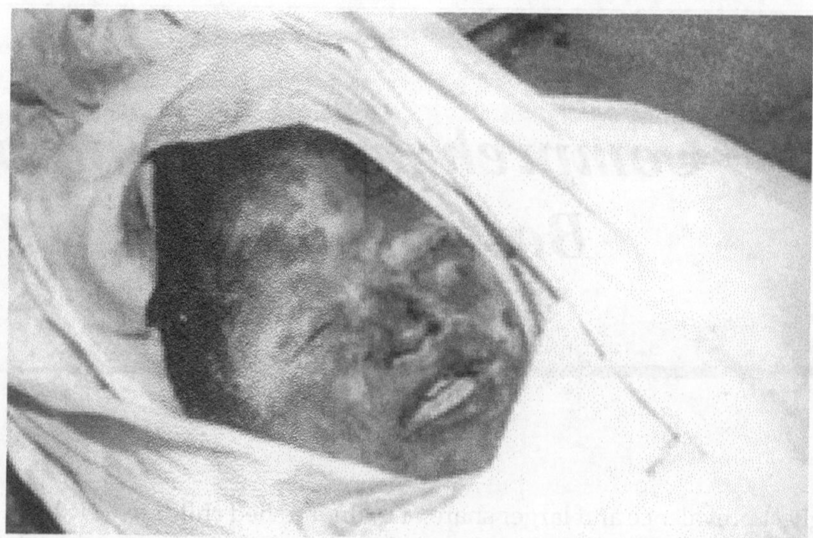

Fig. 12.25: The innocent angel unaware of what is happening and why is it happening and who has done it; precious life before blooming fades away to the ground. The inhuman tragedies caused by man-made disaster cannot be forgotten and forgiven easily. It is challenging and shame on humanity to comprehend, incredible yet the truth of lost life makes you and me thinking *(For color version see Plate 2)*

13 Comprehensive Community Based Nourishment

India has the highest prevalence and larger share of malnourished children, low birth weight babies and anemia levels amongst children and women in the world. Other micronutrient deficiencies such as vitamin A and iodine also constitute serous public health problem. Various government schemes set up to combat these problems have not had the expected impact in reducing malnutrition or micronutrient deficiencies.

This is not only due to low utilization or inadequacy of the schemes but also due to the over population problem together with it not adopting appropriate behaviors to improve their health and nutrition. They need to be provided correct and timely technical advice on nutrition to their client's and their families with adequate emphasis. Whereas when we know that malnutrition contributes about 55% of child mortality. To reduce this percentage the community nurse intervention and advice on health matters is very much important. Because she can play a vital role in preventing and reducing malnutrition by her frequent visits and health education to the families. As for growth and development of client, good nutrition plays an important role in maintenance of health.

The basic cause of poor health is poor nutrition. Food is essential for life; the food that is consumed by every person should include all the nutritional factors that have quantity and quality of food. Animal sources are rich in proteins, they are costly and most of the Indians do not eat meat on religious grounds, plants proteins are cheaper and readily available. So people could be taught the nutritional value which is suitable for each group according to the vegetarians and non-vegetarians. E.g. Soybean milk fortified with vitamins and minerals promotes good growth and good supplement. Food is the important necessity of life. The diet we take metabolized and absorb and assimilate in the body for its growth and maintenance thus body remains fit and fine and healthy.

Certain amount of fatty food is necessary for our growth and it should be reduced in quantity as person grows in age when the digestion slows down. As the presence of fat in the diet delays the emptying of the food from the stomach, bile is essential for the digestion and absorption or it helps for fat digestion. The energy value of foods can be expressed in terms of kilocalories. The energy value of foods is usually determined using the instrument called bomb calorimeter. Food has a stimulating effect. The energy requirements are calculated by energy required for the body for its routine functions adding energy required for work.

If vitamins are not present in sufficient quantities in the diet, vitamin deficiency disease occurs. The body contains about 24 minerals, calcium occurs in the highest amount in the body. Higher levels of proteins in the diet help to increase the absorption of calcium. Water is the largest constituent of the body. Water is lost continuously from the body via kidney as urine, skin via perspiration and sweat, lungs in the expired air, large intestine via feces, lactating women in the milk, water depletion occur in the body leading to change in the body fluids.

Foods differ widely in their contents of various nutrients. For maintaining good health and physical efficiency, the diet should provide adequate amounts of all nutrients. Food consumed at the same time, must have nutritive value. Some people due to lack of knowledge avoid certain foods and eat large quantity of same foods everyday without any variety. A balanced diet that contains the various groups of foodstuffs according to different age group taken in adequate quantity and quality helps to preserve health and prolong life. The increased nutritional requirements during growth of child, in pregnancy and lactation period taken for maintaining good health, which will help effectively in improving their nutritional status.

CHANGE PATTERN OF FOOD CONSUMPTION

The process of aging brings about marked physiological changes in the body, these changes influences in nutritional requirements. As there is decrease in the metabolic and poor digestion, 25% calories are reduced according to body, as there is less of activities. If excess food is consumed, it is converted into fat and stored results obesity. The body weight should be maintained constant at the normal level by adjusting the calories intake. If one failed to follow this rule, it results in signs of diseases and early death.

Food habits are influenced by education, economic level of the community, availability and cost of food practices, once the food habits are established they are handed down from generation to generation. We have to make every effort to raise the level of nutrition, low cost productive food; which is affordable and gives all required benefits. In Indian culture, food is prepared in so many ways in different parts of our country with numerous types of recipes. If client is ill, modification of diet necessary in treatment of different disease; which will sustain him and maintain his body.

Foods that are responsible for allergic reactions are eliminated from the diet. Diet modified to consistency to suit the need of the client. There is different diet such as soft diet; high and low calorie residue diet, clear fluid diet, full fluid diet, and IV fluids are given to the client as per situation. Without proper adjustment of diet will deplete the strength and stamina of client and the recovery will be delayed.

CHILD MALNOURISHMENT

India has the largest numbers of malnourished children in the world not only in terms of the number of children but also in terms of the proportion of children less than five years of age. While India has close to 22 percent of the developing world's population, our share of malnourished children is almost double at 40 percent. In fact, India has the dubious distinction of having the largest proportions of malnutrition at low birth weight rate at over 30 percent, in early childhood 53.4% undernourished by weight for age criteria and 52% stunted that is, by height for age criteria and during adulthood 47.1% of women and 46.4% of men having chronic energy deficiency according to body mass index criteria.

Such unacceptable levels of malnutrition have been persisting for more than twenty years in spite of the country having several good programs such as the public distribution system to distribute foodgrains at subsidized prices, to provide supplementary nutrition through programs such as the

Integrated Child Development Services. Still common man suffers from such a preventable diseases due to lack of it. There are still today people living in such a condition that they do not have one square meal a day. They go to bed hungry with empty stomach. They long if and only if I could get full stomach food, such is a plight of poor people still living with hardly keeping themselves alive and surviving in certain parts of rural and slum areas. We cannot ignore and close our eyes in such a situation. They earn for the day, next day if no work they have to starve or go to bed hungry or eat some leaves or roots from forest.

We have to make every effort in coordinating the total health and nutritional activities, facilitating linkages between nutrition, health and other activities, training the staff and community on nutrition health aspects, to visit and supervise the nutrition centers and to extend feedback with regard to maintenance of centers, upgrading and analyzing the data related to Health and Nutrition program, to develop the linkages between staff and PHC and other health service institutions is vital. To develop linkages to the community with banks and other financial institutions, and thus building solidarity among community.

Community health nurse has to know and learn the different kinds of diet advice according to the needs of that particular group in which she works. Which diet is good in sickness, different types of diet that exists, feeding helpless person on her visit when she meets bedridden or aged person, when person has no appetite what action she has to take; when a client has a feeling of fullness, discomfort, nausea, and anorexia how to act and remedy and find proper solution or the reference to the health center for guidance. Diet is an important in treatment of diseases. A modification in diet or in the nutrients can cure certain diseases. Food we consume gives energy, heat, growth, and development of body. Diet given in diseases as part of the complete care of the person. According to the condition and disease lot of modification needs to be done.

Regular diet or full diet has to be well balanced diet. It is vegetarian or nonvegetarian. This is for person. That does not need to make any modifications. Soft diet is to be provided light and easily digestible foods with minimum residue; simple food with less spices and more easily digestible and lower in roughage. It includes canjee, soft cooked pulses, mashed potatoes, poached egg, double boiled rice, custard, curd, sieved cooked vegetables, ripped banana.

Liquid diet is to provide caloric intake and liquids requiring minimum digestion, it is clear liquid diet; weak tea, black coffee, fruit juice, barley water, sugar and glucose. Milk is given as it contains calcium and adequate protein, Salt free diet, low fat diet, low calories diet; high protein diet, low protein diet varies according to persons illness; such as special diet in diabetics, diet in anemia, diet in acute nephritis and uremia. When she visits families and finds people with such difficulties can help and demonstrate such practices and give advice on diet and food. Faulty diet is the root cause of all illness.

The **National Health Policy,** 1983 aimed at reducing the low birth weight. And yet, progress over the last two decades can be described at best as 'stunted'. To understand why not much progress has been made? Only 51% of India's children are exclusively fed on breast milk during the first three months of life; less than a-third of children receive complementary feeding on a regular basis during their age 6 to 9 months. We already know that a growing infant needs about 1100 kcal of nourishment everyday.

Breast milk even at peak production capacity can meet only part of this need after six months and therefore, it is essential that solid, mushy foods be introduced as additional feeds on a regular basis to all children at around six months of age. Supplementary foods such as cow milk, fruit juice, soft cooked rice, mashed potatoes, dhal water, soft cooked egg, and vegetables and so on. The food must be rich in protein and other nutrients. At the age of one year, the child must receive solid foods consisting of cereals, pulses, vegetables and fruits. Because these children are more active so they need extra calories and proteins. The foods can be prepared at home using low cost locally available foods such as groundnuts, pulses, jiggery etc.

Child of 1 to 4 years has nutritional deficit of about 400 kcal per day. Such deficits are the real reason for malnutrition setting in. A very young child thus loses out on the very important energy needs early in life. If the foundation of the building is weak the building will have less life and may give way to collapse. Much of the deficit is not so much due to a lack of food at household level, but to inadequate feeding practices. Health practitioners are amongst the very few whose advice is sought by parents and other caregiver on matters related to childcare.

Most practitioners meet parents of young children for immunization during the second, third and fourth months of life and critical advice related to feeding and doctors give nourishment. It appears that we are not able to communicate effectively, the urgency and absolute essentiality of quality feeding for all children in this age group. Community health nurse therefore must begin early in their interactions with parents and caregivers with advice on feeding the young child with soft, mushy foods on a regular basis from the 6th month of the child. This persistent malnutrition contributes to nearly half of the child mortality, which has remained stagnant despite improvement in health care delivery in a number of states.

Nutritional stability of the children has been and is one of our major concerns to have satisfactory health. We have to realize that there are so many factors that are adversely affecting though areas of supplementary nutrition which can increase the physical and intellectual capacity of the children. Majority of the children looks healthy and flourished; because through the essential child health information, the families were empowered the health of the children in the villages improved drastically.

The different program has raised awareness regarding health and child development and has succeeded in improving the nutritional status of children to a great extent. Putting today's essential child health knowledge into practice, the children are given appropriate care and the physical and mental growth has been ensured. In comparison with many other children who are outside these schemes or programs, these children have at least reasonably maintained their health. So the additional nutrition is important.

Children under 3 years have inadequate food and frequent infections lead to malnutrition and hold back physical and mental development of children. Children under 3 years have special feeding needs. They need to eat often and adding mashed vegetables, small amounts of fat and oil should specially enrich their food. Malnutrition can cause poor growth, debility and death. Poor child growth is a result of inadequate food, repeated infections and illnesses and inappropriate care. Immunization programs protects against several diseases. Monthly weight recording of the children, regular medical check-ups, supplementary diet, vitamins, de-worming medicines and additional medical care of children who are underweight is vital to prevent preventable diseases at this age.

Children are the second major category of vulnerable groups. As with women, their oppression takes many forms, like child labor, sexual slavery, child pornography, the sale and trafficking of children, prostitution, drug trafficking; the physical, sexual, and psychological abuse of children within families. An increasing number of children are forced to live on the streets, and are deprived of the social and economic support of families and communities. Widespread poverty, lack of access to education and social dislocation in rural areas, are among the causes of the trends, which increases the vulnerability of children.

Poverty is main cause of child labor and efforts should be made to provide necessary incentives like schools and mid-day meals to wean the children away from the labor force. Commercial sexual exploitation of children related the staggering scale of child sex abuse. Children are sexually exploited through prostitution and pornography every year, young as 10, in its sex industry.

MID-DAY SCHOOL MEAL

Childhood is a period of rapid growth and development and physical activity. School meals provide opportunities for nutritional education, food hygiene. The school meals should be a supplement and not a substitute to the home diet. The meal should supply at least one third of the daily calorie requirements and about half of the daily protein requirements. It should be cheap and nutritious. The menu should have flexibility, variety and change. As far as possible, locally available foods should be used, to reduce the cost of the meal. They can be given foodstuffs are cereals, pulses, oils and fats, leafy vegetables, non-leafy vegetables.

When the body does not get the proper kind of food in the amounts needed for maintaining health malnutrition occurs, child looses weight, skin changes, skin becomes dry, scaly or rough, loss of subcutaneous fat, night blindness, hair changes light color, brittle, bones edema, apathy, listlessness, bowing of legs takes place.

Pregnant and Lactating mothers are anemic. They suffer from iron deficiency anemia. Till recent years, women would not go for a health check-up unless there is a serious complication during pregnancy. Now, due to different awareness programs, either they are convinced of its importance from the very beginning of the pregnancy, on their own or with the help of health workers seek medical care. Mother's supplementary diet includes an extra meal herself besides the routine meals that she takes everyday. Antenatal regular check-ups during pregnancy, together with it all the women are advised to have trained person to assist the delivery; recording of weight, immunization against tetanus.

By the completion of pregnancy, if they show any complication they are advised for a hospital delivery, otherwise, they still prefer home delivery. During antenatal clinic, the necessary information regarding safety measures for a safe home delivery is given. As a result, there is a great decline in stillbirth babies, tetanus neonatarum and postpartum complications. The care of newborn babies and the importance of feeding the colostum to the newborn are also has become very much part of their life.

The nutritional program and medical care have decreased the number of low birth weight babies. As number of death and complications are prevented by taking prompt action at home; recognizing the importance of referring the mother and child to a health center in case of an emergency. Proper care of the pregnant women like taking iron and folic acid tablets, regular adequate diet, regular check-ups and immunization with tetanus toxide injections are the steps taken to extend protection to mother and child.

Of the numerous problems facing India's development malnutrition and health are the most dominant. The most vulnerable group affected by this problem is the villagers. The health problems among the villagers can be said to be caused by a number of factors. Widespread poverty, illiteracy, traditional food taboos, a hostile and inaccessible environment, regional imbalances in food production and seasonal variation, lack of sanitary facilities and safe drinking water, inability to seek out health intervention programs – all these contribute to the conditions prevailing today.

Intervention through health care and nutrition programs helps to arrest the fast deteriorating health condition of our people. Women and children being the most vulnerable group, they continue to be our priority in the health and nutrition program. 1st and 2nd degree malnutrition still persists among children. In general, the pregnant and lactating women are anemic and underweight. The health workers still have a vital role to play in animating the health of the community. We need many miles to walk yet to reach high level of dietary health in rural poor areas.

The education program, which includes balwadis with feeding components as well as for the children in primary school education activities; Balwadis are considered as the cradle, where new generation is to be molded up and values of equality, love, unity, sharing etc. are practiced. In balwadis, children learn to seat, eat, play, sing and learn together, respect their parents, and learn to practice truth. The new value system instilled in them will provide a strong base for this growing generation of villages. There itself we can instill in them and the parents the good habits of nutritional foods.

In balwadis, the educational motivation is imparted to the children and parents, is immeasurable. Parents can see the budding talents of their young children through various programs organized. Balwadi is a movement of Liberation. In order to that this movement continues in a proper way, we would have to safeguard some significant factors. Foster an overall and smooth functioning. To select or reselect good, efficient, and reliable cooks, preferably women, who will prepare sufficient and delicious food for the children in time.

The effectiveness and success of the program depends very much on the active involvement of the village community. Over the years through the different programs undertaken the village community is made to realize that the balwadis program is their "own". The entire responsibility of running the balwadis could be entrusted to the village committee. They can manage selection of the teacher, safekeeping of the provision, supply of vegetables, eggs and fruits. They also can look after the collection of the local contribution in cash or in grain and vegetable given by the village people. And be responsible for children's and their community welfare.

For balwadi children there can be once in a while a Van Bhojan that is to have a meal in the forest, to create awareness among the children, for the love of nature, ecology, environment and over and above to create an awareness of belongingness to the nature the mother earth. A meal can be served cooked by the villagers. During these programs people experienced togetherness, unity and friendship among themselves.

An organization of **Bal Melas** every year could also be planned. This is the yearly gathering of all balwadi children. The purpose is to make them experience of togetherness and unity among themselves and among the whole village. For this program, children can prepare the cultural program. The purpose of the cultural program is to bring out their hidden talents of the children, and to make them proud of their own rural culture.

It is children in the villages around whom the whole developmental activity of balwadi scheme could be geared. All the village voluntary health worker, Mahila Mandal women's, village guide, etc. all pool their energies and resources to attend to the children; so that the children can come regularly to the balwadis. Also the village community makes sure that the children attend the balwadis regularly and everyday. It is true that the teachers' and supervisors' primary responsibility is in reference to the balwadis. It is made sure that there is interaction between teachers, supervisors and village community. It is to be made compulsory that the teachers and the supervisors have to pay visit to the houses together with health workers.

Certainly, the children are the focus of attention. Over the passage of time surely there will be lot of difference and village themselves will able to see and test the fruits of the balwadis. Child is progressively becoming the object of more concern in the community. There is a realization growing at some extent among the community that the child is not only the responsibility of the individual parents alone but of the community too. It is becoming increasingly clearer, day-by-day, to the village communities that while the government agencies are interested in the balwadis, their organization and support is important. Without this the balwadis would be meaningless and dysfunctional. Balwadi is definitely a rallying point around which the whole village can come together.

Balwadi provide the children with an opportunity to come together. This opportunity instills into them a sense of oneness as well as belongingness. The tuition classes together with balwadis have fostered the interest and confidence in the school going children. More personal attention and guidance are given to them in their studies. The improvement in the studies can be seen. They come to know themselves and each other better by coming together to balwadis. Different talents are discovered in the process of learning.

Today we are happy to know that the education created awareness among the people. That awareness makes them to think about village development, literacy, unity of the village, health, sustainability, human rights and so on. Steady income to the teachers and cooks in the village has given them a better status economically.

The education of a child does not begin with the alphabet. It starts in the lap of a mother who is considered worth 100 teachers. In this computer age, it is extremely important that children start pre-schooling early with changing times and fast life. It is indeed a boon for the tiny tots. The children then learn the alphabets and numerals in English. They are able to read and write, sing and dance. The children who attend the balwadi regularly easily can get through the examination. Balwadi teaching is a great help in development of the children and the whole community. Bal meals, Van Bhojan and other activities can increased their self-confidence.

The balwadis children are given a full meal while the tuition class children are given only nutrition snacks. The balwadi classes are held in the places provided by the village community. Since parents are aware of the importance of education, they send their children to the classes when the bell is rung. The stock of grain and nutritious snacks is kept in the house of the village leader or one of the houses close to the balwadis. The cooking is managed by the Mahila Mandal women and is remunerated. The emphasis is more on the reading, writing and counting. The teachers make use of pictorial charts, nursery rhymes, action songs and educational games to teach the balwadis children.

The supervisors with the help of the health workers do the weight monitoring of the children every month. Earlier, the weight-monitoring cards were kept with the supervisors. As per the recommendation of last evaluation, the family folder cards are now given back to the mothers. The mothers are taught to read the cards and understand the health progress of their children. The village health worker visits the balwadis every week. They supervise the cleanliness of children, sanitation of the surroundings and the hygiene of the food. Supervisors who are qualified nurses visit the balwadis once a month.

Regular medical examination of children every month is to be continued with follow-up without fail for the progress and continuity. Where the children are given vitamin-A de-worming medicines once in every month. A dose of iron and vitamin B complex is orally given every day for 10 days or so from time to time to all the children of balwadi, a record of which the balwadi teacher maintains. Calcium supplement is given to all especially many children who are with a weak pigeonhole chest. Other medicine dose is given to mothers to be given at home. Special instruction is given individually to each mother of the child, who shows slow progress or no progress at all in health. Mothers of the children in balwadi are also members in Mahila Mandal. They receive health instruction during the

Mahila Mandal meetings as well as through the village health workers and the balwadi teacher who visit their homes on a regular basis.

The balwadi teachers also had some classes on health and nutrition, the main topics of which are related to hygiene and health and handling of and serving food with cleanliness. A general supervision of cleanliness of children, the surroundings, cooking of food etc. is done through the village committee, village health worker and the balwadi supervisor. There are so many factors that are adversely affecting, it is seen very clearly that the children's health situation is improved very much due to good meal and proper medical care. Now people try to change food taboos and local health habits. And this change of attitude positively affected the health of the children.

Objectives of our intervention should be to improve the health status of pregnant and lactating women; to bring down the level of malnutrition among children of 0–3 years old. A report made by "the independent commission on health in India "in 1997 has made interesting studies and has critically analyzed the existing health system. Favor of policies and programs, which genuinely focus on health care system that ensures equity and concern for the deprived and unreached people.

The basic goal of development planning is to eliminate poverty, ignorance and ill health, improve the quality of life of the people and raise their standard of living. Lack of nutrition security is result of poverty, which are enhanced and re-inforced by ignorance, and the absence of health and nutrition education is a small step along the way, helping the people to build up their own strength, though gradually, as we march towards the ultimate goal of elimination of poverty and attainment of nutritional stability.

Breastfeeding mothers should get good nutrition and the mother should be encouraged to eat adequate and balance diet during pregnancy, childbearing period, to be able to store fat in the body as reserver to get sufficient milk later. Does less heavy work to conserve energy. Traditional customs be avoided, e.g. fasting. Proper care of nipples, encourage mother and baby bounding, which will stimulate milk. She should be provided proper privacy and she should be convinced that breastfeed is best natural food for baby.

Meets fully nutritional requirements, protects baby form infection, diarrhea, respiratory infections. Mothers milk is clean and sterile, available 24 hours. Requires no special preparations. It is easily available, digestible, helps space children, and reduces IMR, natural contraceptive – God's gift to humankind. Mother should sit on an easy chair/bed with back rested against wall, holding baby semi-sitting position etc.

There is some common problems in breastfeeding such as emotional feelings like worry shock anxiety which stop the flow of milk and it can interfere. If problem of flat nipples can be pulled gently several times a day also if there is a sore and cracked nipples it could be due to child's sucking very hard or it could be due to dry nipple you can rub with antiseptic cream.

The body requires food to provide energy for organ function, for body movement and to work, to maintain body temperature and provide raw materials for enzyme function for growth, and replacement of cells and its repair. Food is ingested, digested and absorbed to produce energy needed for all these factors. Food provides energy to repair tissues and build body. Food helps in the formation of immune bodies, enzymes and hormones. What is eaten in our day-to-day life affects all aspects of health from conception through old age. Body requires certain nutrients to maintain health. Nurse has to recognize signs of poor nutrition and take effective steps to initiate necessary changes.

Healthy signs of good nutrition are where the person will feel alert, he will have normal body weight, will have normal body built, firm muscles, good torn, some fat under the skin, good color, normal reflexes, psychological stability, good appetite and digestion, normal regular elimination and good sound sleep habits, vigorous appearance, firm, pink healthy appearance, no weakness, looks healthy red.

Signs of poor nutrition person on the other hand will feel listless, apathetic, underweight or obese, humped back, wasted appearance, chest deformity, anorexia, indigestion, constipation or diarrhea, liver, spleen enlargement, easily tired and fatigued, lack of energy, falling asleep easily, tired and apathetic, pale and dull appearance.

What people eat is not calories but food; science of food and its relationship to health is to repair and maintenance of body tissues. Preparation of meals for the well and the sick is vital. The subject of nutrition is very extensive, since our concern is with community aspects of nutrition; we deal with dietary constituents, nutritional requirements, assessment of nutritional problems in public health and nutritional program in India.

Food is important part of human beings for maintenances of his health and avoidance of disease. Due to lack of adequate food person develops nutritional disease. Such disease identified as protein energy malnutrition, endemic goiter, nutritional anemia, nutritional blindness, and diarrhea disease, kwashiorkor, night blindness, xerophthalmia (dry eye) also the association of nutrition with infection, immunity, fertility, mother and child health and family health, coronary heart disease, diabetes and cancer also are well established.

NUTRITIONAL PROBLEM

In public health, low birth weight is high, malnutrition and anemia is significant risk factor of malnutrition. Protein energy malnutrition identified major health problem in India occurs in weak child and is cause of morbidity and mortality. Clinical forms – kwashiorkor and marasmus due to inadequate intake of dietary foods, loss of appetite malabsorption, altered metabolism, weight loss, immunity lost, mucous damage, it is a vicious circle and infection contributing to malnutrition vice versa.

VICIOUS CIRCLE

It is like a web that is interconnected poor environmental conditions with large family size has poor feeding of children has its adverse cultural practices relating to child rearing a weaning, leads to poor mother and child health leads to lack of failure of lactation, results in premature termination of breastfeed and over diluted cow's milk and discarding cooking water from cereals and delay supplementary feeding leads again malnutrition problem. Principal features of PEM are muscle wasting, fat wasting, edema, mental changes, skin hair changes, diarrhea, and hepatic enlargement fat not firm, diffuse pigmentation.

Early detection of PEM with regularly betters to maintain growth charts. Prevention of PEM in community is measures directed towards pregnant woman, education and distribution of supplements, promotion of breastfeed, improve family diet, family planning, home economics, family environment, immunization, periodic surveillance, early diagnosis, treatment follow-up.

Nutritional anemia syndrome caused by malnutrition, a condition in which the hemoglobin contains a deficiency of nutrients- iron, and vitamin B_{12} deficiency. Nutritional anemia is a worldwide problem. The incidences are highest in women and children. Woman loses iron during menses, malaria and hookworm infestation, loss of blood during delivery, severe cases of blood transfusion is necessary and followed up with iron and folic acid supplementation. Hunger and nutrition are problems everywhere and have harassed humankind through history.

IODINE DEFICIENCY

Disorders goiter, cretinism, found in Himalayas known as goiter belt needs iodized salt, and iodine monitoring.

Nutritional factors in selected diseases affects such as cardiovascular coronary heart disease plasma cholesterol, high blood pressure, cigarette smoking, and lack of physical activities, in take of cholesterol of animal fat, extra-added salty diets, dietary fat, and fiber. Also diabetes, obesity, cancer caused due to faulty diet therapy that is either undernutrition, overnutrition, or of imbalance, specific diet deficiency.

Action at the family level and in community needs to be stressed on elimination of harmful taboos regarding foods and dietary prejudices, open to accept the combination of locally available and acceptable foods; by adding supplementary feeding program, midday school meals, Vitamin A prophylaxis will provide palliative, partial or temporary solutions increasing the availability of foods both in quantity and quality – significant improvement of living conditions – in brief a broad socioeconomic development of the entire community.

Action on National level needs to be taken for rural development for nutritional uplift, to increase total food production, at affordable rate, help to increasing agricultural production, with modern farming, together with expansion of cultivated area, by the use of fertilizers, better seeds. Food price policies, irrigation project undertaking, mosquito-offer vector control program, stabilization of population – nutrition related health services, activities, family planning, MCH, could improve the nutritional status.

Action at the International level can be taken through cooperation in time of acute emergencies caused by floods, droughts; which will enhance grains from world food program that will help in keeping safe food. Food surveillance for food hygiene, milk hygiene, infection of animals that can be transmitted to man be done in such emergencies to prevent added burden on people who will have already suffered due to this calamities. Providing safe, clean and pasteurized milk, regularly watch meat hygiene, its inspection in slaughter houses, sanitation of eating places, location floor, room walls, light ventilation, kitchen, storage of cooked food and uncooked food, washing facilities, water supply. Inspect the food handlers and their habits of washing hands to control food born disease.

Nutritional program in rural India is very vital yet how long will a country be able to feed its children who may number 100 million without socioeconomic impoverishment? For that we have to help people to help themselves by other practical means where they improve the agricultural products on large and cheaper rate at affordable prices which will reduce the pressure on the government and common man will be happy with the facilities and means provided to him.

Sufficient food is one of the most essential basic needs of the people. We need nutritious food to sustain our body. The children in big towns and cities get nutritious food and do well in their studies. To study well you need health of body and mind. So nutrition – physical and mental development are closely related. Hunger and malnutrition reduce the physical and intellectual capacity of individuals and impede the economic and social development of people and village. Our purpose of any activities is to improve the food and nutrition of underprivileged children and people of rural village. As we know and it is true that nutrition plays a vital role in the process of education right from the early childhood. To achieve this goal we need to give a full meal everyday, enough vegetables, eggs and fruits to enhance their performance. That means to be malnutrition means not learning enough as a child and not earning enough as an adult later. To do away with the malnutrition in children, give to children supplementary food that contents nutritious at the same time keeping the local diet in mind, in terms of quantity and cost, the staple diet that is "one square meal a day. A child's calorie requirement varies with age. The rest of the calories will be compensated at home in the evenings. There are adequate proteins in our cereals pulses in India. Vitamins are adequate in the green vegetable available in the area. Spices are needed to increase the taste of the food given.

Poor nutritional status and its related problems such as poor body weight and height, poor weight gain during pregnancy, low hemoglobin levels are some of the common problems of pregnant women in rural area. Unbalanced diet intake poses many nutritional risks. Inadequate food, repeated illnesses and infections and inappropriate care make age group very vulnerable.

Growth monitoring of balwadi children within the age group 3–5 is of vital importance. A good weight gain means good health, which in turn means good nutrition. A poor weight gain means, poor health due to poor nutrition. If there are diseases or genetic factors it may be a cause for concern and further investigation. A periodic checking of weight to assess the speed of weight gain is an extremely important fact of assessing this children's health. All the children in the balwadis are weighed monthly. The road to health chart is maintained. De-worming therapy is done for all the children. Vitamin A and D, calcium, iron and B complex supplements are given to children at regular intervals. General hygiene of the children is taken care. Improving the level of nutrition of 3 to 5 years of children, an incentive and encouragement could be fostered.

Keeping this view in mind, we have to be very conscious about the nutritional aspect. That the food given contains enough fresh vegetables, eggs and fruits. That the tuition class children too receive the nutritious snack. Like chana and various kinds of biscuits, which contain enough proteins and sugar, could be provided.

While poverty is multifaceted and manifested in terms of the lack of access to food, health, education, shelter, information, equality and other rights and expenditure associated with food intake. For it is essential that the food consumed have the necessary nutritive value.

Optimal nutrition will demand the intake of wide rage of foods which, taken together and in a judicious combination in a well balanced diet, can provide the essential nutrient that we need. Ensuring good nutrition is not just equivalent to avoidance of hunger. While, we may be immediately concerned about the efforts to stave off hunger among the poor, our long-term goal must be the achievement of a optimal state of nutrition for our people, which will help them find full expression for their genetic potential. Nutrition security is much more than food security.

Good nutrition essential not just for the achievement of optimal physical growth and development, but also to ensure mental well-being, the ability to withstand the inevitable process of ageing with minimal disability and degenerative disease; and the ability to withstand the toxic effects of pollutions. Thus, practically every major dimension of health is dependent on the achievement and the maintenance of good nutritional status. Good nutritional status implies for more than freedom from hunger and starvation, i.e. the achievement of dietary adequacy with respect to calories.

To improve the health of the children is one of our major concerns. Nutrition food and regular medical care can increase the physical and intellectual capacity of the children; thus, they can look healthy and flourishing.

Imperfect nourishment happens because the demands of the body nutrient are not met. Nutrition is a integral part of health and well-being of every individual. Good nutrition is determined by the intake of an adequate diet.

Malnutrition has an adverse impact on morbidity and life expectancy that increases mortality. It shunts physical growth, leads to functional impairment, disability, diminished productivity, and reduces resistant to diseases. The problem of malnutrition is the result of the people and the number of people to share the available food in the family; lack of food availability, food accessibility, lack of the purchasing power.

The aim of health education is to help people to achieve health by their own actions and efforts and to meet the energy requirements at different ages; to identify earliest evidence of undernourishment and to take corrective measures. Despite the fact that food production has increased over the decades, malnourishment is a major problem and a majority of Indian women belonging to the lower socioeconomic status are undernourished. Within households, the available food is distributed according to the status of the individual rather than according to dietary requirements.

Women and female children usually receive what is leftover. Malnutrition not only makes a person tired and weak, but also predisposes one to innumerable infections worsening an already fatigued state. Women continue hard labour till the last stage of pregnancy; in addition to their household chores. Working beyond the limits of physical tolerance their bodies are depleted of essential resources, thus resulting in fetal wastage, still birth, and low birth weight babies.

Importance of keeping food safe—Whatever food we eat needs to be clean and safe for eating. Then only we can keep ourselves healthy and disease free, care should be taken not to take polluted food. Why and how the food get polluted? The food gets polluted because of foodstuff used are not clean, if the food is not kept covered, dust collects over it, if flies sit on the food, if the food has become stale, if the plates and spoons used are not clean, if the food is handled with dirty hands, if the place where the food kept is dirty.

Fresh vegetables contain vitamin C than stored ones. It should be fresh so check for mould and worm infection. Never buy any food in poor condition; over-ripe fruits should not be purchased. If impure food is eaten, diseases like food poisoning, dysentery, vomiting, and typhoid occur in order to avoid these diseases the food should be handled safely. Foods brought from market such as rice, wheat, moong are taken in a sifting pan and winnowed, grass, stone, and sticks and husk are separated from it. Storing food items that are in large quantities, exposed to sun, dried and therefore do not get fungus, use boric power in tin and keep in airy place with airtight lids. Do not keep cooked foods exposed.

The place of cooking should be clean, sufficient light in the kitchen, wash hands before cooking. Cooked food should be removed in as clean utensil, using clean spoons. Allow to cool before covering, place lid half covered over the food, so that dust does not settle down over it. During the summer season, cooked food should be kept in cold water in a large vessel. Freshly cooked food should be used of immediately. Cleanliness of house and the kitchen such as oil in and around the gas be cleaned to avoid rats, ants, small insects nuisance, they spread diseases. Wet garbage disposed properly.

We need to develop **community based nourishment** and health and food security development. Strengthening the human potentials of the community, thus improve the capacities of the staff. Community is capable enough in identifying the issues and addressing the issues through their respective village associations. Staff is also capable enough to initiate community planning, monitoring and evaluations in the development process. Identifying and prioritizing the issues involving people at village level. People themselves do the certain management, by participation, in problem solving capacity with solidarity. People participation in entire program is the key to success.

To handover **management of nutrition program** and help them to increase their own contribution, so as to control the malnourishment. To make aware women's initiative to recognize the nutritive values of locally available foodstuff in order to increase their consumption levels. To motivate family awareness on to preservation techniques of certain seasonal foods, cheap and is easily available. To be aware of the pregnant and lactating mothers on weaning food practices and establish seed banks at each village level to recycle and sustain the gardens. This program could aim to improve the awareness levels among the community regarding nutrition and health aspects. To promote long-term plantation such as papaya, drum stick, beans, guava and banana around the garden.

The nutrition education research provides new knowledge about the process of how people learn, change or adopt new nutrition practices. Majority of health workers in developing countries still rely on face-to-face communication method to carry out their daily routine, as a sole source of information, this approach is too time-consuming. In addition, there is lack of trained workers to handle this approach effectively.

World Food Day is celebrated on 16th October, National Nutrition Week on first week of September.

The food we take shows in everything from our stamina and strength to the shine of the hair and the glow of the cheeks. Eating well helps us to live well and look well. Both body and mind need good nourishment to function efficiently. The emotional dimension of health is closely tied to our eating patterns. Food satisfies one's emotions. Happiness is an emotion and feeling happy often goes along with good appetite. Many people eat food when they are lonely, bored or tensed and eating good food makes them feel better. Food also functions as a social lubricant.

Food brings and holds people together. Kitchen and restaurants become meeting places, supermarkets serve as contact points and picnics and barbecues reunite scattered families and friends. Health, everyone knows that a good diet is essential for good health. We are indeed what we eat. We need six nutrients namely carbohydrates, proteins, fat, vitamins, minerals and water. Most of us eat enough food to get all these nutrients in sufficient quantities.

Changes in lifestyle have altered our eating habits. Many prefer a series of small meals or snacks instead of the set traditional patterns. In this bargain, they eat more sugar and less starch, more fat and less fiber, more meat and less vegetable protein and often much more food energy that they used up. Ingestion of animal protein drives up on one's cholesterol levels. Saturated fats stimulate the liver to produce more cholesterol. All the extra cholesterol that enters the body is left where it does not belong – in plaques in the arteries. Therefore, eating a diet high yet low in fat particularly for breakfast take cereals, which will reduce the risk of coronary heart disease?

Increased risk of kidney stones is found to be more pronounced in people who take decreased quantities of water and insufficient intake of citrus fruits. Thus, it is evident that intake of balanced and varied diets is important in the context of diet and health. Garlic is said to have a thinning effect on the blood and also it is claimed to prevent or cure, cancer, boils, cysts, cuts food poisoning and many more ailments.

Physical activity enables one to cope with the effects of aging to a certain extent. Increased bone strength, increased physical work capacity, increased joint range of motion or flexibility, improved sense of well-being, increased muscular strength, improved glucose regulation, decreased blood pressure, improved sleep patterns and low levels of anxiety, decreased body fat, decreased risk of osteoporosis etc., increased mental ability, decreased depression, improves balance and posture.

Physical activity can be fun and should ideally be conducted in a group-setting with friends, thus increasing social integration. The aging human body generally responds well to physical exercise and improvements may be anticipated in heart and lungs function, muscular strength and endurance, flexibility and one's ability to respond to stimuli. Some changes like those in skin composition, vision, hair, hearing etc.

CHILD HABITS

Another reason for growth faltering usually in the second half of the first year is the habit of children to put every object that they see into their mouths and also the frequent respiratory infections that are seen the young children. While we treat the infections, we fail to give correct advice on feeding, especially the need to give extra foods in the convalescent stages to allow for catch up of weight that as lost during the course of minor illnesses.

An important issue relates to how children are fed within households. While it takes two individuals – the child and the mother or the caregiver to ensure that a very young child of age below three years is fed well, there is not sufficient appreciation of this by both family members and those who give advice. Interfamilial distribution of food should ensure that those who are vulnerable – children and women get adequate amounts of quality foods within the household, for they do not generally eat elsewhere; on the other hand, men and earning members of the family generally tend to eat not only within the household but also outside their homes.

One of the simple ways to determine if the child is growing well is to regularly weigh the child and take the length/height of the child and plot its weight on the growth chart and use the chart to help the mother and care-givers understand the importance of physical growth and the importance of timely complementary feeding intake of the young child.

MICRONUTRIENT

Apart from the protein energy malnutrition, three micronutrient deficiencies are well documented in India – iodine, iron, and vitamin A deficiency. They affect not only young children but also population of all age groups, some more than others. Iodine deficiency can cause irreversible brain damage before birth and is the main cause of mental retardation and increasing levels of deaf-mutes born in certain parts of the country. Iodine deficiency in countries such as ours are rampant partly because of the extent to which environmental degradation is taking place where iodine from the top soil is continuously washed away and our diets are either deficient in iodine or we take other food items which compete with the available iodine in diet.

At present, the Government of India **policy** is to ensure that all salt consumed in the country is iodized and noniodized salt is not sold for human consumption. This will not only prevent iodine deficiency disorders but also prevent the invisible forms of mental retardation that are seen in communities in the form of decreased IQ points in the populations feeding on diets deficient in iodine. Studies have repeatedly shown that there is no part of India, which is free from iodine deficiency. At present only 70% of the population have access to iodized salt.

Iron deficiency anemia is another major micronutrient deficiency that affects very large proportions of children, adolescent girls and women in the reproductive age group. Nearly three out of four children below three years are anemic and over half of women in the childbearing age group are iron deficient. This has important implications for their work capacity, the learning abilities when they get into school, retards their ability to grow well, cause frequent ailments and further contribute to both morbidity and mortality.

India has for years been running a **National Nutritional Anemia Prophylaxis** Program for preventing anemia in pregnant and lactating women. Under the program, till 1992, 60 mg of elemental iron were administered to all women for 100 days. From 1992, the prophylactic dose of iron has been increased to 100 mg of elemental iron. Yet, the levels of anemia are very high and possibly contribute not only to anemia being carried on to the next generation but also have a negative effect on the birth weight of newborns. One of the major reasons for high levels of anemia in this country in spite of a national program is the poor compliance in terms of women not taking the full course of the prophylactic dose that is given to them. As a community health nurse, we have an important responsibility to ensure that children and women are routinely examined for anemia, counseled for increasing iron rich foods in their diet and where necessary give complete treatment for iron deficiency anemia with a special emphasis on follow-up for compliance.

Vitamin A is another micronutrient, the deficiency of which not only contributes to night blindness but also to increased morbidity and poor protection against severe forms of respiratory and skin infections. Studies in certain countries have also demonstrated that they have a role in decreasing childhood and maternal mortality as well, the National Survey of Blindness (1986-89), suggests that prevalence of night blindness in children under six years is around 6% with Bitot's spots having been observed in 0.7% of children through another survey during the same period.

While the government program envisages administration of large doses of vitamin A to children aged 9 months to 3 years, the medical practitioners can contribute to decreasing the vitamin A deficiency states in the community by encouraging their patients and their families to consume adequate amounts of green leafy vegetables and other vitamin A rich foods and ensuring that young children receive 2 lacks of IU of vitamin A every six months (1 lack IU during infancy) from the government health centers or by prescribing vitamin A capsules to children below 5 years and to women immediately after delivery to build adequate body stores of vitamin A for increasing the concentration of vitamin A in their breast milk. In this, community nurse have a major role to play in reducing the very high levels of malnutrition and micronutrient deficiencies in the country.

Specific messages and timely counseling of patients, families and the care-giver of children on breastfeeding, timely complementary feeding of young children, adequate nutrition for pregnant and lactating women, consumption of iodized salts, enriching the diets of families with foods rich in iron and vitamin A as well as diagnosing early the deficiency states and providing the correct treatment can go a long way in decreasing morbidity and mortality of the vulnerable segments of the population.

FOOD SURROUNDING PLACE

The atmosphere in which they live is very conducive to infection and many children as well as adults have complaints of worm infestation, we have take this as a preventive measure to treat the children every three months for worms. They could be given health instruction during the Mahila Mandal meetings as well as through the village health workers and the balwadi teacher who visit their homes on a regular basis.

Healthy lifestyle and a life lived in accordance with laws of nature would keep us protected against such ailments. Nutritional diseases take a heavy toll every year. Thousands of children die from treatable nutrition-related problems. Deliberate and sustained nutrition education seems to be the only long-term solution for eradicating the problem of malnutrition and achieving optimum nutrition for the people. It will also help in the promotion of healthy lifestyles among people.

'Nutritional Education for All' keeping people well nourished are the theme chosen for the 21st 'National Nutrition Week' being observed from 1st to 7th September 2002. Deliberate and sustained nutrition education is recognized as one of the best approaches for prevention and control of innumerable nutritional problems encountered in our country and also for promotion of healthy lifestyles among people. The ultimate goal of nutritional education should be to expand knowledge, create awareness, modify attitudes, behaviour and ultimately improve the nutritional status of population.

Nutrition is the most important factor in promotion and maintenance of health. The human body can build up and maintain healthy cells and tissues, glands and organs only with the help of nutrients. The body cannot perform any of its mental, physical or chemical functions without specific nutrients.

QUALITIES OF FOOD

The foods we consume also contain non-nutrients such as antioxidants, phytochemicals and dietary fiber, which bestow positive health benefits. The dietary fiber present in plant foods is indigestible carbohydrates, which contribute to the bulk and have some useful function in the digestive tract. Foods are now known to be capable of playing not only a health-promoting but also disease-preventing role.

Eating behavior and social aspect of nutrition, of people includes food purchasing, food preparation and food consumption, which are, determined far more by social, cultural, psychological and certain situational factors than by physiological factors. What foods we select, how we eat and even when we feel the hunger is mostly part of a learned behavior. Eating behavior in general and is deeply embedded in social and cultural norms. Food that may be considered a delicacy in one culture is rejected and may be odious in others. It is because each society sets its own limits on what is edible for its members and how the food should be prepared, cooked and served.

Formation of food habits in children are highly dependent on family for their food intake in the early years and many of the patterns of eating seen in adult life are established at this time. A good mother is always viewed as a good provider of food. Palate appeasing functions also play a vital part. It is not fully realized and appreciated that man takes food for his pleasure, is determined by taste, odor, temperature, appearance, structure or texture. People sometimes identify a community by its food. Eating and drinking together during social functions establish bonds of friendship and trust. Food is also a sign of wealth or status. All cultures have prestige foods, mainly reserved for special occasions. The food habits and dietary pattern of a society are never constant. They change with the socioeconomic system.

Malnutrition is seriously retarding improvements in human development and further increasing the mortality especially among children. Nutrition is an important factor in promotion and maintenance of healthy cells and tissues, gland and organs; maintain health. Food build the body, it determines how long you live.

Despite the implementation of several developmental program, nearly half of the children suffer from various degrees of protein energy malnutrition. The child population of urban slums has the lowest proportion of children with normal body weight and records the highest proportion of malnourished children.

Major causes of chronic energy deficiency continue to be inadequate food intake, infections, poor caring practices and poor health care. Low dietary intake in already chronically undernourished women has adverse effects on health and nutritional status of both the mother and the offspring.

Hidden hunger is one of the most severe problems confronting the country. A large number of children, adolescents and adults, particularly women, are affected by this problem. Hidden hunger relates to deficiencies of micronutrient. These deficiencies can lead to serous health problems, including blindness, mental retardation and reduced resistance to infectious diseases and in some cases to death.

The dietary intake of 350 million people is inadequate to meet their nutritional needs. More than 320 million people suffer from iron deficiency anemia, prevalence being the highest amongst women and children and pregnant women, adolescent girls, seriously affecting the health and productive faculties. Over 200 million people suffer from iodine deficiency resulting in a series of mental and physical disorders. O n an average, 13 IQ points are lost on account of this deficiency. About 60,000 children go blind every year due to vitamin A deficiency. It also results in mortality and morbidity in young children. The incidence of low birth weight less than 2.5 kg is alarmingly high as 30% in India.

OVERNUTRITION

The newer health problems like hypertension, diabetes, heart disease and cancers arising due to excessive intake of calories, saturated fats and cholesterol are on the rise among affluent segments of population, especially in the urban areas. You do not heal old age, you protect it, you promote it, and you extend it. Owing to faulty eating habits and a sedentary, relaxed way of living, a vast majority of our population is falling prey to creeping obesity and its disastrous health consequences. With the ready availability of cooking gas, piped water supply and labor saving gadgets and ready transport, there had been a substantial reduction in the physical activity pattern and energy expenditure. However, the dietary intake has not undergone any reduction. In fact, ready availability of fast food, ice creams and other energy-rich food items at affordable costs have resulted in increased energy consumption of these by all members of the family.

Fat person die suddenly. The longer your waistline, shorter your lifeline. Be active and healthy. Extra weight is due to extra eating. Extra fat puts a strain on your heart, kidney, liver, joint of hips, knees, and ankles, so extra calories in diet is deadly. You are shortening your own life at your own dining table. Your ideal weight depends on your height, sex, age, and type of body build. The kind of work you do, the amount of calories you burn up, how active you are according to it either increase or reduce your food intake. It takes real will power to lose weight, but it is worth it. Maintain new way of life stay there, change lifestyle, faulty dietary habits.

Food safety and quality should be adequate not only in quantity but also in terms of quality. It should be free from adulteration, microbiological and chemical contamination. In the wake of globalization, concern over food safety has attained a new dimension. With the increase in trade of food products from one part of the globe to another due to increased marked access, food importing. In recent years, the number of people eating outside their homes has increased. The factors contributing to this trend includes the changes of lifestyles, rapid urbanization, increased number of working women etc.

ECONOMIC CONDITION OF THE POOR

Occurrence of natural calamities like droughts, floods and famines, market distortion and urbanization have worst impact on poorer segments of population, especially on women and children. Inadequate food intake, frequent infections leading to diarrhea and harmful caring practices such as delayed complementary feeding. Poverty and gender inequity are also among the most important factors responsible for the high level of undernourishment. Children who are malnourished are unlikely to reach their physical or mental potential.

The first constitute poverty alleviation programs, we have to stress the schemes to improve purchasing power of the poor, provision of essential food-grains to poor households at subsidized rates through targeted public distribution system to enhance household food availability, supplementary nutrition program, midday meal program also known as nutritional support to primary education, food for work program and integrated child development services program to provide food supplements to pregnant and lactating women and preschool children.

NUTRITIONAL STATUS

India has made substantial progress in human development since independence in 1947. In 50 years, life expectancy had doubled, mortality has fallen by more than half, and fertility has declined by more than two-fifths. Poverty levels have been reduced; however, improvements in nutritional status have not kept pace with progress in other areas of human development, for several reasons. First, nutritional status is closely linked to poverty and gender inequity, both of which remain grave problems in India. Second, most malnutrition is less visible than other forms of human suffering, and hence commands less urgent attention.

At present, there is lack of sufficient focus and thrust in horticulture especially cultivation and marketing of the low-cost locally acceptable green leafy vegetables and yellow vegetables and fruits. Because of this, availability of these vegetables throughout the year at affordable cost both in urban and rural areas has remained an unfulfilled dream.

Nutritional problem can be found in all age groups and socioeconomic classes in all parts. The Community Health Nurse (CHN) caregiver, teacher, a resource person can have perfound influence on the families assessing dietary practices and provide important information. Body built, age, sex, physical activities, influence the daily caloric requirements of a person. Parents are responsible for setting an example of good nutrition for their children. Families from lower socioeconomic class spend greater percentage of their limited income on food, as the cost of food increases, the tendency is to seek out cheaper foods that may not provide adequate nutrition, nurse must assist the poor in making food choices.

Periods of intense growth such as infancy, adolescence, pregnancy and lactation cause increased nutrient needs. Nutritional needs are stabilized during adulthood. Therefore age influences the food intake all through life cycle nutrition needs keep changing in relation to growth physiologic, sociocultural, psychological, religious, economic, cultural life style etc.

Nutrition in adolescent who are undergoing rapid growth and development also are one of the vulnerable group. Early marriage and pregnancy will perpetuate both maternal and child under-nutrition. At the other end obesity is increasingly becoming problem. With onset of menstruation, girls in this age group are vulnerable to anemia and all its adverse consequences. Over half the girls get married before the age of 18 years. Early pregnancy further aggravates under both nutrition and anemia and leads to difficulties in detection and management of obstetric/nutritional problems and result in adverse outcome of pregnancy. With a view to minimize these adverse effects, nutrition education, health education and the appropriate nutritional interventions for adolescents should be taken-up more rigorously under ICDS and RCH programs. In order to reduce anemia, supplementation of iron and folic acid to adolescent is currently being taken up on a pilot basis under both these programs.

The Government of India has promulgated the National Nutrition Policy in 1993. Since nutrition is a multifaceted discipline with multisectoral involvement, a holistic approach has been evolved to tackle different forms of malnutrition in the country. The policy seeks to strike a balance between the short-term measures like direct nutrition intervention programs and the long-term measures like institutional/structural changes and thus create an enabling environment and necessary conditions for improving nutritional and health status.

National Plan of Action on Nutrition has been drawn up to work out the modalities of implementing National Nutrition Policy in to. Several ministries and departments, both under the central as well as state governments and other research institutions, nongovernmental organizations and international bodies have been entrusted the responsibility to implement the policy guidance.

Policies are framed and programs are launched for the betterment of health of the people. More attention has to be paid so as to reach these policies to the decided goals. For that the policy-makers need to involve community, then only we can be sure of their success. The principal objective of National Health Policy, 2001 is to evolve a policy structure, which reduces expenses in terms of availing the health facilities. Implementation of National Health Programs through state government's decentralized public health machinery.

To have an objective assessment of the quality efficiency of the existing infrastructure in the health sector; extending public health services. Involvement of local self-government institutions for effective functioning of the services. To ensure adequate availability of personnel with specialization in the public health and family medicine disciplines. To enhance the health care facilities in mental health care sector. Importance to education and communication emphasized for information dissemination about health. To have a national disease surveillance network for the purpose of timely intervention in the case of outbreak of diseases. Enforcement of quality standards for food and drug; equitable distribution of health services across social and geographical areas. Emphasis on increased budget contribution of central government; to have collaboration with the private sector.

Health policy has been equated with the population policy. This needs high motivation, commitment and political will on the part of the government to succeed and reach its goal. Health care of the adolescents, who are the future citizens of the country to be given importance and cannot be ignored. Problem of anemia, nutritional deficiency among women is to be highlighted which, though is not a disease, is responsible for a number of diseases among women. Provisions for mobile health care facilities need to be kept in mind. To take the note of quakes operating in remote and rural areas who are harmful to the people. Special provision could be made for the provisions of free blood test, x-ray facility and ultrasound facilities at the hospital itself. Together with screening of the health condition of the workers is not sufficient.

Needs focused approach for strategy to help workers. NGOs have to be encouraged to work in the health sector to this support system. Problems of slums need to be considered. Negative effects of globalization have to be taken in to account. Public health and health standards have to be adequate. Health infrastructure has to be satisfactory. Realizations that the attainment of health has to be even across the rural-urban division, and openness of the system needs to be appreciated.

The **acute shortage of food** is a serious problem today. Warning food prices could hamper economic growth faced with unprecedented food prices and a global grain supply crunches the need of government to change its focus urgently. The malnutrition is a national shame. The figures are mind bogging, every second child under three in the country malnourished. Fifty five million that is 35% world's malnourished children live in India, which can be prevented. It affects economic productivity. Malnourishment problem starts long before the child is born; the age at which a woman marries has a bearing on the child. During and after birth of child, her educational status will decide wheather mother goes for institutional deliveries to prevent infection, follows hygienic condition, immunizes child, if not the damage done to a child by the time child reached age two years. So our focus to be on child from 0-2 years of age.

The health services cannot be accessible to all and there is a need to enhance the budgetary allocation to the health sector. This problem can be solved to some extent through alternative resources. Allocated financial resources to the health sector have to be utilized. A policy document to deal with this fundamental issue for ensuring health care services to the people. The risk sharing arrangement implies that those who are fortunate enough to be healthy pay for those who are sick, with the clear understanding that if they fall sick later, their costs in turn will be covered.

Health insurance, which has remained highly underdeveloped and a less significant, segment is poised for a fundamental change in its approach and management. Proper evaluation of the quality of health care services. Time-bound evaluation of health policy and the launch of new policy is needed keeping the changing scenario in mind.

PUBLIC SERVICES

There is a need to improve the quality of the hospitals through a proper and time-bound approach. We do have hospitals, but without the proper infrastructure which is needed at every hospital to ensure quality treatment. It is general observations that visit to public health facilities generally involve considerable out of pocket expenses.

The extent of these expenses is in contrast to the common misconception that services in the public sector are free. Out of pocket expenses may take the form of payments for medicine, laboratory tests, dressing, linen, food or direct payments to the providers. It has to be ensured that all these services are provided to the vulnerable sections of the society free of cost and access to quality health care should be seen as a basic human right, based on need rather than a person's ability to pay.

Else the poor are less likely to access public services. Public financing in the health sector is surely justified for public good – goods and services producing externalities and merit goods. Clean air, potable water and information on health are examples of public goods that no one can be prevented from consuming.

If such services are to be marketed or charged, public health facility utilization is likely to be sub-optimal. Reproductive health and prevention intervention such as the use of contraceptives, safe motherhood, prevention of anemia, adolescent reproductive health programs etc. are goods and services that people are likely to under consume and, therefore, they ought to be subsidized or provided free. Attention has to be paid to the social determinants of health for ensuring quality health care services. More emphasis needs to be on preventive rather than curative measures. Yellow cards need to be issued to vulnerable sections of society so that the health services may be accessible to them:

Doctors can be assigned the duty to serve at rural areas for some years; these doctors need to be given some incentives. Those vacancies in the health sector, which are lying vacant in the rural areas, need to be filled up with efficient and dedicated doctors and health personnel. It needs to be ensured that they have periodic training for skill enhancement along with the medical kits. There is a need to have a proper code of conduct for private practitioners.

Aware generation about seasonal trends of diseases in the rural areas must be made more effective and that can be done through posters, pamphlets, media and dramas. For this, the help of different sections of society can be taken like students, housewives and elderly. It is a general observation that in most of the cases the state-level medical authorities become active only at the outbreak of diseases and that leads to immense expense on manpower and medicines. There is also need to be aware of the information about the available health services, as the rural population does not know what is available.

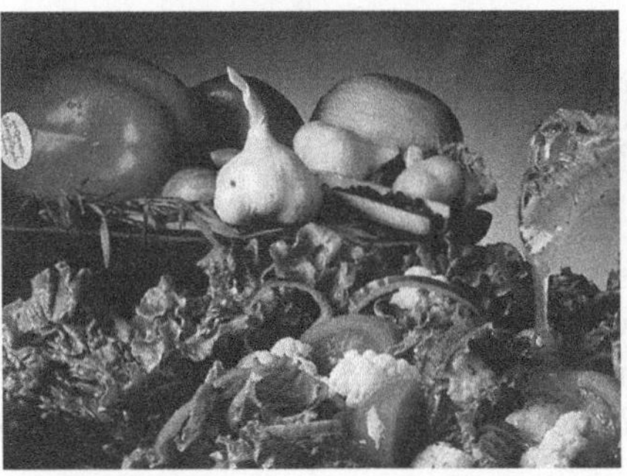

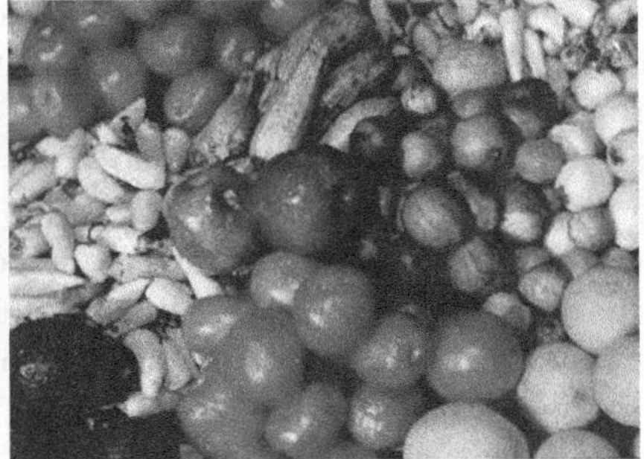

Figs 13.1 and 13.2: The energy value of foods is expressed in terms of calories. Balanced diet is a sufficient number of calories. Adequate amounts of protein, fat and carbohydrate. An adequate amount of minerals and vitamins for maintaining health, vitality and general well-being

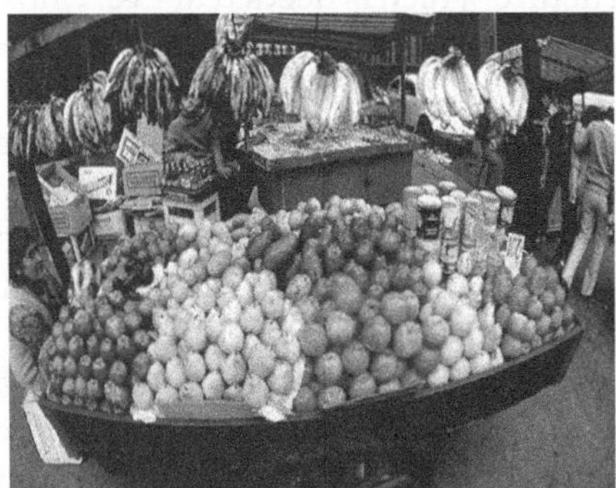

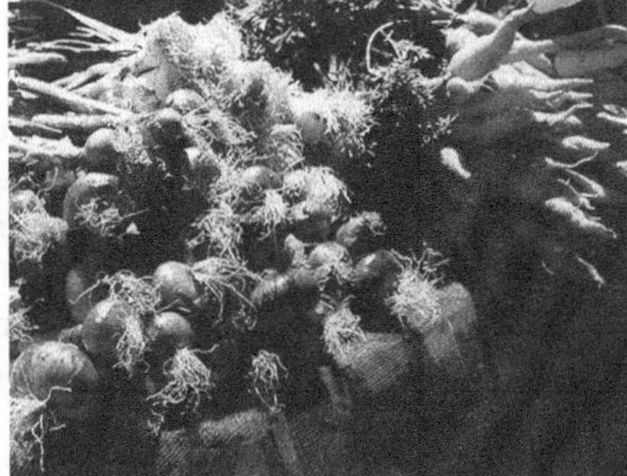

Figs 13.3 and 13.4: The energy producing foods, body building foods and protective foods are needed for growth and development. When a condition which occurs when the body does not get the proper kind of food in the amounts needed for maintaining health; it causes malnutrition

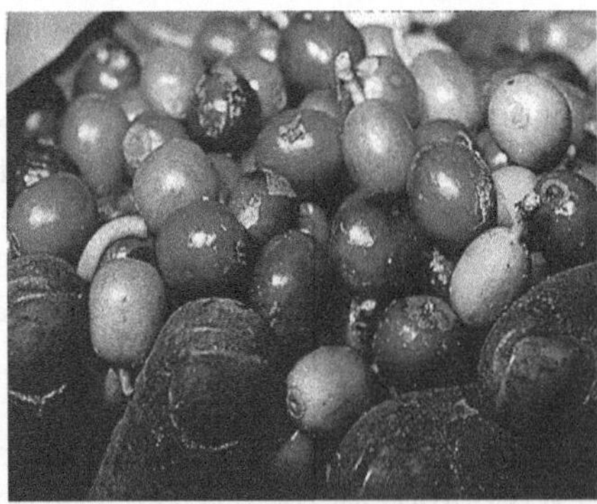

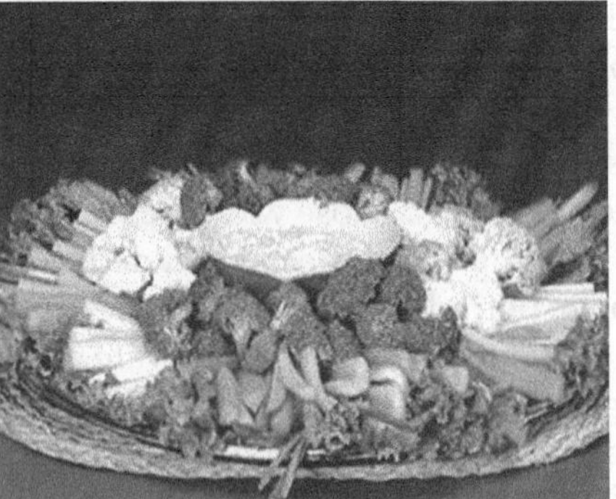

Figs 13.5 and 13.6: Regular intake of green leafy vegetables in the diet is necessary. It is essential for normal vision, skin and mucus membrane. It requires for the metabolism, essential in wound healing, it is essential for transport of oxygen and it is required for formation of hemoglobin. As it contains vitamin A, C, iron etc

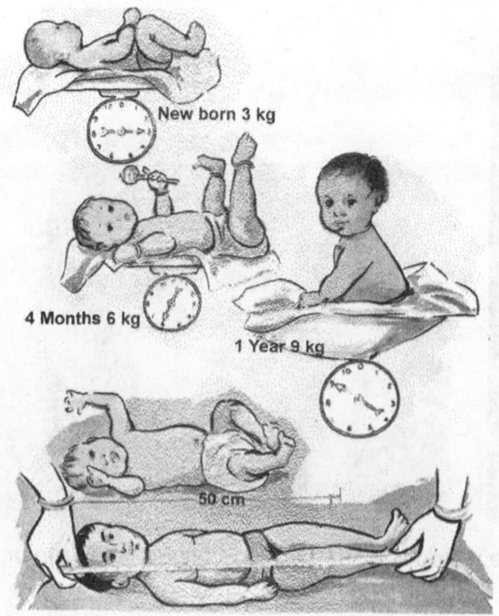

Fig. 13.7: Anthropometry indicates valuable information and status of the child. During the first year of life, growth is very rapid. A newborn infant weighs about 3 kg. By 4 months, the weight generally doubles and by one year, the weight should be about 9 kg. The length of the newborn infant is about 50 cm and by one year, the child reaches a height of 75 cm, i.e. one and half times its length at birth. The rate of growth in the infant is much faster than in the older child. For normal growth to take place, the baby must have sufficient nourishment

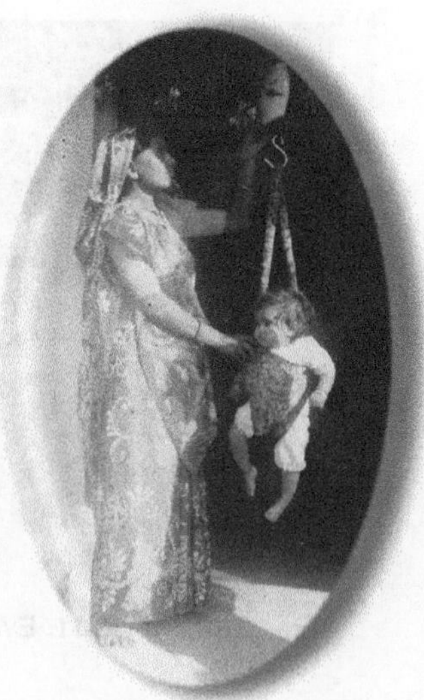

Fig. 13.8: Weight of the child is determined by using weighting machine. To assess the growth of children; to monitor the impact of nutrition and to analyze the reasons for the nutritional disorders

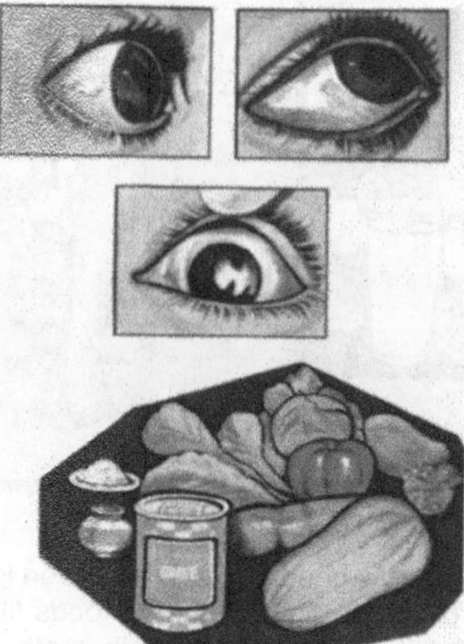

Fig. 13.9: Certain foods like yellow vegetables and fruits such as pumpkin, carrot, papaya and mango and green leafy vegetables; Ghee and butter are rich in vitamin 'A'. This vitamin is necessary for keeping the eyes and skin healthy. If there is less vitamin 'A' in diet the whites of the eyes become dry and wrinkle, the child cannot see in the dark and if the condition is not treated the eyes become ulcerated and child may become totally blind

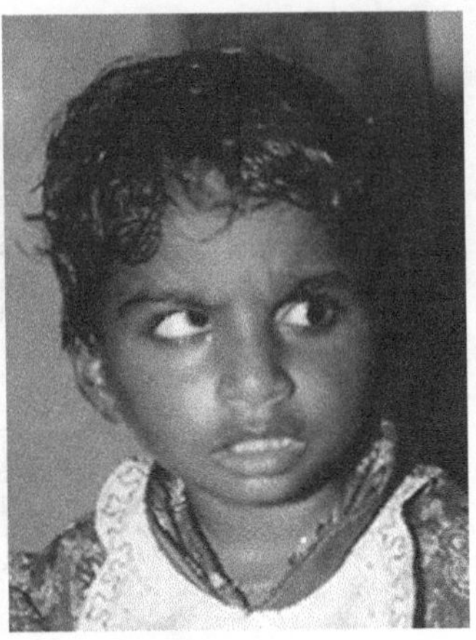

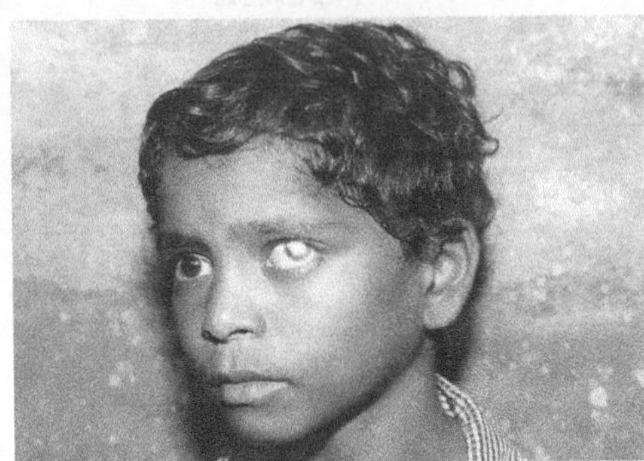

Figs 13.10 and 13.11: Eye is the window of the soul and blindness is major National health problem

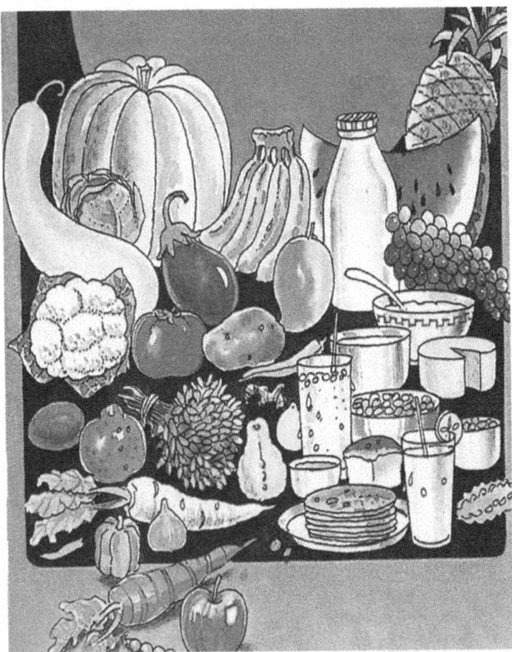

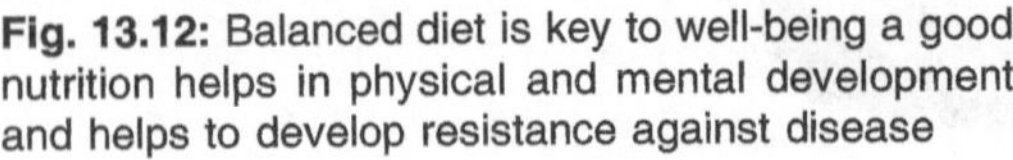

Fig. 13.12: Balanced diet is key to well-being a good nutrition helps in physical and mental development and helps to develop resistance against disease

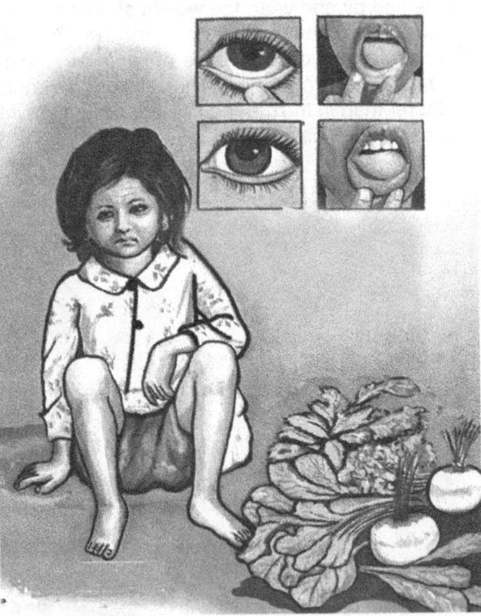

Fig. 13.13: Iron is very essential for the body. This element is found in foods like green leafy vegetables such as spinach, amaranth, methi and the tops of turnips, bit root, etc. If foods rich in iron are not given, the child suffers from anemia. The inner lining of the lips and eyelids look pale and the skin and nails are pale. The child lacks interest in play, is listless and tires easily

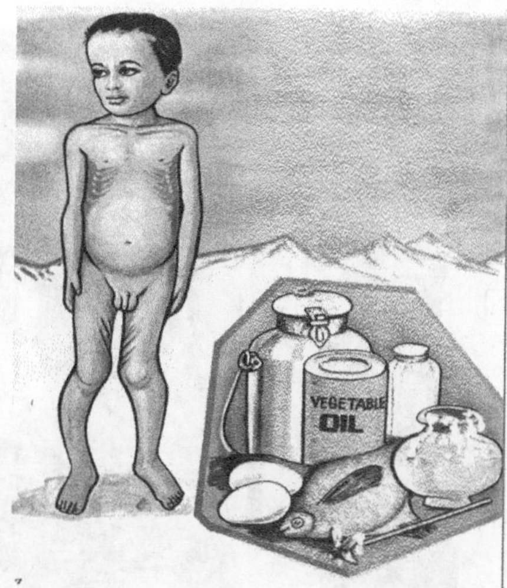

Fig. 13.14: Another condition caused by malnutrition is rickets. In this condition, the child has a pot belly and bony deformities such as bowing of the legs, knock knees, bulging of the bones of the forehead, and knob-like swelling or beading of the ribs. This condition can be prevented by exposure of the child to sunlight which is plentiful in our country and is a source of vitamin 'D'. Certain foods are also rich in vitamin 'D' such as ghee, eggs and fish liver oil

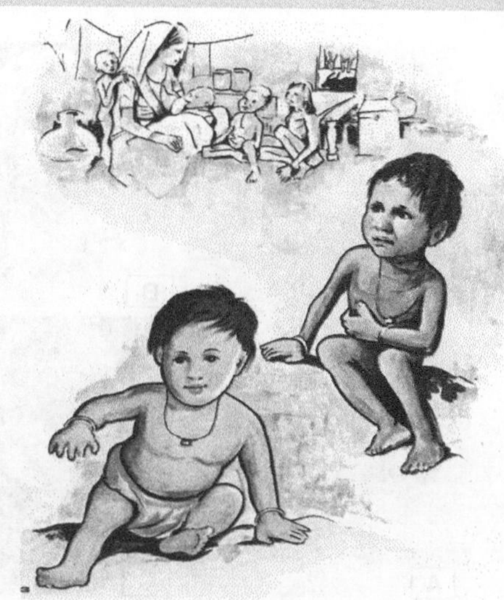

Fig. 13.16: Many mothers do not know that for this rapid growth to take place the baby needs sufficient nourishment. At times, they give the baby foods such as thin gruel or a piece of chapatti to keep the child from being hungry. But these foods are not enough to meet the needs of the growing child. As a result the baby becomes weak, it tends to fall ill, and its growth is stunted

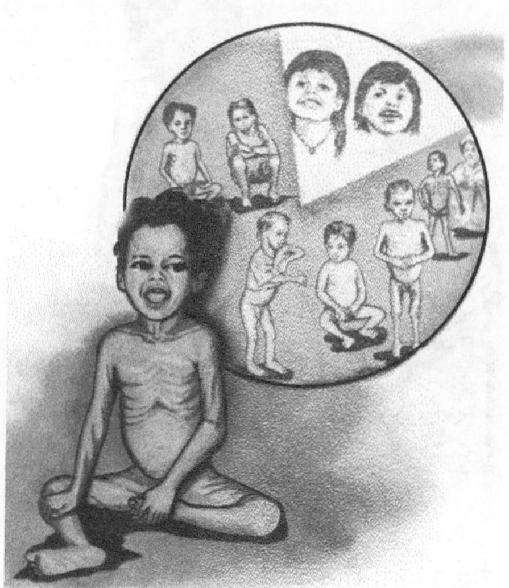

Fig. 13.15: When the body does not get the right type of food; in the right quantity the child suffers from malnutrition. In India, out of every ten pre-school children (below five years of age), eight suffer from some degree of malnutrition. Malnutrition can be of different types

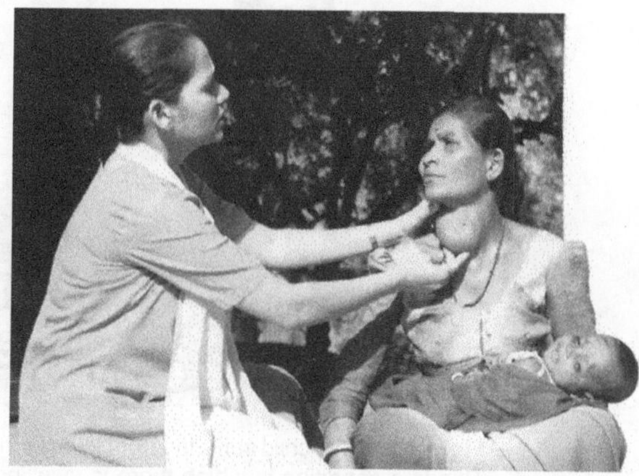

Fig. 13.17: Nutritional related problems, i.e. goiter control community action—iodine monitoring and surveillance

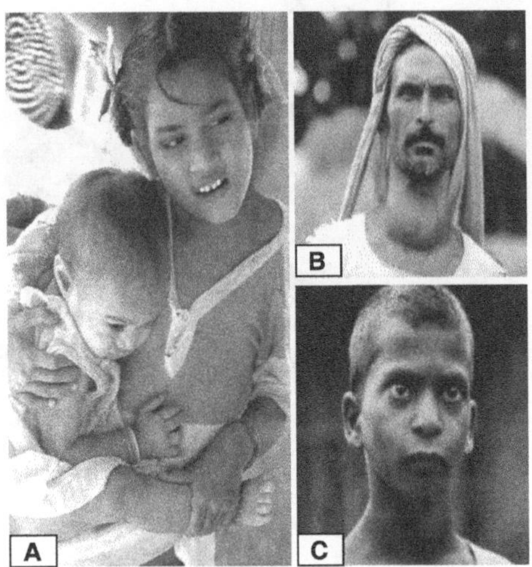

Figs 13.18A to C: Iodine deficiency disorder is another major nutritional problem in India. Till recently iodine deficiency was equated with goiter. It continues to be a serious health problem in many third world countries. There are almost 140 million people estimated to be living in goiter endemic regions of the country. Gonda of Uttar Pradesh is known to be highly endemic. Changing dietary habits, taking iodize salt or iodized oil and with nutritional education, condition can be brought under control

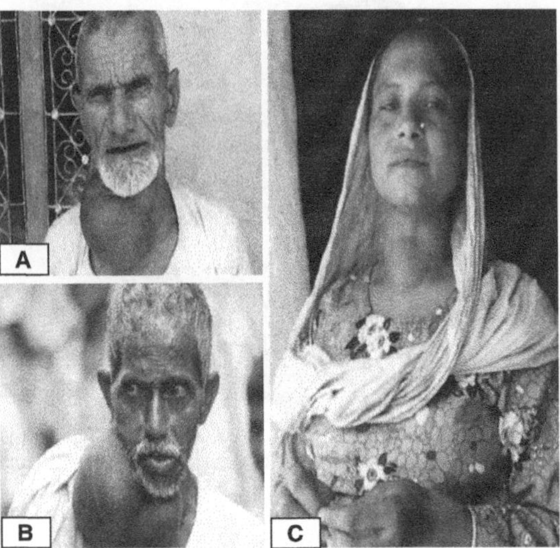

Figs 13.19A to C: Prophylactic for goiter—iodized salt most economical, convenient and effective measures

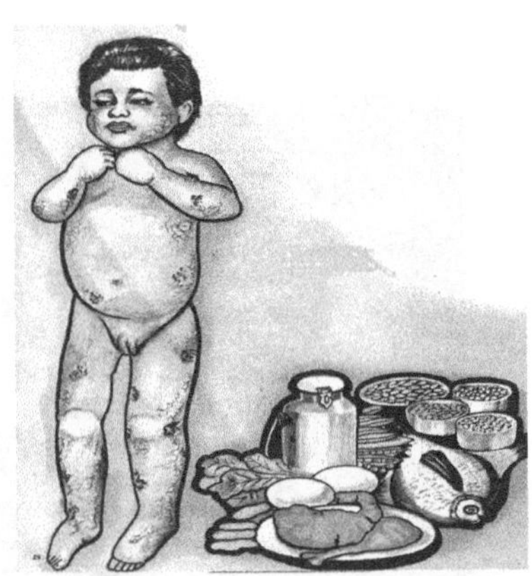

Fig. 13.20: This child suffering from kwashiorkor. This is a condition in which there is swelling of the feet and legs and peeling of the skin. The hair is light reddish in color and is very brittle. The condition is caused by taking a diet which is deficient in proteins. Kwashiorkor can be prevented by giving the child plenty of protein rich foods such as milk, eggs, meat, fish, dals, pulses or nuts

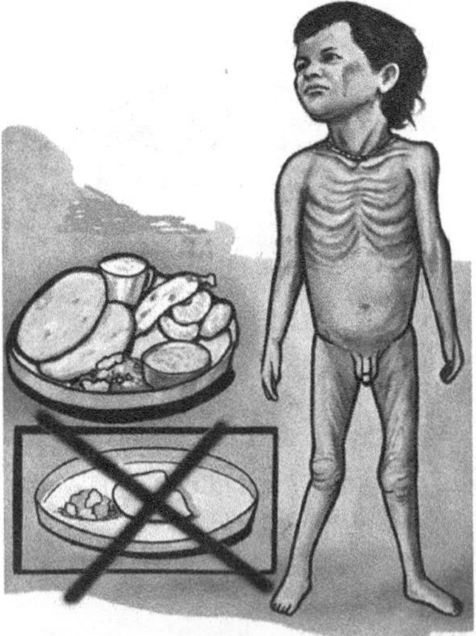

Fig. 13.21: This is marasmus. The child is very thin with the bones showing. The skin is wrinkled and loose, the abdomen is bloated and the child has a wizened expression on the face like that of an old man. This condition can be prevented by feeding the child with sufficient amounts of food. The diet should include foods from the various food groups, i.e. carbohydrates, e.g. chapatti, proteins, e.g. milk and dal, green leafy and yellow vegetables, fats, e.g. oil or ghee and fruits

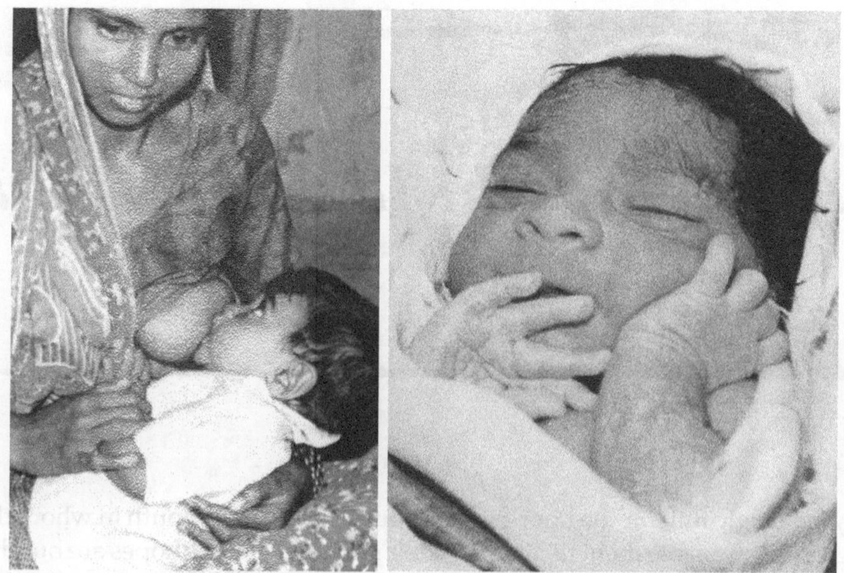

Figs 13.22 and 13.23: Mother's milk is the best for the newborn babies. It usually remains the main food for the baby in the first few years of life. Breast milk is the best food for the infants because it is clean and safe, it contains all the necessary nutrient for the newborn infant, it is easy to digest, it protects the baby from diseases and infection

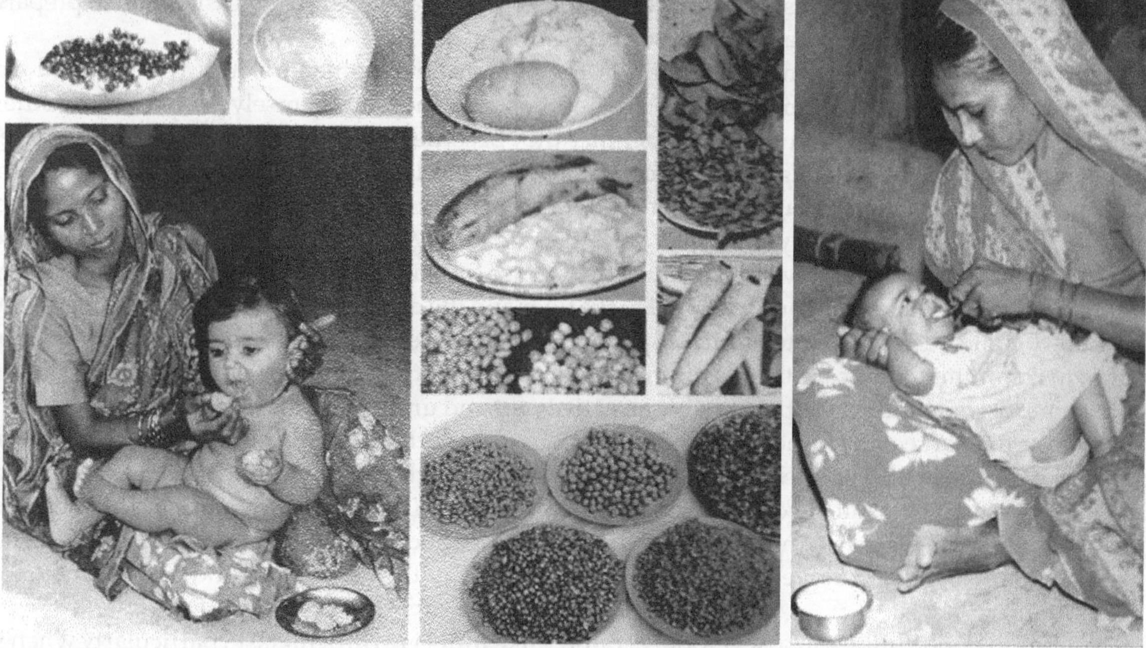

Figs 13.24 and 13.25: However, after 4 months mother's milk alone is not sufficient to meet the needs of the infant. Milk substitutes can also be prepared from vegetable sources such as ragi, groundnut or soyabean, green leafy vegetables made into a soup or fruit juice. These foods contain vitamins and minerals for baby's health

14 Youth: In the Community

A new way of being youth for the unorganized youth. Prepare the youth in whom the freshness of life is bubbling, and will enable them to discover their potential. Future hopes are build on youth of today who are the main actors, the trends that they set, the vision that they have, the directions that they indicate, can have a very great impact of life as it unfolds at the very inception of this new era which we call the beginning of a new age. Youth should re-capture the power to build up a new society in our country. Let every youth of the country commit himself to this task starting from the concrete situation one is placed and lives. Where they can dedicate themselves to build small human communities. To help them to overcome the greatest destructive weapon; discouragement and depression; and to prepare their tender minds to face the challenges of society.

Youth works in solidarity and collaboration for human development. Youth trys to build up community communion. Quite many youth are unorganized, they cut themselves off from the other youth, and they go into their own shells. Sometimes they become indifferent, violent and destructive. They also at times join mafia gangs, support communal riots, and get addicted to vices. They lose their identity, dignity and rights for various reasons. To conscientization and channelizing the unorganized youth for the betterment of society. Youth is a heaven in the society. To be leaven means to transform the whole mass through an inner, invisible, silent activity. Also by being a community of love and sharing. Youth committed to dialogue. Youth devoted to the poor and the downtrodden. All the resources of the community could be mobilized to eradicate poverty and oppression from our communities, not only their own community but from the rest of the human community with which we are related. Unless youth come forward and participate to play an active part and group effort is important.

Youth is a time of search for meaning, for belonging and for achievement. It is a key stage of intense discover of ones self, and of ones qualities and capacities. Youth is not only physical age but also a psychological stage; to instill in youth the correct concept of self. To reflect how youth could contribute towards the implementation of the values of fellowship, peace and truth. To reflect on the social values. To enable youth of India to move towards casteless society. Tap their potentials and prepare them for a better future.

Creating job opportunities in a developing country like India is a difficult task, particularly when it comes to the expectations and aspirations of the youth. In addition, when they are not met with, many related problems like drug addiction, violence and various other concerns arise. Employment will enable our anxious youth to find some ways and means to tackle this important problem of our society.

Youth has desire to become someone in this digital fast forward ultra modern age. Youthfulness either it is urban or rural is time to do something new and different; it is time of full of energy, vitality, and zest. Youth though not yet adult, they wish to be treated as such. All young people need loving and consistent support. He has reached biological maturity, but has not reached emotional maturity. Gaining a separate, adult identity is a youngster's central aim. Physical attractiveness, influenced by films, television and fashion is extremely important to youngsters. Where youngster experiences the way he looks as being unsatisfactory, with onset of puberty, they experience great uncertainty about who they are, what they will become and what they want to become.

Anxiety about identity worries about the future. Choose and develop a career to occupation have responsibility for the health and welfare of others. It is generally described as a difficult period in life. Young people are exposed to various dangers in society including drinking alcohol, smoking teenage pregnancy drug abuse. This will have serious consequences effect on his personal as well as his family. Rectifying such a situation is not easy. Both together have to do something about the problems they are experiencing all young people need loving and constant support. Any rigidity may result in maladjustment resulting in emotional instability and may lead to mental ill health if parents appear to be authoritative they may not cope up and will become irritable.

Youth is energetic, adventurous so they need guidance. Poverty, low economic status, unemployment, can lead them to frustration; measures to prevent give sex education, establishment of youth activities, developing hobbies.

What is your life philosophy? Keep aim, goals at the forefront of your life. Daring in facing difficulties and problems, overcoming obstacles, make your back strong to accept and respond to the challenging responsibilities ahead. You have inbuilt, inner, never ending, unlimited capacity, reservoir, recognize that.

Change is a law of nature. Day turns into night, darkness into light, every moment changes, flowers into fruits and seeds into tree, birth turns into death. Due to this there is change in childhood into adolescent period taking place and this growth and development is natural and normal. Sexuality is God given gift. Body is holy and is a temple of God where he lives. So have to respect your body and keep it always pure. So adolescent has to promote this precious life in healthy way by handling it in acceptable way according to following norms of society in which he lives. Every teenage has to pass from childhood to adulthood.

Not everything shinning all that is glittering is gold. If we are hungry we eat, if we are frighten we run but if we want we can change this thoughts. Drive all your attention in developing hobbies; today there are wide choices in variety of fields and scopes for youth. Flowers do not praise self or put a board, though they know they are beautiful and have nice fragrance. Build your personality with strong determination and inbuilt strength; focus on your target and work hard to achieve your aim and objective with strong will power and single-mindedness. Everyday is challenging. Everyday we are different. Accepting each day as a challenge, there is no limit to what you can do. Rose is rose and jasmine is jasmine both have unique identity and beauty of their own. You are unique become what you are. Obey your parents, elders, and teachers and get in time proper direction and guidance. Build strong moral value based character.

How do you inculcate good sound values in you such as hard work, discipline, punctuality, respect etc? Child by birth is not born as good or bad. You are parents of tomorrow. The future of tomorrow is being moulded and formed in what you do today. Expect future obstacles and difficulties. Do not pretend they do not exist. If you really desires a thing so deeply that you are willing to stake your entire future on a single turn of the wheel in order to get it, you are sure to win. Believe that you will simply find the way to solve your problems. Beliefs have the power to create and to destroy. Reinforce your belief. Challenge all that comes on your way and have courage to be your own constructive critic. It is better to wear out than to rust out.

Trust your highest power and in your infinite possibilities. You are great by your deeds, not by birth. Once you start working on something, do not be afraid of failure and do not abandon it. Learn that being kind is more important than being right. That life is tough, but I am tougher. That it is those small daily happenings that make life so spectacular. That to ignore the facts does not change the facts.

The youth always need a future orientation, if they have to make their lives meaningful. They do not look at the sunrise merely to enjoy the beauty of its colors and shades. They walk towards the rising sun and discover new horizons and new challenges. They become messengers of hope with their lives, builders of the future with their activities. They should realize that if their life is entirely caught up in the present, it would become a tiring experience. It will be like gramophone needle that has been caught up in a particular track of the record, always repenting the same note, so youth needs to move forward.

The elders cannot make very radical changes as they are rooted in the past. Youth is another name of the hope because with their creativity, energy and initiatives, they could make a difference in the current corroded system due to illiteracy, poverty, unemployment, to make breakthrough with collective leadership and take up as a challenge, new approach to life by tackle on priority basis.

Youth reality in India we need to make them more relevant by youth to youth approach. Give youth not only what youth like but also to provide what they need, the concrete issues affecting their lives.

Perseverance is great force, which guarantees success. No obstacles hindrance stands your way once you make up your mind to attain your objectives. You must decide your aim, objectives, and priorities and try to pursue them with hard work, regularity and discipline. Your smile adds value to your face, kind word adds value to your action and you live.

Learn from your mistakes. We learn from our experiences of daily life. Education moulds your character, shapes the destiny of the nation, influences the mind and directs your lives. Develops knowledge and wholesome attitudes towards life.

With advance materialism and globalization life has become mechanical, fast paced and consequently stressed out. All professions have become commercialized. In competitive world requires not just an excellent academic record, but courage and confidence to overcome situations. Dream dreams, strive hard and be the master of your own destiny. Prove your worth. No matter how much time you fall, get up, rise and walk.

Once you make up your mind with strong determination you can achieve your goal. It is a state of mind; you can only if you want. The final decision is made up by your mind. It is your own choice. Be positive in life. Toil for it. You have ability, the capacity to challenge and to change. For that you need strong determination, endurance, tolerance and constant perseverance.

So excel in all walks of life. Love the work you do. Competition exists in every level. Train your mind towards it, and be rooted. Make things happen to you by turning on your side. Tap your individual capacities. Stand up for yourself, take initiatives, and be responsible for your action.

Do not waste your precious moment either brooding over the past blunders or making castles in the air. Do not waste today in fretting over yesterday and daydreaming about tomorrow, which is yet to come. Time is your most precious possession. Opportunity never knocks twice.

Perseverance is a great force, which guarantees ultimate success. If your enthusiasm is dipped at the first sign of failure can never achieve goal. No obstacles/hindrance can stand in the way of a person who makes of his mind to attain his objectives.

We need good leaders like you to take us forward to 21st century. What do you want to be in your life? Are you aware of the hidden potentials, talents you possess? You become great by the use of opportunities, surrounding in which you live in. Values incorporate and cover all dimension of your life. It helps you all round development. Honesty enriches all other qualities. It is never too late to mend. He who would climb the ladder must begin at the bottom.

Think everyday that today is the last opportunity and I have to live intensely. Let not any opportunity pass by, spend each minute, invest each valuable resource, overcome every obstacle.

Destiny is not a matter of chance, it is a matter of choice. It is not a thing to be waited for, it is a thing to be achieved. The world of tomorrow belongs to the youth who has the vision today.

Swami Vivekananda fascinated the youth irresistibly during his short span of life; therefore youth who know him adores him because his message opens up new dimensions of ones own personality. The future of India largely depends on how earnestly the youth of India responds to this call. First of all, our young men must be strong. Stand up, be bold, take up the whole responsibility on your shoulders, and know that you are the creator of your own destiny. All the strength and succour you want are within you.

Learn the importance of time. Use your time constructively. Remember time and tied waits for no one. Your today will decide your tomorrow. Hit the iron while it is hot. Dig the mud while it is soft and wet. Who will decide for your happiness or sadness? What is the center of focus of your life?

Build self-esteem; focus on your potential instead of your limitations. Determine to know the truth yourself. Distinguish between who you are what you do. Where there is an open mind, there will always be a frontier. Every adversity carries the seed of an opportunity that can be transformed into prosperity.

This is important phase of your life and carrier. You will have to build your own future. Search your own road, walk your own path, discover your hidden strengths. Prepare yourself for responsible parenthood. Life is Gods greatest gift to humankind. Live it in its fullness, in its totality for the purpose God has created you for. Find meaning and purpose for your life and be a role model for coming generation who will look at you and follow your footsteps.

Youth who is firm and resolute will mould the world to him. There exist limitless opportunities in every industry. Youth becomes great exactly in the same degree in which he works for the welfare of his fellow man. Every challenge or adversity carries the seed of an opportunity that can be transformed into prosperity. Empower your life and work enthusiastically. Motivation is one of the greatest diving forces for success in life. Pride of mind is the most dangerous disease and the most difficult to cure. Remember no one makes it alone. Have a grateful heart and be quick to acknowledge those who helped you.

Take charge of your attitude. Don't let someone else choose it for you. Remember that 80% of the success in any job is based on your ability to deal with people. Don't burn bridges. You will be surprised how many times you have to cross the same river. Become the most positive enthusiastic person you know. Never give up, miracles happen everyday. Always accept an outstretched hand. The heights charm us, but the steps do not; with the mountain in our view we love to walk the plains.

You are Gods image and are a unique person. He has a plan and purpose for your life. You possess lots of hidden talents and potentials. Younger youth are facing conflicts and dilemma at every turn and stage of life. With the impact of modern living and breakdown of joint family there is an erosion of culture and ethical base and strengths in our multicultural society, it is important to instill and reinforce values, for to face the modern society they live in. It is vital to mould youths character that is higher than anything else. This will enable them to blossom into courageous, morally strong, better persons and confident citizens.

It means being on time and doing things in time. Use well your time, if you waste time you will have great loss. Be on dot, do things in time, time lost never returns. Do not waste precious moment brooding. Build your inner personalities and it will help you to grow in maturity to handle your life successfully. Path is paved by walking. Dream the impossible dream, fight the unbeatable foe, run where the brave dare not go, and may this be your quest. Success comes from repeated efforts. It is a blend of hard work and good luck. No one knows what he can do until he tries. Every great achievement was once impossible until someone set a goal to make it a reality. You feel never alone if you are accompanied by noble thoughts. You must be melted before you can be moulded. Success is not the key to happiness; happiness is the key to success.

You are unique, no one is like you or you are not like the other. Whatever you are, you are you. Sometimes we try to become like other—hero worshiping, wearing a mask, hiding our own self. Remember whatever you are God loves you just as you are with all its strengths and limitations. So become what God has designed you for.

In family, in school, through your friends, parents, teachers you get lot of negatives. Then you think of your negatives and ignore your qualities, you do not pay attention to your positives. While doing this you do lot of harm to yourself. To achieve your goal first be aware of your abilities, capacities, and potentialities. Not all get opportunity you have to create your own opportunity. Change yourself and change the world.

Be a creator of your career. Miracle of hard work and strong willpower pays you at the end. A youth when encountered with obstacles and difficulties does not get frustrated, discouraged and disappointment but when determined achieves greater things in life. Work hard even you have to struggle be ready for it. One day you can create a revolution you will find these examples in history ordinary men turning and reaching extraordinary achievements.

What do you admire in your best friend? Friends are like the branches of a tree. Friendship helps the weary, cheers the sad and drives dark clouds away; the one who shares your smile as well as tears. So try to get good motivated challenging good friends.

How do you deal with conflict? Do you try to handle ugly situation in a peaceful creative way? Recall a time when someone insulted you? Have courage to be you. Because we are so different from each other we have so much to share. What you resist you persist, what you accept transforms. Accept it and owe it.

Our time here on earth is very limited. Your hidden powers are super. Your own attitudes can become your greatest medicines in the world. You are what you choose for yourself. Our minds are capable of storing an incredible amount of data. Your mind is your own, and you have a terrific capacity. You will perceive, think, and feel in your unique way. The strongest person in the world is the one who stands most alone. If you want to achieve your own greatness, climb your own mountain; you will have to use yourself as your first and the last consultant.

Believe in yourself. Believe stimulating power within you. Change your thoughts and ways of living and believe in God. Since God and you form a strong undefeatable combination. You are a product of what you choose for yourself. Flash out the negative out of your mind. When you get into storm you know that it will not last forever. There is fair weather ahead, see life big, let not your thinking detoriate you.

Be vibrant with life, filled with energy and dynamism so that difficulty becomes your motive force. Life is elimination of all sense of deadness. Your life is meant to be fully alive. Alive in every element of your being; Life should be perpetually fascinating.

Set behavioral goal to act differently then you will ever do before. You are sum product of your choice. Learning from your mistakes is healthy and necessary part of growth. You are a tower of strength; you are not going to collapse or fall apart if you encounter something new. Have internal security, trusting you to handle anything that may come down. If you equate your worth with failure and success, you will be doomed to feeling of worthlessness.

Remember your abilities are not better or worse but simply different from others. Be your own hero. Become a person whose external action correspond to an internal conviction is called a authentic person. Drop your false ideas. A problem exists in human mind. Yes, you will glimpse of the sky some day, and you will fly. Your self worth is located within you. By changing the inner attitudes of the mind, you can change the outer aspect of your life. Keep your face to the sunshine and you will never see the shadows. A tree cannot forget its roots; its life depends on them. A person cannot forget his parents and his rootedness in his family.

No one is born by birth as a doctor or an engineer. All have to work hard towards making it. You can become great by the use of opportunities offered to you by society, family and all that surrounds you. Be particular in keeping your time. Success is both blend of hard work and perseverance. He who climbs the ladder must begin at the bottom. It is better to get an egg today then a hen tomorrow. Sow the seed of hard work in all that you do and you will reap the harvest of good results with excellence. Invest and spend each minute of your time fruitfully today. Make up your mind and start today as day one. Wake up, this is the day made for you here and now.

Destiny is not a matter of chance; it is a matter of choice. It is not a thing to be waited for, it is a thing to be achieved. The greatest thing in life is to keep your mind young. Winners do not do different things they do things differently. Do not wait for what you want to come to you, go after it, keep going when you feel like giving up. Every great achievement was once impossible until someone set a goal to make it a reality. Consistence and hard work is the key.

Today human beings living in rocket age and they are becoming and living more and more mechanical, money wealth has become there life's top most priority, and man is attracted by passing glamorous world. He wants to become rich by hook or crook, no matter which way – either using shortcut, by illegal dealings, by cheating, or kidnapping. Be aware of this kind of ways that will tempt you and may one day lead you to doom where you may land up in jail or never to rise again.

Be honest and sincere in all that you do that will pay you at the end. Work hard because it is not money that counts, or how rich or poor you are but how happy you are, the art of living that life has taught you is important. Select good quality friends, who will show you the right direction, accompany you and walk with you showing and guiding you on right path. One wrong decision will ruin your future life. Be a good friend to yourself. Good friends are like mirror where our own personality gets reflected. You will be known by the company you keep. Friends introduce you to others, and friends give strength and courage. And give meaning to our existence we feel life is worth living because of this good friend. Have positive thinking, new thoughts, learn the art of living and art of silence, keep your emotions under control with hard work you can get fire out of stone. Keep high hopes, high ideals and go after it.

Life is precious, there is possibilities of growth, let your life bloom and blossom, face the defeat, do not run away, fly high with courage, accept the challenges, you have to build tomorrows society, coming generation will look at you, your children will have to face still rough and tough competition ahead. Only those who have courage will swim across. Your today will decide your tomorrow.

Do not waste time, be serious in what you do, all have to go through rough times to become someone, without struggle no one can become what they are today, all have faced the turmoil and rough seas. Have strong willpower, determination, and single mind, focus on target. Diamond is polished then only shine comes, gold is tested in fire, when the night is dark you see the stars shine and twinkling, strong willpower and perseverance is key towards success. Every one does not get everything in life. You become what you decide, think; ask what do I expect from my life? Plan your time and your work.

Adolescent health—Health nurse in modern times has a significant responsibility in effectively carry out sex education guiding the youth especially in rural areas. Health nurse can be of immense help in guiding to handle younger ones, when problem faced she can use services of experts such as psychologist, counselor. To work with the youth is a challenging and difficult area yet it is necessary in modern times if the youths are to be given proper direction for the benefit of the nation. They have to be physically and mentally fit.

Those turbulent teen years growing up are not easy. Changes always raise serious problems. Confusion and uncertainties, what to do? Expect some mistakes; unfair competition. Rapid growth brings many changes and under friendly guidance they are willing to accept suggestions. We are able to help them in their troubled minds. And show them the brighter side of life by doing something constructive. The youths are the future of the country and we need to pay closer attention to them.

To keep abreast with things in the world trend that is slowly evolving. Many are still groping in the dark. They need to come together and define their roles and functions. Have we empowered them sufficiently? Do we trust them with skills and competencies? Are we making the voice of those who labor under the yoke of injustice, heard? What should we be doing to usher in more just and humane society where the values prevail? What should we be doing to revive that spirit? What special activities/ programs should we undertake? Are we afraid to face the challenges that confront us? For that we have to move with single mindedness focusing in a union of heart and mind moving towards tomorrow together.

What's holding you back from living your dream? Most of us have a dream, wheather it's a better home, good relationships or career, often we are our own worst enemies when it comes to achieving them. Each of your action takes you step ahead. Your hard work is more productive and less stressful. Time is precious, therefore use it intelligently, working smartly requires you to innovate, optimize, learn, be aggressive, work as a team member and strike a balance between work and life.

Become from transforming persons to transforming communities and culture; By taking the whole village community into confidence. How participative is the movement? Is it a movement based on youth? How do we approach youth? With respect that they have a right to self-determination? Understanding them, their belief systems, culture, etc? All of us feel called upon to seek differences, pool resources together to fight. We can no more remain mute onlookers, must gather all men and women of goodwill in the struggle against those who are bent upon destroying national integrity and social harmony of our country.

You are designed for accomplishment and endowed with the seeds of greatness. You are the only one who can use your ability. You are capable of getting health, wealth, and happiness. And the foundation is honesty, character, faith, integrity and loyalty. E.g. if you want to become weight lifter you will have to develop muscles, it is the same way you have to develop your talents work hard to win. By choice and by training you become what you wish. Your success starts with you. You have the ability to become successful. If you do not use it you lost it.

Who am I? Youth has explosive power within if he gets proper guidance he can re-create himself describe your best quality as a human being? What is your memorable moment; what is one thing you would like to change yourself, why? If you were given a choice to be re-born what you would be? Why? What is to be youth according to you? If you have three wishes, what would you ask for? Where are you at this stage?

Discover yourself, who you are, discover your identity? Do I bring happiness where I am? How do I see myself as ME, am I growing? How much of the world ambition, prestige, reputation has crept into my life? Do I accept myself, forgive myself? Do I admit weakness? Do I then feel worthless? Who is God for me, a punishing God, a judging God, a God who demands gifts, bribes to grant his love and favors?

Do I hold God responsible to or at least I think that he permits it when anything goes wrong? Can I relish my preciousness especially when I discover my weakness? Can I relish the preciousness of others even when they appear disgusting? What are your parent's expectations about you? What are your hobbies? Your likes and dislikes? Do you adjust to your family? Do you want to be known as a good person?

What is your motto-ideal in life? What carries you forward in life? How much time do you spend with your family? What is the home for you? According to you who are the good leaders? What are you looking for in life? Do you use your talents fully? Why? What are your desires and plans for future? To achieve if there comes obstacles how do you face them? How do you come across to people? What is there opinion about you, why do they think about you this way? Is life worth living?

The youth are the prophets. They are dynamic, creative and capable of dreaming the impossible and struggle towards its realization. They can change the face of the society. Stand for yourself, dream dreams and achieve it, discover what you are good at. Do not get attach and attracted to what is meaningless and useless. You are the backbone of the nation; you are the sing board, and master key. Due to self-confidence, lion though smaller than elephant, with his roaring this big animal starts shivering. One spark can burn the mountain of cotton.

Every morning a deer wakes up, it knows it must run faster than the fastest lion or it will be killed. Every morning a lion wakes up, it knows it must run faster than the slowest deer or it will starve to death. It does not matter that you are a lion or deer, you had better be running.

A winner never quits and a quitter never wins. Empty your mind of failure thoughts. I can, I must, I will excel. There is always a reason behind everything that happens. Very often reason for failure or losses, tragedies is human error. We make the mistakes and then we blame some unseen force. Life is not meant to be fritted away in hustles and bustles of life purpose are forgotten. Money seems to rule everything and becomes the aim of life. Give your best in whatever you do. Make right choices and believe in it. Just three steps to success work hard, work harder, work hardest.

Get educated, it will mould your character, shape and direct your life. To become good leader develop team spirit, cooperation, service mind, going out of self, open to new ideas, ready to change, be confronted, give importance to others, impartial, hard working, sincere, lead the group to unity, bridge builder, respect others, promote peace, strive to be good listener.

He who would climb the ladder must begin at the bottom. People always like to go to the top most position in life quickly and easily. Those who are in top position, if you ask them you will know that they had a humble beginning. It is a blend of hard work and good luck. The world is like a mirror if you smile, it smiles back at you. You get back what you give.

Every economic activity involves a risk. Short-term, non-formal, modular courses of 3–6 months duration can be made available to youth. Multi skill training may be offered to make self-employment viable in the rural economy. Providing basic skills, knowledge and attitude for self/wage employment in their own village or nearby areas. Offer skill upgradation programs in their own fields. Society in both urban and rural areas specifically women, minorities, school dropouts, street children and physically handicapped. NGOs, voluntary agencies, village panchayats and retired teachers, engineers and other reputed persons should be involved in the process of multidisciplinary skill training.

Improve their quality of life, productivity and energy efficiency. Offer upgradation of existing technologies used by villagers. This needs to have proper delivery system by providing backup technical support to the panchayats. The villagers also need support of other kinds for their professional improvement to widen the scope of their activities, and to enhance their productivity.

The kind of support needed may vary widely from a mere psychological boost in some cases to complete guidance in acquiring loans, supply for raw materials, acquisition of necessary know-how, development or marketing and distributing facilities to others. All communication media such as leaflets, brochures, filmstrips, video films and other audio visual aids could be used. Providing information through exhibitions; organizing youth clubs, community workshops, and seminars.

Identify, orient, motivate, train and assist the rural youth to take up self-employment. Employment generation in rural areas, deceleration of urban migration capital formation in rural sector, awareness of self-employment opportunities.

Be your own boss, start your own business: Be a job creator, make creative use of your talents and skills, increase your family income, option to learn at your own place and time, get counseling support throughout, follow-up support, opportunity, become eligible for getting loan.

Project for the youth organization and development of the socially and economically marginalized communities to be made available with subsidized rate.

Set up a library where they can read different newspapers, magazines, which will keep them in touch with the world. Take care of the training and organization of the urban as well as rural youth. Through camps and leadership training program, plan to make them aware of the social situation and their responsibilities to transform the existing unjust situation.

Where is the Indian youth today? How I see the youth today? In many ways the situation is changing, we have some picture in mind when we speak of "youth" today. Whom are we talking about?

Adolescence and young adulthood has always existed as a stage of psychosexual development – but not quite. In most rural, pre-literate societies, the average life span was short, 45 to 50 years, and childhood was immediately followed by adult responsibility. Rather, childhood it included minor responsibilities in running the home or the farm. This is still the case with a considerable number of adolescents in rural India today.

Many of our boys and girls help at home and in the fields even from their childhood. The childhood is followed by a prolonged period of time when one is neither a child nor a grown-up with adult responsibilities – the period referred to now-a-days as "youth". In rural communities, a boy's or girl's work was wanted and needed by the family. Adolescents and even children contributed to the family income through their work. This is by and large not the case with most young people in urban and semi-urban settings today. Adolescents and young adults are a big financial burden on their families, because of the expensive education and the nonavailability of jobs for unqualified people.

Our population is basically young. Unlike the graying populations of the affluent west, a greater part of our population is below thirty.

As a culture gets saturated by mass media, something else happens, too. The new generation gets warped messages of instant gratification, easy money and sensational achievements.

Adolescent health has always been overshadowed by children's health. However, adolescence is a crucial bridge between childhood and adulthood. Any holistic approach to improve the health status of India's children must therefore, address adolescent health.

Low levels of educational achievement; persistent gender disparity in school enrolment and in labor force participation, high level of participation in the labor force, high unemployment rate, early sex, marriage and childbearing, poor knowledge and use of contraceptives, unwanted pregnancies and abortions, short birth intervals and unplanned births, poor nutrition and antenatal care, lack of information and adequate access to health services.

Diseases such as diabetes and anorexia are becoming increasingly common among adolescents in urban areas and are a major public health challenge. Moreover, the stress faced by adolescents these days surfaces in disastrous and often, unthinkable ways, including suicides, murders, deviant behavior and substance abuse.

Consequences of early marriage and early sex: India has a population of more than 200 million adolescents, of whom 36 percent in the 13-16 year age group are married. As many as 64 percent of those in the age group of 17 to 19 years are already mothers. Early marriage has significant health repercussions; and while the problems faced by adolescent girls have received some attention, those encountered by male adolescents tend to go unrecognized. Sexually active by the time they are 18. Most adolescents reach sexual maturity before they are ready to handle or grapple with their own social, emotional and psychological development. Moreover, there is widespread lack of information among adolescents on reproductive and sexual health issue.

National economic development of any country depends on effective organization. For an effective organization, it essentially needs updated trained skilled manpower. We have to train our youth for their need of achievement.

Youth are interested in doing something new and unique, they have desire to influence others, desire to take initiate, ready for acceptance of challenges, have high hope of success. Ready and willing for moderate risk-taking, and show willing openness to constructive feedback. Learning from experience, can develop positive self-concept, will boost their high level of aspirations and emotional commitment. That will seeking help can change get the problem solving ability; self-confidence and belief in others that environment. Keeping creative mind, with time orientation, independent in thoughts and actions, ready for hard work, concern for improving performance, concern for doing better than others, researching the environment for entrepreneurial opportunity, take personal responsibilities.

Thinking skills necessary to put knowledge to work, personal qualities that make them dedicated and trustworthy, the ability to manage resources, creative thinking and problem solving, interpersonal negotiation and teamwork, organization, goal setting and leadership all this follows step by steps. Thus, integration of rural youth into national economy and joining them to the mainstream is an urgent need.

With this skilled training at the doorsteps of the rural youth their arms can get extension. Skill development training programs relevant to community needs. Identify problems, which need intervention of other outside agencies and NGOs. Community mela should be considered as one of the important activities of the scheme. Number of youths to be trained, number of technologies to be transferred in villages, support services to be provided in various areas. Closely interact and understand the problems of the rural community. Assess periodically the progress, discuss problems in implementing and find appropriate solutions to overcome them. Keeping the objectives of monitoring is to achieve the physical and financial progress of the community, analyze strengths and limitations of the systems as a whole as to areas where the intervention and the support of the government is necessary.

Facilitation of various activities under the scheme, to review from time to time the activities of the scheme and to respond appropriately to ensure effective implementation, with timely submission of reports. Planning, organizing and supervising the activities of the scheme, coordination with various departments, review the work done. To analyze and propose solutions to problems encountered in planning and implementation of the programs for community development; by monitoring the scheme of community youth.

Community development is a gigantic task and it cannot be implemented in isolation. Coordination, collaboration and linkages with other agencies involved in rural development. Village youth, local NGOs, voluntary organizations and other government agencies are needed to be involved at different stages of implementation of the scheme to have allround development in the area; where information sharing, commitment to the task, credibility, good rapport, and good delivery with other agencies.

Indicating the difficulties faced, conducting socioeconomic surveys, job potential surveys with the view of introducing new trades at existing extension centers, rotation of trades amongst the extension centers and the feasibility of establishing new extension centers. It is a time consuming process of conducting the feedback surveys.

After conducting a detailed survey and taking into consideration the socioeconomic and technical feasibility and resources available. Provide some appropriate training to the physically disabled. They put up a brave struggle against the odds and calamities of which they are constant victims. Preservation of food and vegetables, purification of well water, earth water filter and cooler, solar cooker soak pit; integral, as the word implies, political and economic situation of our country.

Income generating through new trades; skill development and training programs; non-formal agro based skill like bee keeping, boring/drilling mechanic, fruit/vegetables preservation, mushroom cultivation, civil engineering rural latrine and soak pits. Agarbati making, bag making, bamboo work, basket making, brick making, candle making, chalk making, cloth printing, cutting and tailoring, embroidery, mat making, rope making, toys from waste material, wooden articles making, night soil biogas plant, portable gobar gas plant, community type chulha, maintenance of rural roads, drains, sanitation and water supply, tree plantation, drinking water facilities, rural house building, improvement of village environment, electrification of street light, wiring, plumbing, repairing mobiles, follow-up and maintenance of various technologies could be installed.

Promotion of community health through legal aid also needs importance as the world has become too small with technological advancement, administrative efficacy. Still certain strata of the society are deprived of their right to have dignified advanced livelihood because of the unawareness and less accessibility of these systems. The time demands for awareness building in youth of the society.

Human dignity and human rights belong together. The poor are often deprived of their lands. Moneylenders adopt extortionist methods and some debtors even become bonded laborers. The poor and the marginalized are often oppressed precisely because they belong to a particular weak class of people. Their rights to their sociocultural identity must be recognized. Denial of this right cuts at the root of human dignity and welfare. Thus to bring transformation in the society, to work for the establishment of a free, just and fraternal society. To enkindle faith in the youth and build up self-confidence among the oppressed, to organize them and to enable them achieve economic self-reliance and social identity.

To provide legal aid and assistances to needy youths especially those belonging to the socially and economically backward communities, organize and conduct legal literacy programs, workshops, prepare and distribute material connected with legal literacy, disseminate information about the constitutional and legal rights and duties of citizens. Conduct programs aimed at imparting information and education about political process in the country, voters' responsibilities working of government machinery and fostering of democratic values and national integration.

Emphasis is given to hard work, the process of accountability, serious study and reflection. Apart from the normal activity, team members are expected to meet regularly – for sharing, reporting, evaluation and planning. Every member is expected to give selflessly his/her maximum in service. Nature of works is more of a commitment and a responsibility than a task. These entail regular meetings, camps, seminars, training sessions and exposure programs which go beyond the confines of a time schedule. Each employee is, therefore, expected to give the maximum time possible.

To foster, organize and conduct independently or in collaboration with other similar government or nongovernmental educational institution courses; conferences, seminars, remedial programs, radio and TV programs; campaigns and competition for the removal of illiteracy; adult education, rural and agricultural development, motivation of youth, promotion of justice, community health and other similar programs aimed at promoting or completing education which is not, or cannot be, provided through the formal channels of education and to award prizes, scholarships and certificates.

According to the demands of the hour we firmly believe in the power of the young dynamic student group emerging in the rural land, that each rural youth will ever work for the alleviation of all the ills faced by the exploited rural masses in their home land. He or she will never shy away from the groaning of rural people. We hope that in all circumstances he or she will make every effort and struggle to maintain the cultural identity, honour, growth and well-being of the rural people. We envisage a rural society where there will be a collective responsibility and leadership and each dynamic young rural youth will play his or her role to transform the rural society for better future.

Regularly organized camps, seminars and workshops for the suitable young rural boys and girls to help them develop their skills in writing and journalism in order that they in turn become the voice of the exploited rural masses.

Recognizing the powerful alternative media of the people in the street play, it will now and then organize the street theater, workshop so that it may become the means of conscientization among the rural exploited masses. It will work continuously for the unity and solidarity of all the rural youth. It will make every effort to keep and uphold the rural cultural identity. It will try to inculcate rural culture values among the rural that have given up practicing them. It will make all efforts to maintain environmental balance in the rural regions. Students studying in the university who in turn will provide leadership and guidance for rest of the youth. Team member, which will enable them to move ahead.

Make youth think critically and achieve a critical consciousness. Instill discipline and life liberating force into youth. Make them all conscious that the destiny of India is now being shaped in the classroom.

Impart skill-based information, knowledge education. Let subject taught have some social relevance. Which will develop productive skill? Youth could be given work and employment orientation. To link education with development in the sociocultural, economic, political scenario this will bring social change. Make conscious effort to give value orientation, which will make them aware of social reality outside. Helps youth for allround integral development, which in return will help them in their natural and social environment. Where they will be equipped with compatibility for creative work and will have faith in life.

It will increase their efficiency level, end results in attitudinal change, desired change, and need fulfillment, and only through constant training you acquire it. Let not the victory enter neither your head nor the failure your heart. This has been the success formula of great people. Self-discovery, self-development and self-awareness. Values to be recognized and clarified. Resources to be discovered and developed. Traits to be found out and classified. Abilities to be tested and used. Skills to be matched with our aptitude and trained. New ways of perceiving oneself and the world, new concept, ideas and values, new awareness, new understanding, new attitudes, new determination, new motivation, new intentions. Do your best to complete task, assume responsibility, maintain harmony and be a social reformer. Exploring new pastures, people oriented.

One of the primary developmental tasks of young people is to find their identity. To have positive self image. The real world does not substantiate the idealized, romantic worlds presented to the young people by the media creating in them frustration and despair. The energy, enthusiasm, and dynamism of youth can be tapped to transform our culture and society.

The youths are very faithful; if you trust them they are ready to do anything. If they are trusted, respected and given responsibility, often they are proved to be responsible, sincere and hardworking. If they are given activities they are ready to give their time and energy. If they are made aware, they are ready to change. If you love them they will love you.

Dream dreams; dreams rescue us from harsh reality. It is our dream that push us forward; destiny is a winding, unpredictable road that constructs itself as you move on. Heaven is a dream, no one has seen it, and no one can verify its existence and those who are there cannot tell us what it looks like. It is unimaginable to comprehend to human mind. Do I foster my dream, or do I follow the crowd, do I bear with silent patience, or speak out aloud? About this, why not anyone warned me? The world suddenly seems to have grown 10 times bigger. Life is no longer about adventure and fantasies, from here on all about responsibilities making ends meet and by now, you have family to share your risks.

Dreams do not put food on the table. Did we make right decision? We have the right to dream. I do not know what is stored for me, trust in God and commit and life in Gods hands wheather I live or die God is with you. Sometimes, you ask for flower and you get cactus ugly with thorns, but wait on Gods time the cactus will bloom into beautiful flower that you had asked for.

Youth found into three categories.

One is the youth belonging to the elite class, with more than sufficient resources for further their career and have an enjoyable life. If there is any aimlessness in this category, this spring from having more than plenty. Latest fashions, lavish parties and maximum comforts are their concerns. Study in English medium school.

Another group belongs to the middle class, who needs to struggle to climb the ladder of development. They are trying their best to excel in whatever career they have chosen. This class has no time to waste. There are other groups of youth who hail from the soil. Their parents have struggled hard and have come up economically. Today their children, today's youth, have all the comforts of life, live luxurious and carefree lives.

The third class of youth belongs to the rock bottom of society. They see no future for themselves. There lives consist to trying to make both ends meet. They never dream of climbing the ladder because it is beyond their reach. They are the migrant laborers, brick kiln workers, rag pickers, shoe shiners, tea stall errand boys and other such category of youth. They get lost in hustle and bustle of city civilization. They are left to fend for themselves. Some degree at hand but no hope of any employment. Educated unemployed youth faces crisis, frustration and get into bad habits like consuming tobacco through smoking and eating and doing harm to them. They waist there precious time and energy in unnecessary things.

Because of lack of proper guidance and lack of knowledge results depression. They lack ambition, they look for easy life. They lack adventures, they are afraid of going out for jobs and develop negative attitude towards life, I cannot do this, suffer from low self esteem, no encouragement from the parents or elders. If they want to do something for society they do not get cooperation and there opinion is not taken into consideration. They are easily falling into love affairs, physical attraction and make mess of their lives.

Faced with this reality given number of solutions to live life to the full and challenges ahead. We have to take up this task and live no stone unturned to establish—

Self identity of youth is strength. They are talented and skilled. They are adolescents, who are in search of an identity. In this age of mass media, high-tech, the true image of human being is being corroded. Having is being to be is to have is the philosophy propagated by the consumerist society. In this situation, we have to pledge to help the youth discover their self-identity and self worth as children of God.

Each and every youth has a dream. They want to achieve something in life. But for this the youth needs to undergo wholistic formation that will prepare them intellectually, emotionally, socially and spiritually in such a way that together with self-enhancement they are able to contribute to the betterment of society. Value education is an essential component of this formation.

The youths are a force to reckon with. The potentials they possess are enormous. These need to be recognized, nurtured and developed. But today's consumerist and competitive world, survival of the fittest is the order of the day. Such a scenario calls for the organization of the youth for awareness. Awareness of the exploitative reality and its consequences on the depressed classes, the environmental degradation they are facing, and the consciousness of the grim future that awaits them. This realization, we hope, will lead them to a reflective action that will slowly change the face of the earth and build a world more humane and where every human being lives a dignified life.

There are thousands of youth in the urban streets, slums and shanty dwellings in the cities. Loosing the sense of direction they take up to various vices like drinking, drugs and other forms of unhealthy practices. With little effort we will be able to recognize them, engage them in constructive endeavors and change the course of their lives. Like the other youth, the unorganized urban youth too respond to challenges laid out before them. Instill self-identity in them. Work for their integral formation. Help them make life's choices like career, organize them for awareness and collective action so that they safeguard and promote their culture heritage and social identity.

To unite them so as through mutual cooperation and encouragement they take up their own problems and needs, effectively and they become good citizens, they carry out the responsibility of building up a just society. The mind is most powerful weapon. You get out of something what you put into it. Give and you shall receive. Once you have gained a true understanding of something, the knowledge will be with you for the rest of your life. To excel, one has to focus all energy on the task. Stay focus on one thing. Not to take more then you can handle. Live each moment to the full. Having a big ego gets you nowhere. If you believe in yourself, that a higher power is on your side, you can accomplish anything. You can change your destiny. You are who you perceive yourself to be.

Only you know who you are. Reality is ones perception of reality, nothing more. Preconceived ideas and prejudices always prevent us from seeing the truth. You should open your mind before you open your mouth. Be open to new experience, there is still more to learn. The more you know, the less you know. No matter how much you know, there is always someone who can teach you more. The journey is more important than the destination.

You have to accommodate yourself to life and get used to dealing with your problems as they come. You must learn to cooperate. Because nature is so much more powerful than we are, we must become one with it in order to survive. Ok with what life gives you and you will survive. Put your life into Gods hands and you will be ok. His will help you come out on the top. You should take control of a situation before it takes control of you. If you have faith, things will work out. You don't know what you've got till it's gone.

Without God we are nothing. Just being is the hardest things in life. Knowing yourself is most important thing. Life is not static, change occurs all the time. There are good days and bad days. Being alive has its ups and downs, rain and sun, illness and health, laughter and tears. Nothing bad will last forever. Nothing good will last forever either. Time is mighty force that wipes everything out. Life is a process, not a conclusion. Your road through life may be filled with an assortment of ruts and rocks, but it also has pleasant stretches of pavement. Time heals all.

Nothing is permanent, enjoy, stop complaining. God controls our lives. We may not understand his purpose, so just accept what happens. Nothing occurs by accident. Everything happens for a reason, and worry about what will happen will not help. If you take life just as it comes, one day at a time, eventually you will be able to see the big purpose to it all. If you think positive about events in your life, they will turn OK. Stretch out your wings and fly. Believe in yourself in the power you have to control your own life, day by day. Believe in tomorrow and what it will bring for things will work out if you trust and believe, there is no limit to what you can do.

Youth has explosive power within; if he gets proper guidance, he can recreate himself. Believe in yourself; do not be carried away by worldly values. You are designed for accomplishment and endowed with the seeds of greatness. You are the only one who can use your own abilities.

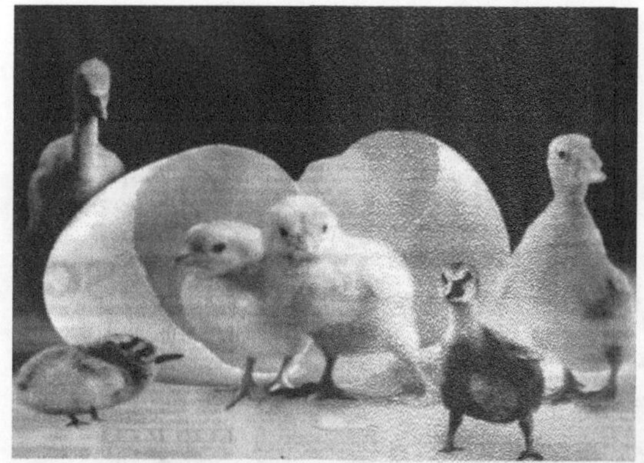

Fig. 14.1: Youth and self discovery. Grow and bloom unto the fullness

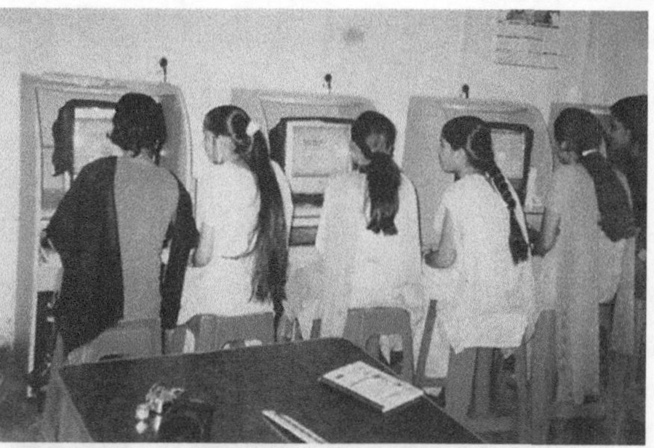

Fig. 14.2: Skill development and training programs

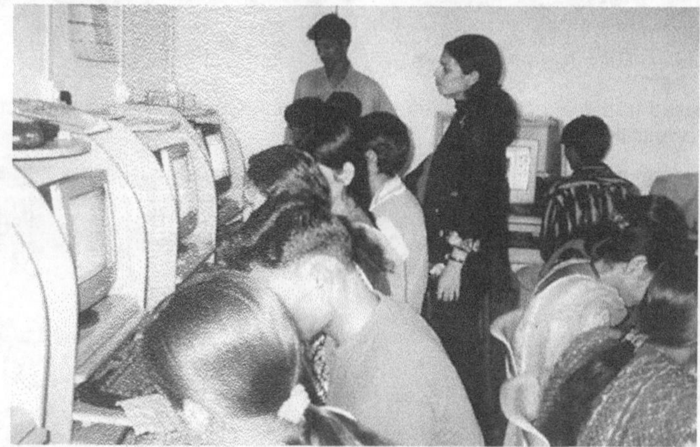

Fig. 14.3: Computer training

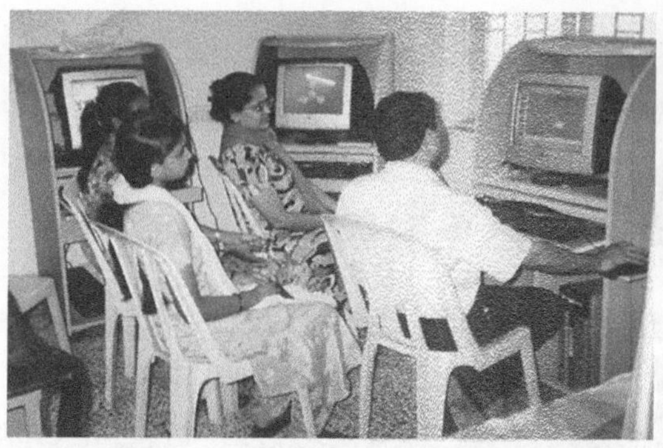

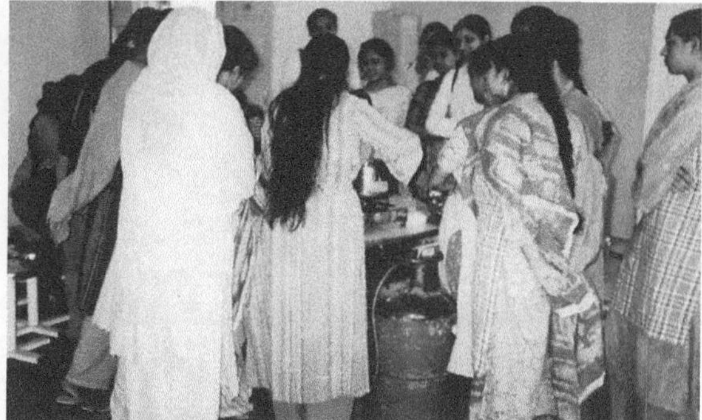

Figs 14.4 and 14.5: If our nation has to rise how it can do so if half of women of the nation lack behind and remain ignorant. Women's organization for capacity building.

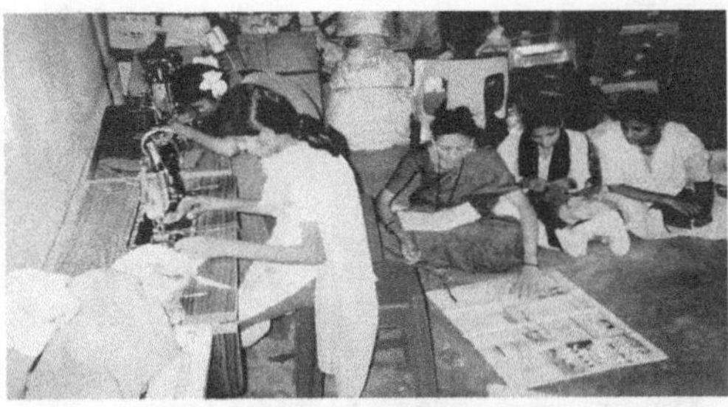
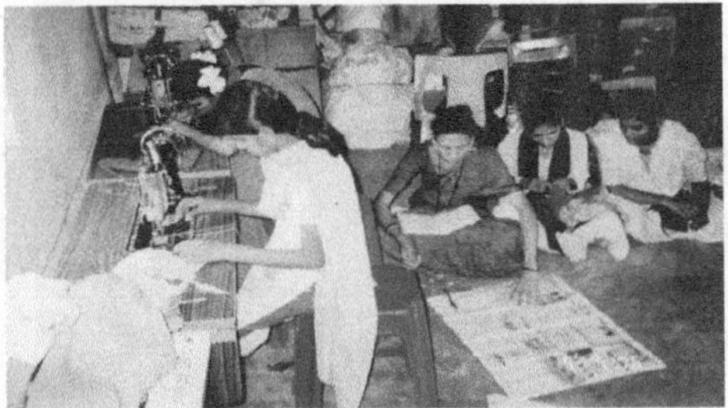

Figs 14.6 and 14.7: Training youth for tailoring. Self help employment creation

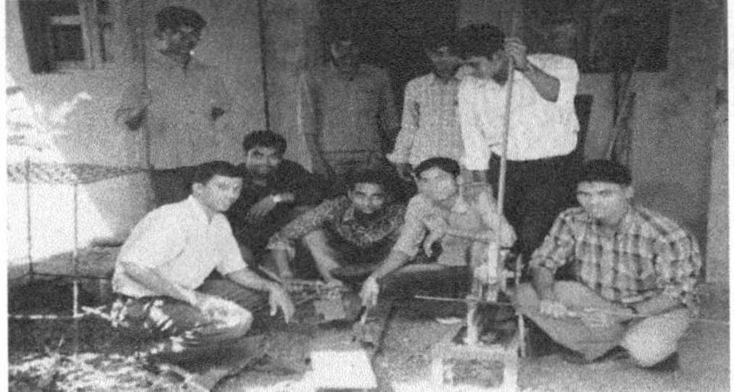

Fig. 14.8: Agro-based trades, electrical trades, mechanical trades

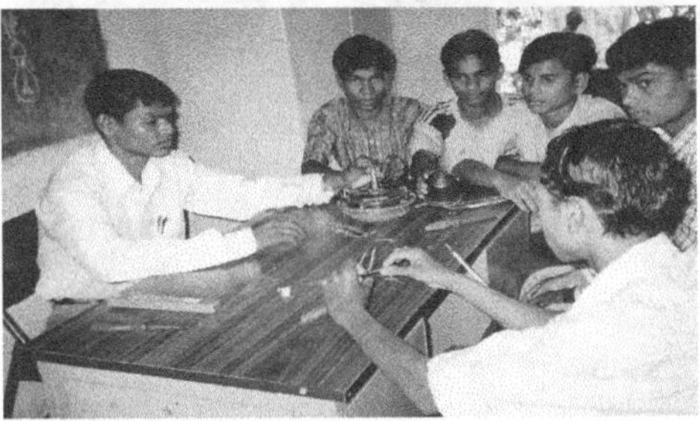

Fig. 14.9: Guiding and giving direction to youth

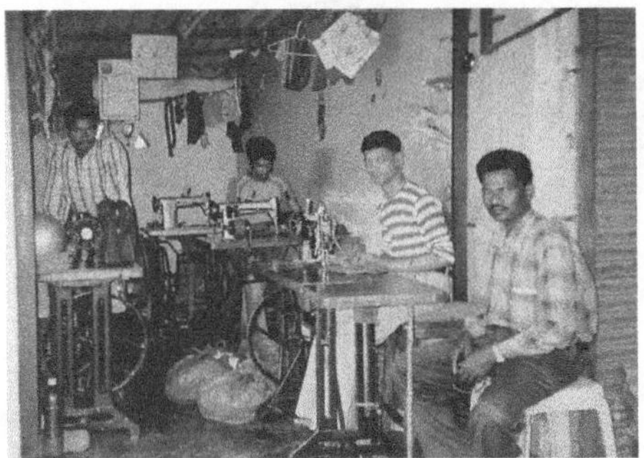
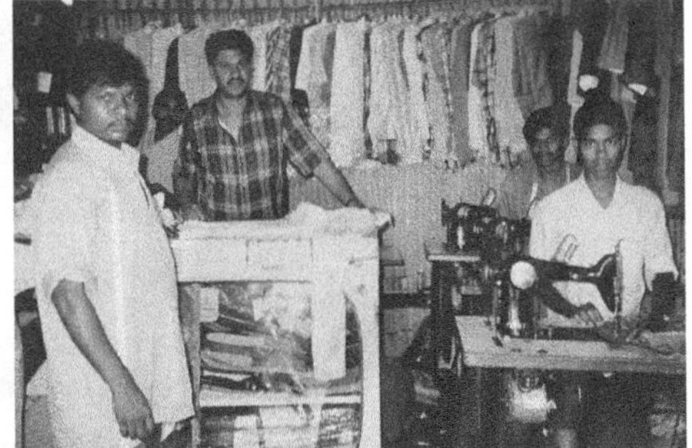

Figs 14.10 and 14.11: Livelihood; After training, working independently

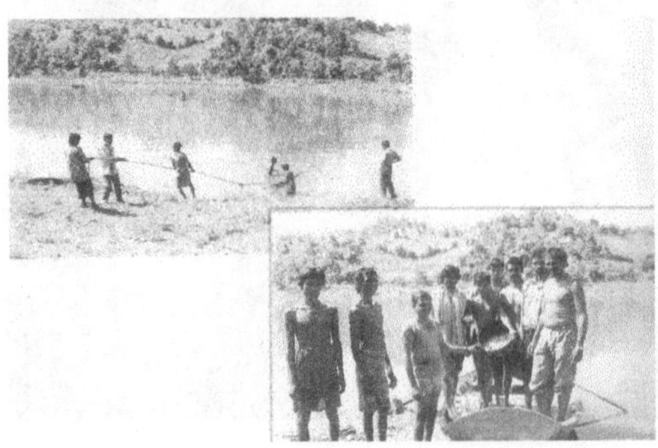

Fig. 14.12: From basket to fishing

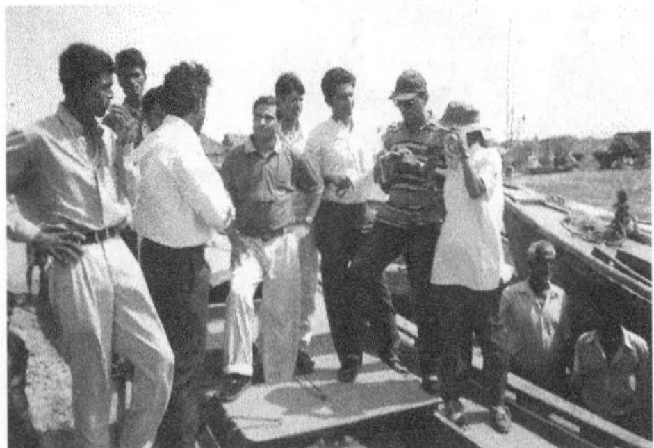

Fig. 14.13: Youth with zest and vigor. Allround development

15 Malaria: A Community Health Problem

Malaria continues to be major scourge in India including metropolitan cities. It is a protozoal disease caused by infection with parasites plasmodium and transmitted to man by certain species of infected bite of female Anopheles mosquito. A single dose of chloroquine may save the life by averting complications.

Malaria is a tropical disease, which occurs, in hot, moist climate. Malaria is most widespread disease of the world. One of humanity's greatest scourges transmitted anopheles mosquito female species bites a patient who has malaria. She draws up a small quantity of blood containing the parasites. These parasites then pass through several stages of development within the mosquito's body, and finally find their way to its salivary glands. There they lie in wait for an opportunity to enter the bloodstream of the next individual the mosquito bites.

About 10 days after the mosquito has injected these parasites into a personal bloodstream, many more parasites can be seen under a microscope. Most of them are now within the RBC of the victim. There they grow until they eventually replace all the hemoglobin within the cell. Although probably only one parasite attacks cell. As a cell breaks up, these are released. Each tiny parasite then attacks another RBC, thus repeating the cycle every 2–3 days.

Many of the parasites are destroyed by the defense system of the body, WBC in spleen, liver, a bone marrow. But enough of them survive to cause plenty of trouble. Good nursing care essential. The patient should be given plenty of fluids, fresh fruits, juices and a balanced diet. A personal precaution is to sleep under a mosquito net. Children's beds should be screened by nets.

Typical sudden onset of high fever with rigors and sensation of extreme cold followed by feeling of burning heat, leading to profuse sweating and remission of fever by crisis thereafter. The febrile paroxysms occur every alternate day. Headache, bodyache, nausea, may be associated features. In children depending on the degree of temperature, complications such as convulsions, dehydration and disorientation may be present. A typical attack comprises of 3 stages such as a cold stage, a hot stage and a sweating stage. The clinical features vary from mild to severe and complicated according to the species of parasite present; the client state of immunity, the intensity of the infection, malnutrition.

Malaria is one of the oldest recorded diseases in the world. Most widespread, a major public health problem in the tropical developing world. Among all infectious diseases, Malaria continuous to be one of the biggest contributors to disease burdens in terms of death and suffering.

Greatest risk of dying are children under age 5 years in Malaria endemic areas, pregnant women, people moving from non-malarious zones for reason's of work, migration, refuge, war or tourism, travelers who visit endemic countries and return home with the disease. Malaria kills more than 1 million children (Africa), many women in malarious regions are anemic, 25% babies born low birth weight. Over and above the economic loss due to not going to work and medicines cost.

Malaria affects all ages. Male more exposed due to outdoor life. Malaria is a mosquito-borne disease, and is characterized by fever with rigors and profuse sweating, enlargement of spleen and anemia. It has a tendency to relapse. It is a public health hazard as well as major mortality rate problem in India.

Complications of *P. falciparum* malaria: Hyperpyrexia, severe anemia resulting in hypoxia, cerebral involvement, pulmonary edema, renal dysfunction, hypoglycemia, hemoglobinuria and jaundice may occur.

Individual cases, house to house survey by health visitors to survey and detect cases. Administration of chloroquine to all fever cases. Collection of blood films of fever cases, laboratory examination of blood films collected from survey for confirmation of malaria. Blood smears should be made from all clients reporting with fever, if suspected for malaria.

Method of blood smear—Third finger of the left hand of the client should be held with left hand between thumb and finger by blood slide collected at the first phalangeal joint. Wipe fingertip with swab dipped in spirit savlon solution. Allow the fingertip to dry. Hold the pricking needle in the right hand and prick the finger. Allow the blood drop to ooze out. Take a clean slide. Take the three drops of blood. One cm from the edge of the glass slide. Take another drop of blood one cm from the first drop of blood. Take another slide with smooth edge and use it as spreader. Make thick and thin smears. Allow it to dry. Put the slide identification number/name on thin smear with lead pencil.

Measures against mosquitoes by screening of windows/doors of house. Proper clothing, use of mosquito repellent, use mosquito net, do not allow water to stagnate in the house or surrounding the house for more than 7 days. Dry your cooler every Sunday with complete change of water. Spraying of insecticide against adult mosquitoes. Larvicidal operations to eradicate growth of larva. Community surveillance to find out active and passive cases. Source reduction measures such as elimination of mosquito breeding places in and around houses. Facilities of health services such as diagnosis, medicine and health care. Health education of population regarding preventive steps and treatment of malaria.

NMEP/National Malaria Eradication Program was launched in 1953, the incidence of malaria from 75 million dropped into 2 million cases in 1958. In 1977, it was modified. A health worker is assigned the detection of malaria by signs and symptoms. Health worker is allotted to population of 10,000 or 2000 houses. He is required to visit them regularly during visit to enquire, give single 1st dose of chloroquine, blood films taken and laboratory shows/proves malaria, he returns to the patients for radical treatment till patient becomes normal. National Eradication Program depends on cooperation of voluntary health workers, follow-up cases.

All confirmed microscopically positive cases of malaria are to be given radical treatment with Primaquine, which ensures a complete cure from malaria in the positive case and makes him non-infective to mosquitoes. Cases are given radical treatment for 5 days. The adult dose is as follows:

A single dose of 600 mg of Chloroquine 10 mg/kg body weight and 15 mg of Primaquine 0.25 mg/kg body weight on the first day followed by 15 mg Primaquine daily for next four days.

Caution to be taken and infant and pregnant women are not to be given Primaquine.

In case of falciparum malaria, a course of quinine/plus tetracycline for 4–7 days has been recommended.

Do not give antimalarial drug on empty stomach. Do not use corticosteroids, do not give IV manitol. Do not use heparin as anticoagulant. Do not administer adrenaline. Do not overhydrate.

PRESUMPTIVE TREATMENT FOR MALARIA

Age in year	*Single dose of Chloroquine 150 mg*
0–1 year	75 mg (½ Tab)
1–4 years	150 mg (1 Tab)
4–8 years	300 mg (2 Tab)
8–14 years	450 mg (3 Tab)
14 and above	600 mg (4 Tab)

Referral of malaria cases—Persistence of fever after 48 hours of initial treatment. Continuous vomiting and inability to retain oral drugs. Headache, which is continuously increasing. Severe dehydration, general condition is too weak. Changes in sensorial that is confusion, drowsiness, blurring of vision, photophobia, disorientation, convulsion or muscle twitching, severe anemia, jaundice, hyperthermia, bleeding, clotting disorder, pulmonary edema, hemoglobinuria. Transfer the client to the hospital.

Prophylaxis—People traveling to malaria zone and desiring to protect them are put on chloroquine therapy, e.g. 2 Tab of 300 mg once a week. They should start 1 week before and continue for 6 weeks or till they leave malaria zone.

Setbacks—Technical problem such as resistance of mosquito vector to insecticides, and malarial drugs was serious obstacles. Administrative failure, rising cost and shortage of drug, operational failure of schemes inadequate surveillance, in adequate coverage leaving many houses unsprayed, undue reliance of basic workers who were unprepared experienced people leaving job.

Toxic hazards of drugs—Side effect of chloroquine: Nausea, vomiting, blurring of vision, headaches, retinal damage, should not be given on empty stomach, toxic manifestation involving the CNS, gastrointestinal cramps, cardiovascular cyanosis, warning sign, treatment stop.

New drugs in malaria such as melfoquine and halofantrine and Chinese herbal remedy known as artemisnin drugs, clear the blood faster than other drugs. Mass drug administration WHO emphasizing control/eradication best method for curbing of transmission with extensive antimosquito measures. Chemoprophylaxis is still desirable to pregnant women causing low birth weight, anemia, high-risk life threatening malaria attacks.

Malaria is a complex disease and its intensity of distribution varies from place to place. Vaccination against malaria is a burning issue today. Vaccines are designed to arrest the development of parasite and reduce transmission a synthetic cocktail vaccine for *P. falciparum* called SPF 66 development recently.

Presumptive treatment means that all fever cases are assumed to due to malaria. This is often the only practical and effective approach in a community-based program.

In 1950s, it was number one health problem. In 1953, National Malarial Eradication Program was launched. The initial success was spectacular. Vectors developed resistance to insecticides therefore the program was upgraded in 1958. One disturbing trend was observed, i.e. the gradual increase in falciparum malaria during the same period. National Malaria Eradication Program for *P. falciparum* also was launched.

Primary Health Centers (PHCs) are involved in the collection and examination of blood smears from fever cases through multipurpose workers. The program in the rural and remote areas relies on community participation. The drug distribution centers are manned by panchayat members, forest officials, village health guide, teachers, forest revenue officials.

Insecticide spraying supervision done by District Malaria Officers. In 1994, malaria action plans to identify most affected areas, hard-core tribal areas, epidemic prone areas, project areas, urban areas was given serious thought. Guidelines of the action plan included the Management of serious and complicated malaria cases. Prevention of mortality with particular reference to high-risk groups. Reduction of morbidity. Control of outbreaks/epidemics. Reduction of *P. falciparum* incidence, and containment of drug resistant malaria. Maintenance of low incidence statue.

Malaria health education inculcates individual/community protective and preventive habits within socioeconomic and environmental context. Malaria week observed before the onset of monsoon, i.e. 1st May to 7th May every year. The main objective is to create awareness among the masses about malaria and its prevention.

CONCLUSION

Many diseases are seasonal infections like dengue, leptospirosis, and now chikungunya were not prevalent in our country. Changes in the environment and urbanization, lack of proper garbage disposal and unhygienic conditions has resulted in this illness getting a foothold in India in epidemic proportions. Pools and puddles of stagnant water serve as breeding sites of mosquitoes. Different mosquitoes spread different diseases. Malaria is transmitted by anopheles mosquito bite, Dengue by Aedes, and Chikungunya by Aedes agypti and an albopictus mosquito bite.

Malaria is caused by *P. vivax* and *P. falciparum*. It destroys blood (RBC's) in the body. *P. falciparum* can enter the brain (severe cerebral malaria) it causes fever with chills, headache.

Dengue is caused by many different strains of dengue virus. It leads to a spectrum of illness from mild to very severe dengue fever-dengue hemorrhagic fever-dengue shock syndrome.

Malaria and dengue can be fatal if not treated promptly.

Chikungunya is caused by viruses (togavirus-alphavirus) causes fever with chills, bodyaches, leg swelling, joint pains, headache and extreme weakness. Fever generally lasts for 2-3 days but may last longer. Fever can be recurrent, bodyaches, and leg swelling and other symptoms may persist for weeks. May be very debilitating, chikungunya is not fatal. Consult doctor immediately. Prompt and early treatment prevents complications and death.

Prevention measures—Use of mosquito repellents, nets at home. Each residential society should ensure that pools, puddles of stagnant water are filled up with mud. Spraying of insecticides. Plants kept outside windows serve as stagnant water pools and important breeding sites for mosquitoes. Tiers stacked in a tire/puncture shop accumulate water throughout the year and serve as breeding sites for mosquitoes. Proper waste/garbage disposal.

How healthy is a community? Responsibility for health, on one hand personal responsibility and other hand a major public concern. It involves the joint effort of the whole social fabric that is the individual, community and state to protect and promote health. It has to be earned and maintained by the individual himself. By self-care preventing their own diseases, limiting their own illness and restoring their own health, individual can get information, technical knowledge and skill observing simple rules of diet, sleep, exercise, weight, alcohol, and smoking. Attention to personal hygiene, healthy habits, lifestyle, selective medical examination, screening, accepting immunization and disease prevention measures carrying out.

The individual and community responsibilities are complementing. Active involvement of families and community that is planning, implementation, utilization, operation and evaluation of health services, people's participation. The health requires the cooperation of government, national and international help to elevate and to remove injustice that disturbs health services, social causes such as poverty, hunger, malnutrition, illiteracy, unemployment, human dignity, and human welfare.

To make health insurance as health assurance. Environmental health is an important component of community health. Safe wholesome and adequate drinking water is therefore a basic to community health service. It should be free from harmful pathogenic bacteria. As health may get affected by the ingestion of such water cause water related illness.

Historical rise and fall of disease pattern in community never constant, new infections keep adding to it, the pattern changes, interruption of transmission- breaking interruption of chain is an constant effort. From time immemorial man interested to control an ivory of disease, down the ages in history we see ever changing concept, goals and objectives theories are at the background of today modern medicines.

Earlier we had traditional healers, ayurveda and many other indigenous practices. Since India became free, several measures undertaken by national government to improve the health of the people. Which have been launched by government to control and eradicate communicable disease rising started of nutrition, control of population, improving rural health and various international agencies provide technical and material assistance. Dawn of scientific revival of medicine, sanitary awakening, rise of public health. Today modern medicines are more costly and complex.

New York researchers have developed a new technique that is much faster and cheaper than the rapid diagnostic tests. The technique uses magneto optic technology to detect hemozoin, a waste product of malaria parasite, in the blood.

Its goal is not merely to treat illness but prevention of disease, promotion of health and improving quality of life of individual group and community.

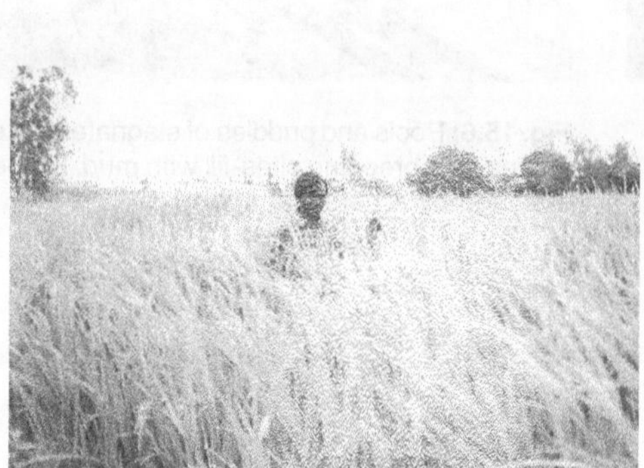

Fig. 15.1: Mosquito breeding: spraying pesticides for control

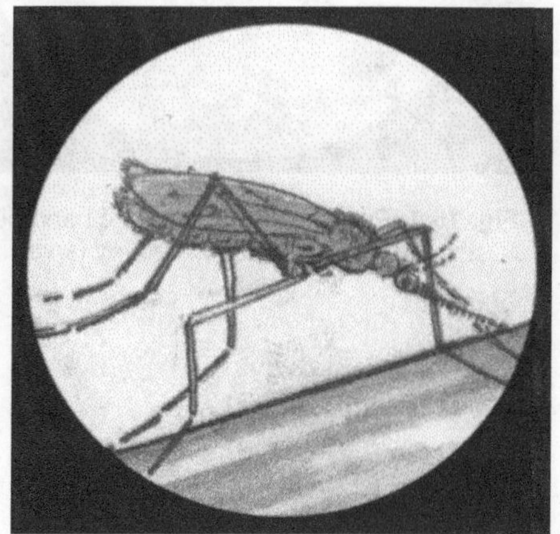

Fig. 15.2: The malaria germ is carried by the anopheles mosquito, when biting this mosquito assumes the position showed in the drawing

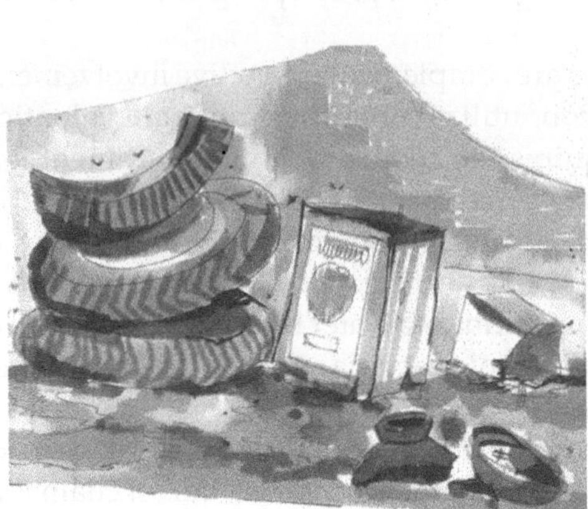

Fig. 15.3: Breeding ground of mosquitoes: To keep malaria under control, keep surrounding clean, and do not allow water get stagnated in tiers, stacked in tire puncture shop, accumulates water etc

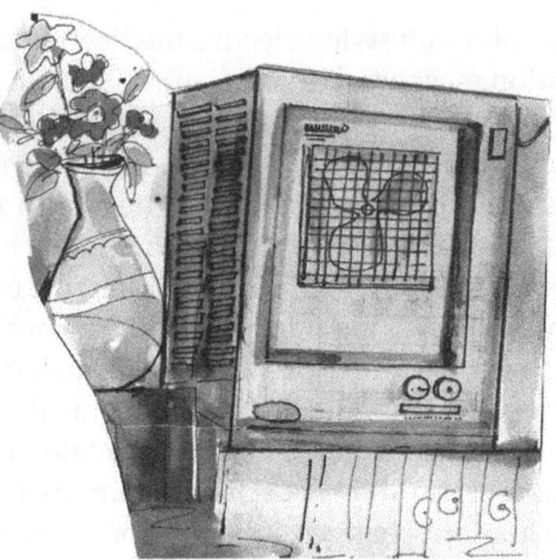

Fig. 15.4: Change water from flowerpots and keep toilet clean

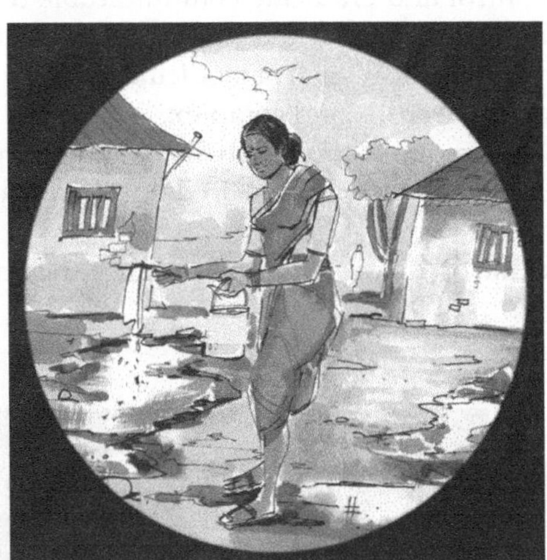

Fig. 15.5: Put kerosene or crude oil and burn the top level of water to destroy larvae

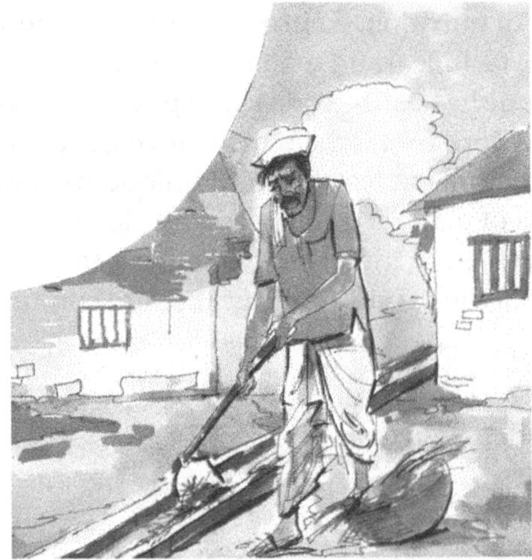

Fig. 15.6: Pools and puddles of stagnated water serves as a breeding sites-fill with mud. Proper drainage by a personal effort

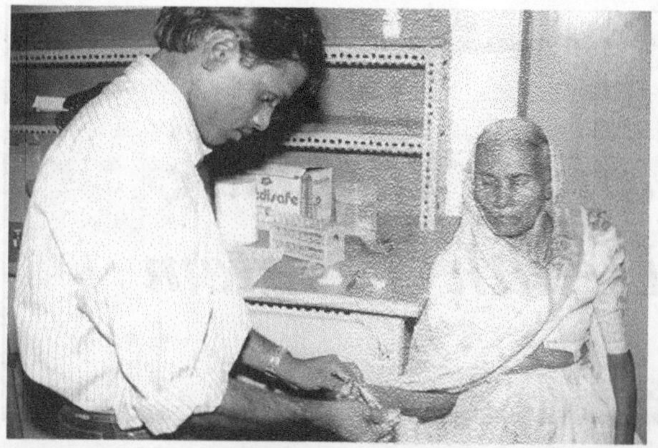

Fig. 15.7: Taking malaria slides for detecting parasites

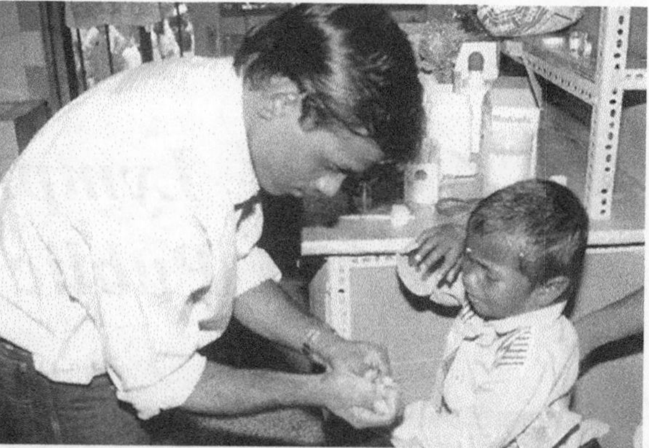

Fig. 15.8: Lab: Blood test

16 Lymphatic Filariasis: Public Health Problem

It is mosquito born disease caused by filarial parasites. It is transmitted by the bite of culex mosquitoes. It is manifested as lymphangitis, lymphadenitis, and elephantiasis of genitals, legs and arms. Pulmonary eosinophilia, filarial arthritis. Though not fatal, the disease is responsible for considerable sufferings, deformities and disability.

Filariasis is a global problem. Millions of people are at risk and get infected in the World. China, India, and Indonesia are more prone area. So it has become public health problem. The problem is increasing day by day. Heavily infected areas are found in UP, AP, Bihar etc. in India. Two types: *W. bancrofti* and *B. malayi*.

There are 8 species of filarial parasites. The adult worms are usually found in the lymphatic system of man, which finds their way into blood circulation via lymphatic. There is a mosquito cycle in stages – larva that penetrates in the stomach wall and in later stage becomes infective. The parasite is small thread-like worm.

All ages are susceptible to infection. It is found in infant age less than 6 months old, social factor responsible like urbanization, industrialization, migration of people, illiteracy, poverty and poor sanitation.

Climate is important factor to influence the breeding, bad drainage, sewage disposal, lack of town planning aggravates problem, pools, soakage pits, septic tanks, open ditches, burrow pits etc.

Infected bite the parasite is deposited site of puncture. It passes through the punctured skin and reaches the lymphatic system. Clinical incubation period is 8–16 months or longer. Although their blood is positive they may remain without symptom. In some instances they are hidden/dormant many years. They are an important source of infection in the community. These carriers are usually detected by night blood examination.

In the first months and years there are recurrent episodes of acute inflammation in lymph glands and vessels. The clinical manifestations comprise filarial fever, lymphangitis, and lymphoedema of body epididymo-orchitis in the man. The chronic stage envelopes 10–15 years from the onset of the first acute attack due to fibrosis and obstruction of the lymphatic vessels causing permanent structural changes. Hydrocele, elephantiasis of legs, scrotum, arms, penis, vulva and breast gets affected.

1. Mass blood survey (night blood collection) 8-30 pm to 12 midnights.
2. Clinical survey – people are examined for signs and symptoms

3. Entomological survey – general mosquito collection from houses – study.
4. Control measures – full regimen of treatment chemotherapy DEC (Diethylcarbamazine) is the only drug available at present. It is both safe and effective, 6 mg/kg for 12 days. DEC is rapidly absorbed after oral administration, reaching peak blood levels in 1–2 hours.

It is also rapidly excreted.

Side effect such as headache, nausea, vomiting, dizziness. These reactions disappear spontaneously without treatment.

DEC carried out in mass therapy in community [DEC mass treatment control program]. This requires mass intensive health education.

- DEC medicated salt (common salt medicated) 1–4 gm of DEC used in some of the areas. No drug toxicity noted.
- Vector control would be elimination of breeding places.
- Environmental measures: Filling up ditches, pools, drainage of stagnated water, adequate maintenance of septic tanks and soakage pits etc. Environmental management is the most efficient approach to the problem of controlling mosquito breeding.
- DDT, HCH resistant – so discontinued.
- Pyrethrum as a space spray is a temporary means of personal protection.
- Personal prophylaxis – preventing/avoiding of mosquito bites by using mosquito nets, combine integrated methods can be used for control of filariasis.
- The village health guide is the key person who should be trained at village level. A single dose of DEC also is equally effective.
- Insecticide sprays on seal latrine and rooftop water storage tanks to eliminate and reduce culex mosquitoes.

NFCP: National Filaria Control program launched in the year 1955.

After independence several measures were undertaken by government to improve the health of the people. Special control/eradication of community disease, improvement of environmental sanitation raising the standard of nutrition, control of population and improving rural health.

Various National, International agencies, WHO, UNICEF have been providing technical and material assistance in the implementation of the program.

Filaria recently estimates about 420 million exposed to risk of infection, 19 million manifest diseases, 25 million are in the blood which do not show symptoms. To control recurrent antilarval measures and antiparasitic measures to be taken.

Surveys are in progress in different districts; units set-up clinics and training conducted also continued research being held, to reduce transmission, annual single dose is given door to door delivery and the day mass drug therapy is given is called 'Filaria Day'.

Disease spread by various ways and each disease has its own phenomena such causative agents are viruses, bacteria, fungi, and protozoa.

Certain disease due to heat, cold, pressure, and radiation. Some others are due to electricity, metals, fumes dust, gases, and chronic friction.

There are diseases in certain age, sex, heredity, nutrition, occupation, customs and habits, human behavior, due to poor environment, unsafe water, contaminated soil, poor housing, lack of disposal facilities of human excreta, lack of education, food habits, poverty, personal hygiene, incorrect cooking practices, cultural practices, poor availability of health services. So it is a web and a vicious circle, which leads one to another.

To eradicate common effort needed, initiative and interest also is of vital importance, for that we need relevant, reliable, apt knowledge. Appropriate methods to identification of needs and steps to be taken for effective care. Develop good observation and rapport with people to gain their cooperation, gain effective and positive responses, local resources used by respecting peoples opinions. To gain kills, make people to think for themselves of the consequences and outcome, develop reflective behavior through health teaching and awareness motivation by instilling knowledge. Assessment and systematic collection of data, then set goal on priority of need encountered, implement with regular monitoring and time to time evaluating the outcome.

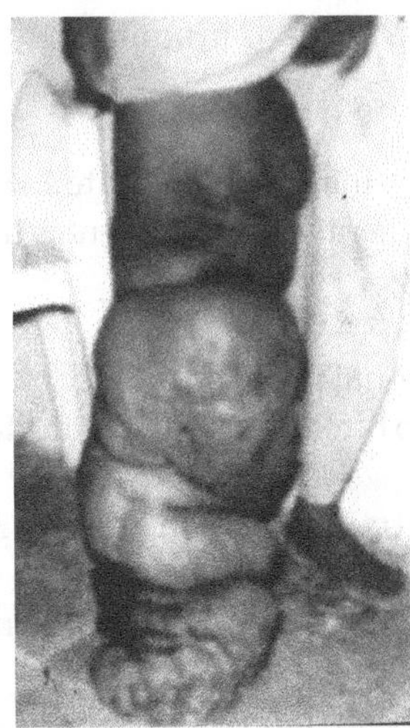

Fig. 16.1: Filariasis is caused by a tiny worm which invades the lymphatic system and connective tissues. Filaria National health problem

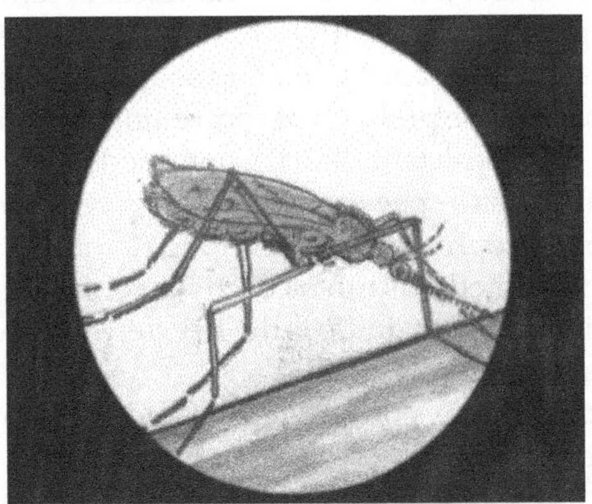

Fig. 16.2: Filariasis too caused by culex mosquito bites. Blood samples taken at night to detect the diseases

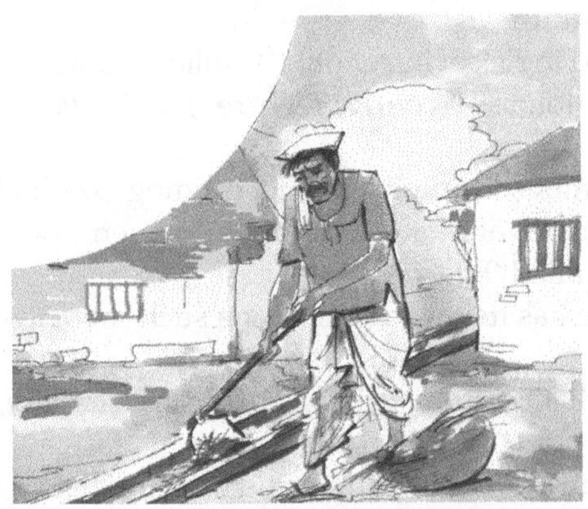

Fig. 16.3: Gutters keep flowing and do not allow to stagnate. Keep the surrounding clean and do not allow free ground for mosquito to breed

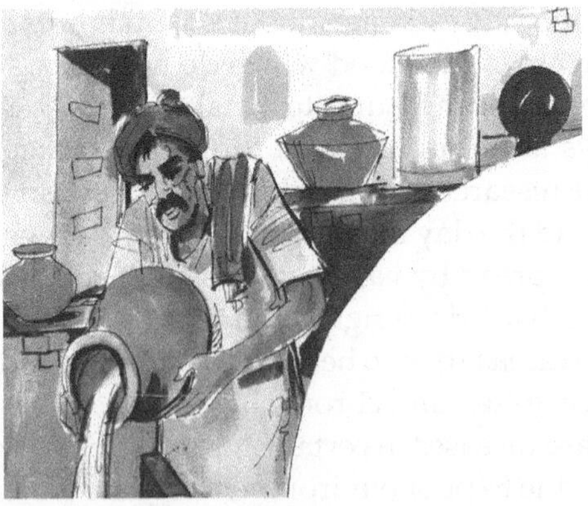

Fig. 16.4: Different mosquitoes spread different diseases. Drinking water should be kept clean by filling fresh water

17 Deadly Disease: Tuberculosis

Tuberculosis is the leading communicable disease of India, and continues to be major health problem. Four people out of per 1000 population have bacteriologically confirmed the disease. It mainly affects lungs. It also can affect intestine, meanings, bone and joints, lymph glands, uterus, skin and other tissues of the body known as extrapulmonary. Tuberculosis is worldwide public health problem despite causative organism discovered more than 100 years ago and highly effective drugs and vaccines are available making tuberculosis a preventable and curable disease. The disease primarily affects the chest organs and causes pulmonary tuberculosis. To make global situation worse tuberculosis combines with HIV. The *tubercle bacillus* may remain dormant for many years and then can reactivate and produce clinical tuberculosis infection which continues a life long relationship between humans and dormant, organism may remain alive in the host for life; it is known as walking time bomb.

Breathing is the first law of life. No one can live more than few seconds without an adequate supply of oxygen. We must have fresh air to stay alive. Tuberculosis makes over 75% of women who suffer from tuberculosis, thousands of children, on the other hand drop out of school on account of parental illness; while over 20% of them take up jobs in order to supplement income over 35% clients admitted to not being able to afford to buy adequate food, clothing and books for children due to loss of income. India has 3.8 million tuberculosis clients at any time. It is estimated 3% of all new cases are multi-drug resistant tuberculosis. To date 6.7 million clients in India have received Dots treatment averting more than 1.22 million deaths. Over the last 10 years 20 million clients have been placed on effective treatment globally. But the diseases still kills 4400 people everyday over 6 lakhs Indians are unaware that they suffer from tuberculosis. India and china account for an estimated 28% of all undetected new cases.

Tuberculosis is one of the oldest diseases known to man. Tuberculosis may attack any part of the body, but it is most frequently found in the lungs. Coughing and sneezing usually spread about its germs. They can ride on particles of dust or water droplets floating in the air. One cough from client can spread many thousands of germs into the air, so that other person inhaling them may become infected with this dreaded disease.

Danger signals undo tiredness and fatigue, progressive weight loss, chronic cough, spitting up blood occasionally, chest pain, night sweats, an afternoon fever, or loss of appetite.

Surgery—Severely damaged lung tissues should be removed by surgery if possible. Healing is quicker and more complete if such tissues are removed and if the client is able to stand the surgery.

Medical control and prevention of fetal disease is very important. TB is number one killer diseases. Identification of patient through health personals house visits, diagnosis and regular follow-up could be done according to doctors' order. So they can benefit accurate diagnosis, cheaper prescription and less overloads of drugs. Problems of spread of drug resistance and dropouts are on increase. Drug resistance remains high; poverty economic recession and malnutrition make population more vulnerable. Drug resistance is threat worldwide. Incomplete and inappropriate treatment makes the situation worse. No single country in the world has succeeded in reaching the point of control.

Every month, one-day specially kept as a TB clinic day. Client is registered in clinic and special case paper kept for a record. Clients too provided with a number card so that they remember when to come and how many month treatments one have to take. As when they come regularly, weight is recorded and needful advice is given. Also personal and in common health education is given. They are made aware of the seriousness of the decease. They are explained in detail the advantages and disadvantages of the course of the treatment. Otherwise if the course remains incomplete the consequences on self, family and in society they live increases and the drug resistance they develop is harmful for them and the family.

In the villages, people casually brushing off that chronic cough as simple chest congestion that has struck them for little long and do not come for treatment. But many times it is very risky. Given the fact that around 50% of the country's population suffers from TB of which one patient succumbs to the deadly disease in every-single minute, it is quiet probable that these patients might also be coughing this way to death.

The TB scene in the rural areas is even more threatening as the intensity of the damage done by the killer disease is not known even by the government who does not carry out survey to find the exact number of TB cases in the villages. The district TB officer has estimated certain number, which could be much higher as private doctors and a large number treat 40% of patients, goes undetected.

Caused by the *Mycobacterium tuberculosis* or the *Tubercle bacilli;* TB spreads through air and by casual contact. The major source of infection is however in the case in which bacilli is shed in the sputum that remains alive for weeks in the dust particles. Inhalation of such dust is the principal mode of infection in villages observed. Other factors came across are poor living conditions, lack of diagnostic facilities and poor knowledge of such facilities. Observed that this disease occurs at any age groups and affects any organ of the body. However, lungs are the much affected, as 90% have is pulmonary kind.

When seen patient coughing more than 3 weeks, chest pain, sudden breathlessness, loss of weight, fever, spitting in blood, take the patient immediately for investigations, like x-ray chest, ESR test (erythrocyte sedimentation rate test), which helps in diagnosis, presence of the bacilli in sputum is a definite proof of the diseases.

Tuberculosis is a chronic and stigmatizing disease. Revised National TB Control Program (RNTCP) that is Dots (Directly observed treatment) a short course treatment lasting six months and the defaulter rate is much less and more effective manager of TB. On an average 5, 00,000 people die of TB every year in India. It is because TB is a poor man's disease. TB is still the number one killer communicable disease, which can be controlled by human effort. One patient dies of TB every minute in India. It is estimated that 2% of the population is having tuberculosis of which 0.4% are sputum positive for AFB that is the stage of spreading the disease to the other in community. TB prevalence and diagnosis shows that 60% uninfected with organism AFB. 40% infected with AFB. 2% with diseases. Out of 2%, 1.6% sputum negative is diagnosed only on x-ray. 4% sputum positive can be diagnosed only on sputum examination under microscope.

The lungs are one of the most vulnerable parts of the body both structurally and functionally, since they have to exchange gases they are necessarily exposed to the wide variety of environment agents such as smokes, fumes, and dusts. The presence of foreign particles in the lungs affects its normal functioning, and the person develops respiratory diseases and disorder.

Difficulties: Apathy towards treatment not inclined because one is not getting well as fast as one wishes. Drugs as soon as started relieve of symptom problems the patient to stop the treatment in the middle. Patient continues other habits like smoking or drinking. Socioeconomic conditions, which give rise to problem, which the patient cannot handle. In chronic cases when the patient is still with cough or breathlessness as ones lung is destroyed or more than half lung destroyed the patient often will not stick to the treatment and change the doctor or hospital leading to a different drug regimen.

Under such circumstances where Community Health Nurse play vital role in motivating the patient and the family. Community Health Nurse tell them in advance this is the danger and the temptation, also most of the patients are from the villages where Community Health Nurse visits regularly and is in touch, Community Health Nurse keep asking, checking and inquiring about the patient. Community Health Nurse's main thrust is to given regular intake of drugs, completion of therapy and achieving cure in every sputum positive patient. Her continuous insistence and giving due importance to uninterrupted free supply of drugs, nutritional milk, eggs, vitamin supply, free laboratory test and other X-ray, screening, traveling fare, health education can lessened the dropouts. TB is too expensive for the poor who are malnourished, underweight and unable to work hard. The shortest course of treatment is say 6 months and the longest 9 months or more. Therefore, total drugs may cost big amount if added the amount needed for traveling, diagnosis, nutrition that would bring the cost Rs 5000. The poor are unable to buy drugs, which sometimes sleep without food, and fall victims such patients need urgent attention to free them from this clutches of infectious diseases.

After few weeks of treatment, the cough and some of the symptoms begin to disappear. Therefore, there is a natural tendency for the patience to stop the treatment, which is resulting in dropouts from the program. Irregular treatment leads to patient developing a resistance to the drugs. It is not easy to convince them of the seriousness of the disease and the importance of curing it. The constant efforts of the Community Health Nurse have made things easy with health education and motivation in this matter. It is heart warming to see so many of them cured of the diseases and living a healthy life. Many of them come for a regular check-up for some months after they have finished the treatment. They are advised to take additional nutrition and whenever they come for a check-up regular weight is done and recorded.

Thus, it helps to extend hands and join for common cause. Where patients are restored back to normal life, with added smile, and warmth with integrated holistic approach, which elevates and restores their confidence.

Tuberculosis remains a major and increasing problem in the villages. Family and community action is taken to reduce the occurrence of illness and death from tuberculosis. As this prolonged illness places a serious burden on the family resources. Good nutrition is important in resisting TB infection. As patient who is under care and follows the advice of drug regime and diet can get completely cured.

The development of health is a holistic process related to the overall growth and development of social, cultural, economic, educational, political and environmental factors. Health also depends on many supportive services such as water supply, sanitation, nutrition, public health and medical services and human resources.

The grim tale of poverty and under development of millions of our citizens is brought home now and again, and inspite of numerous unimaginative economic development schemes of the Government, their socioeconomic condition remains overwhelmingly distressing. A report made by "The Independent Commission on Health in India" in 1997 has made interesting studies and has critically analyzed the existing health system. We need to identify the critical areas in field of health care, which call for a through reconstructing of the health delivery system and above all a rethinking.

The prolonged monsoon also affected the harvesting and many indeed suffered from acute scarcity of food at home. The harvested crop is what they count on, but many cannot harvest on time due to heavy rains, and when harvested later much of the grains get either rotten or sprouted. It is very distressing that the poor always the victims of the natural calamities.

Tuberculosis is still among the top 10 killer diseases of India. In every Indian village there are at least two or three TB cases, which can be proved by sputum examination. These cases are dangerous to others as they can spread the diseases. Children are commonly infected as a result of contact with a TB case. TB is curable and in fact it can be prevented. There are signs and symptoms, which should alert one when he/she is infected. Immediate check-up to confirm or to deny the infection is a must. Early detection and immediate treatment ensures certain cure. It is essential to undertake proper and full treatment for TB without break as this cures TB and controls its spread, incomplete or interrupted treatment can actually harm the patient and delay complete recovery.

However, if treatment is discontinued the disease becomes active again and the symptoms and signs reappear. Irregular treatment leads to the patient developing a resistance to the drug, that is, drugs become ineffective and often-stronger medicines may need to be prescribed. Due to lack of money, nonexistence of health facilities for proper check ups and diagnosis, remoteness of their place of residence etc delays the diagnosis and treatment. Their lack of proper information about the disease, the nature of treatment and the negative effect of interrupted treatment make the implantation of this program very difficult.

If the patients have still slow grade fever, cough with sputum, breathlessness, asthma, debility, weakness, low weight, chest pain and malnutrition, added attention could be given. Confirmed kocks cases are referred for x-ray, screening, ESR, and sputum test. Every three months all the patients are send for recheck up in different hospitals. Once a complete check up is done according to doctor's order a course of treatment is completed. A special attention could be paid to patients who have still habits of smoking or drinking and serious warning is given. A special advice on diet and nutrition is given.

A special nutritional protein could be provided every month. Also daily eggs and milk could be given for a month from the clinic. Necessary antibiotic, vitamins and tonics together with AKT multi-drug therapy is provided free of cost. Most of the patients who get TB are bilateral pulmonary kocks. So follow-up becomes easy. Once chest is clear, weight increased, no anemia, appetite improved, patient able to walk a few kilometers and does daily work without getting too tired is a sign of cure. Also patient's facial expressions and smile returns and oneself feels total well-being.

People who are poor physically, mentally, economically, educationally and in every sense poor even deprived. It is very challenging, lot of sacrifices needed to keep up daily life. Sufferings of people help to understand the others pain. Let us have confidence in us, in God and in people. God is ultimately a physician and healer. He touches us first and we touch others.

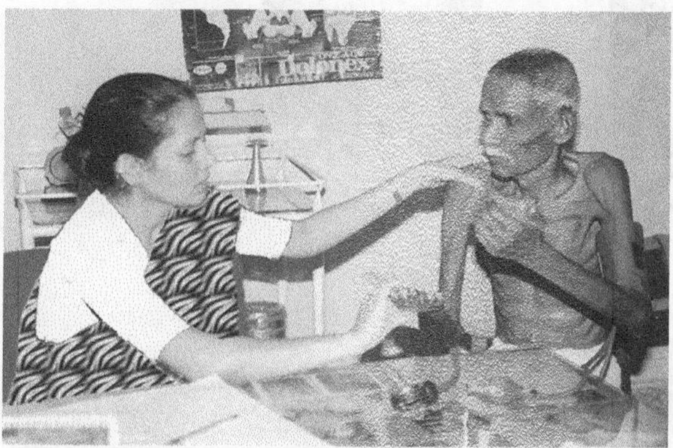

Fig. 17.1: Tuberculosis: National health problem

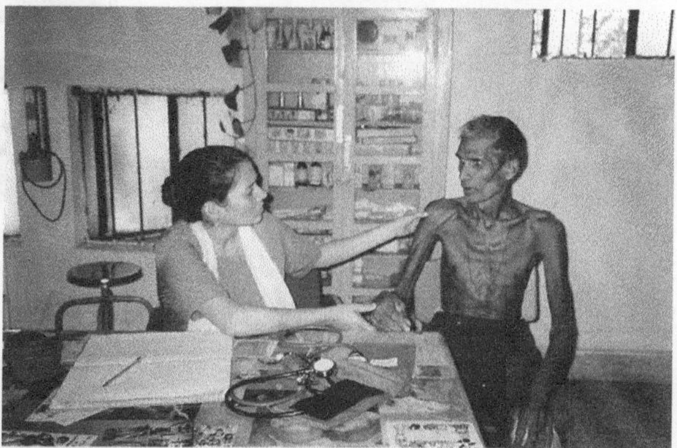

Fig. 17.2: Regular check-up and treatment for tuberculosis

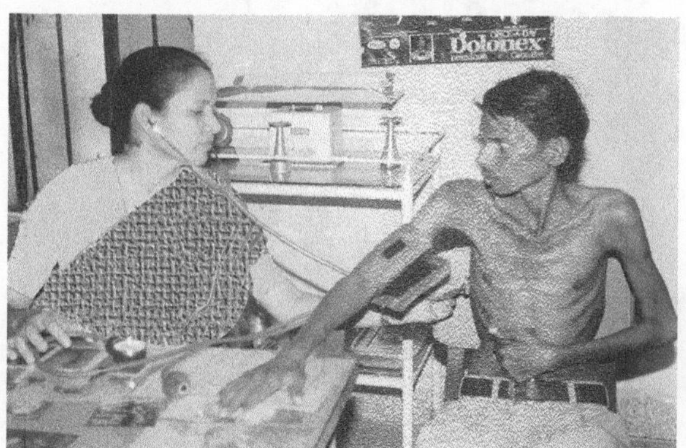

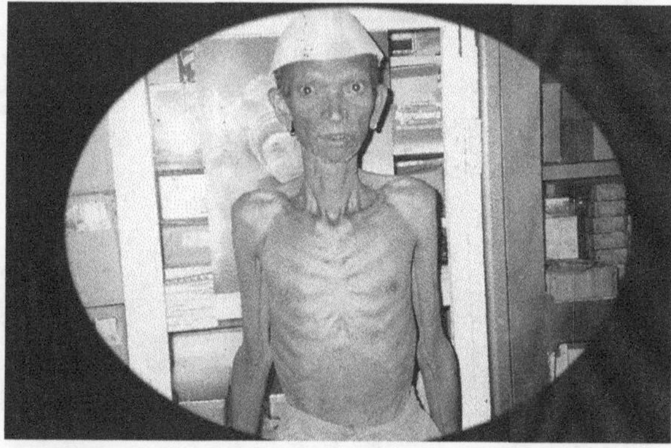

Figs 17.3 and 17.4: Tuberculosis defaulter. Re-emerging infectious disease. Tuberculosis with HIV. Underweight and pulmonary tuberculosis. Factors responsible—illiteracy, ignorance, low socioeconomic condition

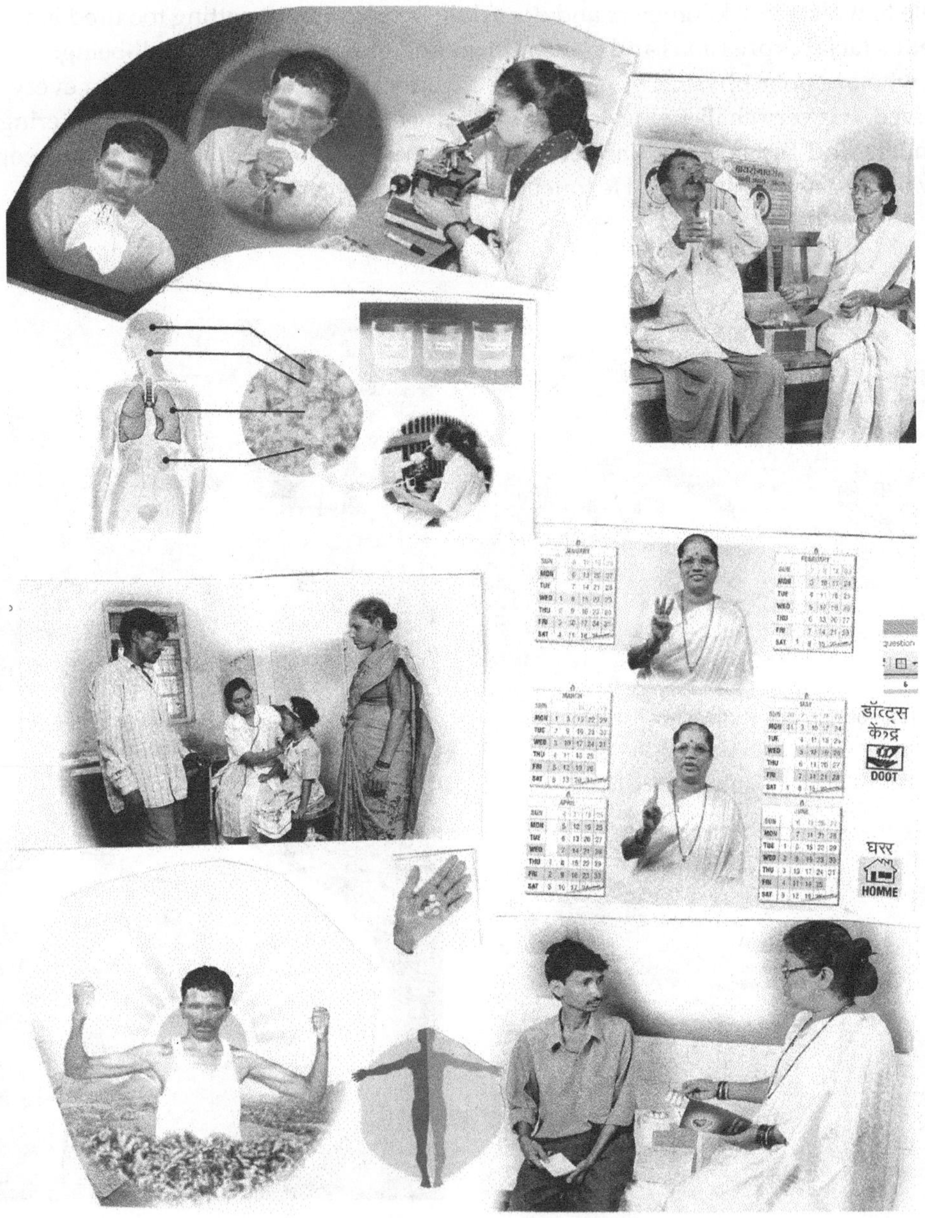

Fig. 17.5: Revised National Tuberculosis Program—RNTP, DOTs—Direct observed therapy; Short cause, prevention by public awareness

18 Sexually Transmitted Diseases : STDs

What is sexually transmitted disease? Any infection that is passed from one person to another during unprotected sex is called a sexually transmitted disease.

People who want to be healthy and strong will naturally avoid all contact with prostitutes from red light district as many of these women are infected with soul-destroying sexually transmitted disease. Physical intimacy can also lead to infestations like body lice. Getting on sexually transmitted disease increases the chances of being infected by HIV nearly five times and could cause other complications if the sexually transmitted infections is left untreated. There are those, which cause ulcers and lesions, and those, which cause a secretion or discharge from the genital organs. It needs to be treated.

Sexually transmitted infection can sometimes be painful or the symptoms can disappear after the initial signs. If left untreated can get into the bloodstream and cause serious damage to your body like infertility or even death in rare cases. It produces highly infectious skin lesions. STDs can pass from person to person during any kind of sex in the vagina, mouth or in the bum. STDs live in blood semen and vaginal fluids. STDs sores on the skin. Burning when you pee, sores, blisters in bumps, near penis, vagina. There is itching, unusual discharge with odd odor. STDs do not go away on their own. Change your careless living on the part of many young people the disease is spreading rapidly today inspite of advances in modern medical science. Public health authorities are doing their best to stamp out this infection. Person must be on guard continually against possible infection.

Sexually transmitted disease constitutes a major health problem in India. It is one of the greatest scourges ever to hit the human race. Within a short time the disease had spread like a plague. It is a dangerous venereal disease. The germ are transmitted from one person to another through sexual contact, in few cases it is acquired through contaminated material and even through injections or blood transfusions, if the germs are present in the blood. If a mother is infected the germ finds their way into the child's body before birth. Over 20 pathogens have been found to be spreading STD. They are group of communicable diseases that are transmitted by sexual contact and it is caused by bacteria, viral, protozoal and fungal agents. They are known as syphilis, gonorrhea, chancroid, lymphogranuloma venerum and donovanosis.

Earlier reproductive maturity and expanded longevity have resulted in a longer sexual life span. Greater sexual freedom, changing role of women, changing in the institution of marriage of the family, decreased social control by religious institutions increased emphasis of sexuality by media, increase leisure time, inexpensive travel, urbanization changed, value system, exploration of new form of sexual conduct.

STD is generally found in divorced, single and separated person, lower socioeconomic group, prostitution, broken homes, unhappy atmosphere, sexual disharmony, strained relationships, to get easy money, emotional immaturity, type of life style due to urbanization and industrialization, long working hours, changing behavioral patterns, social stigma do not revealed and it keeps on spreading.

Syphilis is transmitted sexually. It can cause a painless, single, hard sore on the genitals, mouth or around the anal area. The sore goes away and later becomes a rash, which is non-itchy. It also causes painless swelling in the groin. In the female, there may be a sore deep in the vagina, because there is no pain the woman may not be aware of it. Most cases of syphilis are contracted from prostitutes. Later they invade the bloodstream and are carried to all parts of the body. Blood test of VDRL can help to detect syphilis.

The nervous system is often affected with disastrous results. In this disease, the germ attack the nerve roots coming from spinal cord. Lightening pains, sharp and stabbing, may be felt in the back and lower extremities. Severe gastric ulcers are common. Large ulcers may develop on the toes, heels, and soles. These may also occur in the inner organs of the body. Treatment should be started the moment it is suspected. This must be treated under expert medical direction. Large doses of penicillin will usually destroy the germ. It can be prevented in some extend by use of condoms. It becomes harder to diagnose and treat in-patient who have HIV.

Chancroids are caused by unprotected sex and the symptoms are painful multiple and dirty soft sores on the genitals accompanied by painful swollen glands in the groin. Chancroids can be treated with antibiotics.

Genital herpes is a very common viral infection, causing itching, tingling, redness, pain, blisters and superficial ulcers usually around the genitals and anus. It is transmitted by skin-to-skin contact and unprotected sexual intercourse. It often becomes chronic. Early treatment can relieve pain but will not prevent recurrence.

Gonorrhea is a bacterial infection that may or may not cause symptoms. It is almost always transmitted by sexual contact. It is caused by a tiny bean-shaped germ called a gonococcus. In same cases, it can be contracted from contaminated hands, instruments, clothing, contaminated toilet seats, and even bath water. A thick discharges/pus from the urethra/anal region or pain during bowl movements, burning when urinating or a sore throat are symptoms to watch out for. Sense of urgency and frequency of urination, and in addition, a profuse, greenish, yellow discharge is noticed. In the male, the end of the penis may be red and swollen. In the female, the glands around the opening to the vagina may be hot and swollen, and there may be a thick yellow discharge present during the acute stage. There is great danger of a newborn infant contracting the disease during the process of birth. Unless the infant is properly treated, he may become completely blind later in life. In many cases, sterility results from this serious infection. In the female, the fallopian tubes may become closed by an abscess and the inflammation may spread to the female pelvis. It is also passed by oral sex.

Regular screening, early detection-linked with HIV progression. Penicillin is still the best drug for treating this serious disease.

Genital warts viruses cause warts that are usually visible and painless, and appear all over the body and specifically on the genitals or around the anus. Warts are transmitted through skin-to-skin contact, can be surgically removed, but can come back. Treated by freezing with liquid nitrogen using chemicals.

Genital scabies/Pubic lice: Cause itching in and around genitals, anal region. Spread by skin-to-skin contact. Maintaining personal hygiene, medications and skin lotions can be applied.

Due to sexually transmitted infections patients can get infections such as Urethitis, Cervicitis, Epididymitis, Salpingitis, Pelvic inflammatory disease, Neonatal conjunctivitis, Genital herpes, Genital and anal warts, AIDS, Vaginitis. Many of the patients go unnoticed and the true incidence never comes to know due to inadequate reporting and secrecy that surrounds them. Most of them are not even notified. WHO estimates gonorrhea 62 million and 333 million new cases other than HIV occurrence.

However, information of the sexually transmitted infections is not available. The highest rates of incidence are observed in young people who are in sexually active age. The most serious morbidity is observed during fetal development and in the neonate. Its overall morbidity rate is higher in men than women but it is severe in women. This disease is mostly also found in rural to urban migration, lower socioeconomical group.

Social factors that are responsible for these infections are prostitution, broken homes, death or separation of families, which are broken, sexual disharmony, reflection of poverty, which provides occupation for earning easy money. Lack of female employment, emotional immaturity, urbanization and industrialization, long working hours, isolation from family, social disruption caused by disaster, wars and civil unrest, international travel, changing behavioral patterns in modern society, the value traditionally set on chastity is in conflict with more resent ideas of independence, freedom from supervision, social stigma due to that non-detection and more of going to quacks treatment, self-treatment alcoholism may encourage prostitution, prostitution may boost the sale of alcohol.

Due to sexual transmitted infections there are certain complications of pregnancy that is congenital syphilis cause of stillbirth infection with neonatal gonorrhea, which causes blindness, trachomatis can cause conjunctivitis, fatal pneumonia, PID, infertility, ectopic pregnancy, carcinoma, sarcoma, AIDS. It has shown the serious complications that may develop if appropriate treatment is not given.

To control some infections we need to have seroepidemiological survey, establishing priorities group categorized based on age, sex, place of residence, case detection, screening of pregnant women, blood donors, industrial workers, army, police, refugees, drug addicts, prostitutions, convicts, restaurant and hotel staffs, availability of appropriate test. Cluster testing from the area of the patient where sociosexual environment blood testing could be done and treatments to patient's of contact tracing of the sexual partners after diagnosed patients and after interviewed, patient himself must disclose all sex contacts voluntarily. In some parts of USA, contacts are sought quickly by phone, telegram, and other rapid means of communication. The STD clinic conducted for them and treated. In India those facilities not available so it becomes difficult as cases remain hidden and they do not come to surface.

Health education is very important to help and motivate the individual to alter their behavior. STD clinics set up for consultation, Lab services, and PHC health team to be involved. Information service notification, surveillance, and treatment to be given. Checking the reports of how many cases were interviewed? How many villages were visited? How many cultures were examined? So it is easy to screen high-risk group. Notification and prevent immoral traffic who are exploited sexually for commercial purposes. To take social welfare measures, as sexually transmitted disease is a social problem.

Rehabilitation of prostitutes who is affected, to do provision of recreation facilities, in the community provision of decent living conditions, marriage counseling, prohibiting the sale of sexually stimulating literature, pornographic books and photographs, blue films etc. Constant monitoring and ongoing evaluation is of importance. Do not self medicate, treat in time, do not take antibiotics, or apply cream without consultation and do not shy. Live clean and wholesome living. Life can be unbelievably beautiful when there is a close relationship between husband and wife. This should be a goal of all young people. In seeking for it, they will lay the foundation for happy homes, which they can enjoy, the rest of their lives.

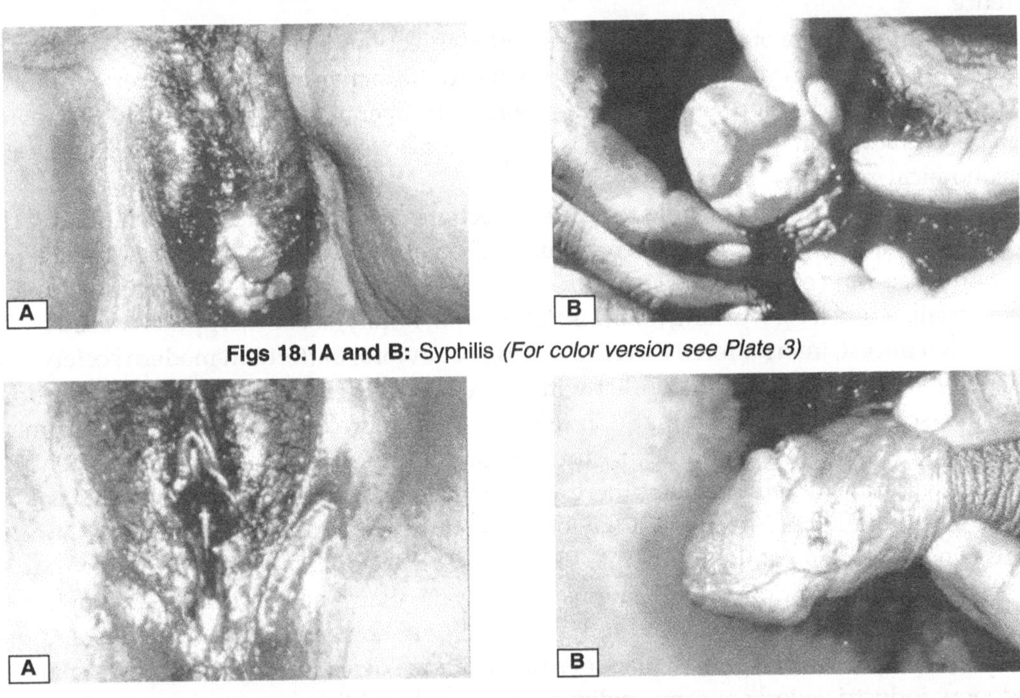

Figs 18.1A and B: Syphilis *(For color version see Plate 3)*

Figs 18.2A and B: Chancroid *(For color version see Plate 3)*

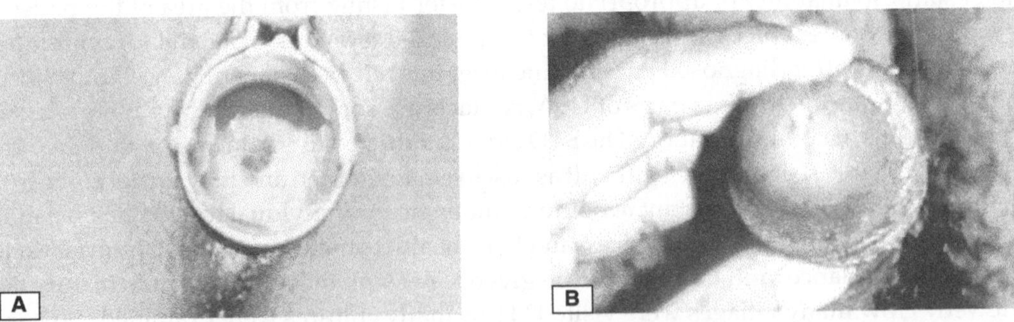

Figs 18.3A and B: Gonorrhea *(For color version see Plate 3)*

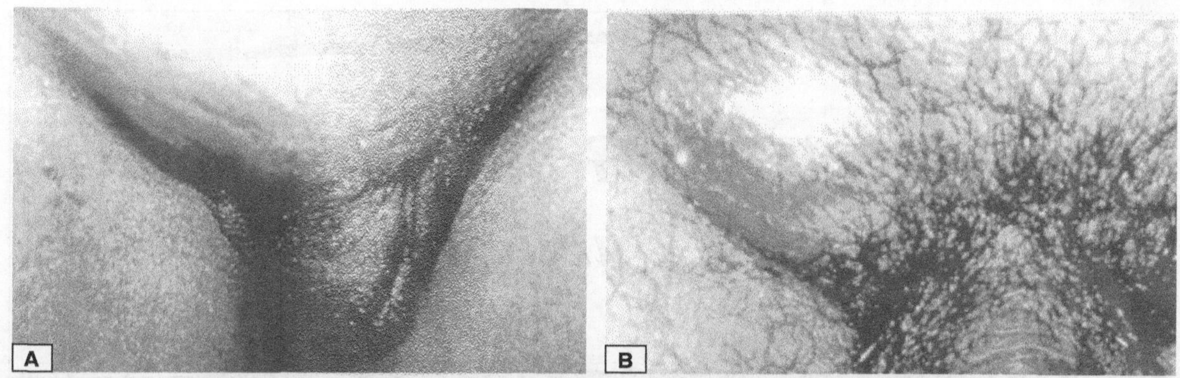

Figs 18.4A and B: Lymphogranuloma venerum *(For color version see Plate 4)*

What is AIDS? AIDS is an Acquired Immune Deficiency Syndrome, which is a growing threat for humanity today. AIDS is a combination of many illnesses resulting from a failure of body's immune system. AIDS is caused by a virus called HIV. This virus destroys the body's immune system, lowers its resistance and its ability to fight diseases.

AIDS was first reported in USA in 1981. In India, it was reported in 1986 in Tamil Nadu. It is spreading from urban to rural areas from high-risk behaviors group to general population. 89% of the reported cases are from sexually active group of age 15 to 49 years. AIDS virus once injected, it is sure that a person will be infected for life.

It has spread rapidly to all the countries of the world. In India it has reached every state. India has the highest number of persons with HIV infection. Soon we may find people infected with HIV amongst our families and friends. We not only need to prevent ourselves from getting infected but also need to care and support the people who are already infected. AIDS is a disease without any treatment or vaccine, but it is preventable with awareness, knowledge and change of human behavior. We can prevent the spread of AIDS.

The immune system is the defense mechanism which protects our body from various infections. It can be compared to the military system of a country defending against enemies. In healthy individuals, infections are kept at a distance because of an array of defenders, which constitute the immune system. The important components of the immune system in the body are the white blood cells, especially a cell called the CD4+ T lymphocyte.

In case of HIV, the virus attacks the CD4 cells, destroys them and multiplies within them. This leads to breakdown of the immune system our defence mechanism. It takes 8 to 10 years for this to happen. After which the persons contract various common diseases, which are cured in normal person but [illegible] HIV infected person due to poor immune system. This leads to weakening of the immune system and as a result, the body cannot fight infections or diseases that it is in normal condition. This leads to the development of certain diseases, which usually affect people with HIV infection, and are labelled as cases of AIDS.

19 AIDS: Growing Threat to Public Health

What is AIDS? AIDS is an Acquired Immune Deficiency Syndrome, which is a growing threat to humanity today. AIDS is a combination of many illnesses resulting from a failure of body's immune system. AIDS is caused by a virus called HIV. This virus destroys the body's immune system, lowers its resistance and its ability to fight diseases.

AIDS was first reported in USA in 1981. In India, it was reported in 1986 in Tamil Nadu. It is spreading from urban to rural areas from high-risk behaviors group of general population. 89% of the reported cases are from sexually active group of age 15 to 49 years. AIDS virus once injected, it is sure that a person will be injected for life.

It has spread rapidly to all the countries of the world. In India it has reached every state. India has the highest number of persons with HIV infection. Soon we may find people infected with HIV amongst our families and friends. We not only need to prevent ourselves from getting infected but also need to care and support the people who are already infected. AIDS is serious as it has neither treatment nor a vaccine but it is preventable with awareness, knowledge and change of human behavior. We can prevent the spread of AIDS.

The immune system is the defense mechanism, which protects our body from various infections. It can be compared to the military system of a country defending against enemies. In healthy individuals, infections are kept at a distance because of an array of defenders, which constitute the immune system. The important components of the immune system in the body are the white blood cells, especially a cell called the CD4 – T lymphocyte.

In case of HIV, the virus attacks the CD4 cells, destroys them and multiplies within them. This leads to break down of the immune system our (defense mechanism). It takes 8 to 10 years for this to happen. After which the persons contact various common diseases, which are curable in normal person but not curable in HIV infected person due to poor immune system. This leads to weakening of the immune system and as a result, the body cannot fight infections or diseases that will as in normal conditions. This leads to the development of certain illnesses that typically affect people with HIV infection and are labeled as cases of AIDS.

What is the Difference Between HIV and AIDS?

All persons with AIDS are infected with HIV. It is the last stage of HIV infection. It takes 8 to 10 years for a HIV infected person to develop AIDS. HIV infected people can lead a healthy life with proper care and support, good nutrition, exercise and rest.

How HIV Spreads?

Of HIV infection virus that causes, AIDS is transmitted from person to person by:

1. Intimate sexual contact with it or opposite sex who is infected.
2. Transfusion of blood or blood products, tissues or organs.
3. Infected needles, syringe and other instruments.
4. From an infected pregnant mother to her child before, during or after birth.

How HIV Does not Spread?

It will not spread from everyday social contact with an infected person like:

1. Shaking hands, hugging or kissing.
2. Sharing utensils, clothes, bedding and toilet.
3. Coughing, sneezing.
4. Mosquito and other insect bites.
5. Playing with an infected person.

How Can One Know if He is Infected with HIV?

History of risk behavior like indulgence in multiple sexual partners, injecting drug use, transfusion of infected blood or blood products. Blood testing from HIV from an authorized laboratory.

What Should You do if Found HIV Positive?

- Though a terrible blow, one need not despair.
- There are many other diseases in the world for which there is no cure.
- Consult your doctor for further advice.
- Lead a healthy lifestyle with good nutrition.
- Watch out for symptoms of AIDS, which may take many years to develop.

The following symptoms are commonly seen such as:

Fever prolonged more than 1 month, white patches in mouth, 10% loss of body weight, double vision, chronic diarrhea for more than one month, difficulty in swallowing, breathing problems, persistent headache, skin rash or itching, reduced vision.

Consult doctor immediately if the above symptoms appear.

Is There a Test to Detect HIV?

ELISA test detects the antibodies formed by the body against HIV. If turns positive from 12 weeks to 12 months after infection. There are other two tests too to confirm the diagnosis (Westen blot and Tridor).

Prevention

- Youth – Not to have sex before marriage, Sex only with one uninfected partner after marriage.
- Do not share needles, use only disposable or sterilized needles and syringe.
- Insist on use of HIV free blood and blood products.
- HIV positive women should avoid pregnancy and if pregnant to consult a doctor to reduce the risk of transmission of infection for the baby.
- Patient's centered counseling, non-threatening and non-discriminating environment, care of STD, transmission of HIV.

Medical Management of HIV/AIDS Cases

- All cases should be treated in general hospitals.
- Confidentiality and privacy of the clients should be strictly maintained.
- Counseling should be an integral part of management of cases.
- Family members should be trained to take care of the clients when hospitalization is not necessary.
- Referral linkages with community care centers and existing health care system should be strengthened.
- There should be no identification marks or boards displayed in the bed head ticket or near the client's bed.

Home Based Care

- Due to long asymptomatic period people with HIV/AIDS requires proper management for long periods without requiring hospitalization. Home based care becomes necessary for these clients.
- Family members must be trained on how to take care of these people at home.
- If necessary referral network may be developed with the NGOs and other voluntary organizations working in that area.
- Family members and volunteer NGOs must be oriented towards simple tasks of dealing with body fluids like blood, urine, stool and sputum, use of bleach solution for disinfections may be enlarged.

Community care – where clients are provided care and support in home like settings, free from discrimination or stigmatization.

Protection of the Care Provider

Family members or other community volunteers taking care of the HIV/AIDS case must be trained of proper infection control procedures like –

- Hand washing with soap and water.
- Disinfections of bed linen if soiled with body fluids.
- Use of bleach solution for disinfections.
- Feces and urine do not carry HIV and they should be disposed of as usual.

Care of the Dead Body

In case of death of a HIV/AIDS client, the body should be disposed off as soon as possible following the prevailing religious practices.

- Religious sentiments should be respected and the rituals should be kept to the minimum.
- Too much of handling of the dead body must be avoided.
- Wound on the body should be properly covered.

Role of the policy makers and the community leaders—Councilor of Corporate, social workers have crucial role in the care and support of people living with HIV/AIDS. These leaders must ensure that the HIV/AIDS case is treated at part with other members in the community. They should be allowed to take part in normal social and other family activities. A positive response from the community will encourage the person to develop a positive frame of mind and adopt safe practices, which would not transmit the infection further to his spouse or other members of the community.

Local NGOs and such initiatives can be supported by the District AIDS control societies.

Religious leaders should also be encouraged to be involved in such initiatives. Ignorance and myths about the disease must be clarified in the community in order to help client lead a longer and comfortable life.

VCTCS/Voluntary counseling and testing centers in the cities for easy excess and all who need to get themselves tested for HIV/AIDS, STDs, VCTC takes extensive sensitization and training, conduct program, educational material and community program. STI treatment services are set in Mumbai KEM, SION, GT, JJ hospitals, as well other cities etc. Today there is lot of hope for people living with HIV/AIDS. They can live longer and healthy life if they follow basic guidelines and draw advice. Due to new effective medicines the quality and span of life can be improved and disease can be put under control.

If a person is HIV positive, the first reaction is anxiety and fear. This is normal and natural. Do not fear. Now the treatment options available are not curative but can help to lead a long and productive life. The virus can be contained and controlled.

Counseling helps—It is available at municipal government centers called as Drop-in-Centers (DIC). Clients are counseled on a one-to-one basis in strict confidence. All questions are answered and individuals helped to cope with the disease emotionally, socially, physically and occupationally. Counselors help to deal with the day-to-day problems that might be encountered. Client is helped to disclose their status to their partners motivate them to meet the counselor, elimination of doubts and misconceptions, guidance, care, support.

What is Antiretroviral Therapy (ART)?

ART consists of drugs used to contain the virus. These drugs work by inhibiting the multiplication of the virus when given in combination, thus improving survival and quality of life. These medicines available for adults and children. They need to be taken life long. It is therefore, important that they are properly administered and client comply with treatment and family instruction. All do not need ART. Doctor will decide when and what treatment to be started after necessary tests and examinations.

The Benefit of Taking Regularly Medicines: How do Anti-HIV Medicines Work?

CD4 cells in our body's immune system help to protect the body from infections and diseases. HIV attacks these cells and multiplies within them, thus leading to their destruction. Over a period of time, the virus count in the body increases while the number of CD4 cells drops. As a result the body loses its ability to fight infections and diseases as before. This leads to AIDS.

The medicines work by blocking the virus from multiplying, thus protecting the CD4 cells from destruction. Keep the viral load low. Keep the CD4 count at a healthy level.

Take the correct prescribed dose at correct time in right manner with food; your doctor decides the course of treatment for each individual. Taking another person's medicines can be dangerous. Do not miss appointment with your doctor. The amount of the drug in the blood is continuously kept at a level that effectively blocks the virus from multiplying. If the level drops too often, two things happen – the virus starts multiplying rapidly again and destroys more CD4 cells. As a result, the viral load goes up while the CD4 count goes down – worse, the virus develops resistance. This means that even when the amount of the drug goes up again, it will no longer be able to block the virus from multiplying. Drug level drop when Client forgets, or not taking several doses correctly. Total 100% faithfulness to family and the treatment. If this fails below 95%, the treatment not effective, may not work. Client feels so many pills, it is causing side effects, can't cope, feel better, embarrassing when other people see me taking medicines, medicines are over, I want to start some non-allopathic medicine, I vomit are some of the reasons given by client and discontinues the treatment.

The virus is 1/10,000th of a millimeter in diameter. The virus is easily killed by heat, can be inactivated by either, and is resistant to ultraviolet light.

AIDS stands for Acquired, e.g. not born with, Immune – the body defense, Deficiency – decreases or lack of, Syndrome – collection of symptoms. This disease affects both men and women and found in all parts of the world. A healthy WBC acts like an army and kills all attacking germs. When a person is infected by the germs that cause AIDS the WBC gets unhealthy and dies. Because of that the body loses immunity and can no longer fight against infections by other germs and thus gets sick. They may also get some tumors. The end result of AIDS is death. However, during the period when the virus is destroying the body's defense, the person stays healthy.

How Does the Virus Spread?

The most common route is through sexual intercourse with an infected person. Since you do not know who is infected, the chance of infection increases in one has many sexual partners – homosexual men who practice penetrative sex are at risk of getting infected. They are greater risk because a greater tissue damage during penetration. HIV infection can spread from an infected mother to her child in the womb and during and immediately after childbirth. HIV can spread through blood.

Using drugs intravenously raises a possibility of an infected person's blood going into the body of another and thus passing on the infection. Routes of HIV transmission, which is present in the body fluids of an infected person, entering the bloodstreams. Surgical that is through transfusion of blood, surgical instruments, not properly sterilized, sharing of needles and drug addicts, who inject.

Semen and vaginal fluids enter into other person's bloodstream through cuts, bruise through mucus membrane by capillary action. At present there is no medicine to cure it or a vaccine to prevent HIV infection. HIV/AIDS is not contagious disease like a common cold. It is not spread through casual contact. One does not get through using toilets, soap, towels or clothes used by an infected person. It is not spread by causal contact, like shake hands, hugging or even by kissing. Mosquito's insects do not spread not transmitted by sneezing, coughing, sharing food or utensils used by an infected person.

Although, HIV is sexually transmitted, it differs from STD/VDS in many ways. Only if these are an STD with ulcers, in the genitals the risk of getting HIV infection is higher.

Condom offers protection against both HIV/STD. After use, hold the base of the condom and remove without spilling the contents. Dispose it appropriately. Do not reuse condoms. Expel the air from the tip of the condom roll it all the way down. Using a condom during sex with an infected person reduces the risk of transmission, provided it is used properly. Take a fresh condom each time, put in only when the penis is erected or stiff. Check that it is not past expiry date.

Today everyone is at risk and nobody is safe. HIV spreads only certain ways. Refrain from sexual activities before marriage, marry an infection-free person and the live in complete fidelity to each other, careful hospital and surgical procedures, and receiving blood from donors, who also understand the importance of a clean and moral lifestyle, virtually eliminates the threat from blood transfusion and surgery. The only one really at risk is those who indulge in high-risk activities, injecting drugs, premarital and extramarital sex, and homosexual relations.

Unless treated for HIV, the young men and women who are HIV positive will fall victims to AIDS at their most productive age. Not only education but also intervention is important to tackle AIDS problem. A time has come to suspect, test and eliminate possibility of HIV in recurrent cases.

People living with HIV/AIDS need your kindness and compassion.

A day has come when every doctor is compelled to be a HIV specialist, willingly or unwillingly.

AIDS we cannot talk about it in isolation as only medical problem. This is the disease with profound medico-socioeconomic implications. It not only affects patient, but also has impact on his family, community and nation. Management of HIV disease is not single drug or therapy but comprehensive, clinical management is one among them. Other components like counseling, nursing care and social support is equally important. Social support is needed in the form of emotional and moral support. Financial support for medicines, support for education of children legal services, transport facilities, support of rehabilitation, networking of different organizations, self employment facilities, access to affordable therapy, home based care, community care, cremation facilities, maintaining dignity of death. Palliative care of terminally ill.

Counseling Can Make a World of Difference

Counseling is an integral and essential part of HIV and has special place as infection with HIV is life long and one can avoid acquiring or transmitting it by change of behavior. There is tremendous stress on the minds of patient; they tend to live in the shadow of fear, fear of impending death, fear of stigmatization, fear of sickness, fear of discrimination, fear of uncertain future.

Being HIV positive is not an end of story. We have to help them learn to live positively. To live a good quality of life with change of life style. With antiretroviral therapy, one can give hope, their will to live and live life fully must be encouraged. In spite of counseling there are lot of misconception in the minds of patients and people and their family members. Afraid of casual contact so they need assurance. Counsel them about authentic centers and warn them against quackery false claims as they are exploited, ruined and misled by them. To minimize health care discrimination is our responsibility. HIV being life long, one must have long-term planning about resource conservation and financial aspect. There is possibility of falling sick very often and hospital admission is repeatedly required. If more than one in the family is infected; then all of them too investigation and therapy should be ensured. Prevent transmission, advice safe sex and no exchange of fluids.

Change of lifestyle, abstinence from alcohol, smoking, and tobacco. Washing of hands before and anger food, maintenance of oral hygiene, avoid a junk and spicy food. People come to us not only suffering from damaged bodies but with bruised minds and lacerated conscience broken hearts. They need a helping hand and not a pointed finger.

Let's know it, understand it. HIV prevention and AIDS care is our responsibility. The rapid spread of AIDS growing threat of AIDS, in India it is terrifying and fastest increasing. Mumbai is capital of the world for AIDS. The infected person loses resistance to disease, and becomes vulnerable to other infections. Various system fail, there is much suffering, and the body wastes away till death comes. AIDS is incurable. Billions of dollars have been spent and billions more are being spent, to develop a vaccine and cure. AIDS is 100% fatal. AIDS is costly and unaffordable. Treatment slow downs the progress of the disease, delaying the day of death. Drug used are expensive, costing about 50,000 per patient every year. It can wipe out the state's entire health budget. The AIDS like time bomb with a very long fuse. Most people are reluctant to take an HIV test, so the infection remains undetected for years. Till then, the infected person looks, feels a functions like anyone else. Such a person can continue to spread the infection for 8–12 years, until the symptoms of the condition show.

The social cost of AIDS means social rejection, difficulty in finding employment, and the advancing shadow of death. When one spouse is infected, the other spouse is almost infected too. Much of the discrimination is rooted in public ignorance and fear, but is very real.

The economic cost: Sexually active age group forms a major part, the HIV positive population, which includes teenagers. Majority suffers are work force of the nation, the economic engine of production. AIDS destroy the backbone of the economy. In many villages, the producers are either dead or dying, while the survivors are the children and elderly, dependents with nobody to depend on.

How safe is 'safe sex'? If the man wears a condom during sex it will prevent the transmission from infected man to uninfected woman. Condom can fail, burst, slips off so promotion of condom how much reliable? As sperm do sometimes get through the pores. There is high-risk and may provide false hope and may expose more people to HIV 100% fatal, there is no cure, no vaccine, infected persons can spread infection, stay away from drugs.

Nutrition: High calories and high protein value should be advised. Healthy and balanced nutrition should be one of the important goals. Maintain the weight and strength, replacing the lost nutritional ingredients improve the immunity prevent the food induced infections.

Always use boiled water. Do not eat raw or uncooked food. Always try to eat fresh cooked food, do not eat overripe fruits, wash hands every time before eating, if possible use spoon, have milkshake cereals, whole grain, potatoes, keep nutritious snacks at hand like nuts, seeds, fruits, biscuits, intake of fibers, apples, bananas, green leafy vegetables.

Eat small amount of food at short intervals. Food helps in improving immunity if extra care to be taken following signs appear. Common reasons for eating problems are loss of appetite, feeling full, soar mouth, throat, and difficulty in swallowing due to conidial esophagitis, nausea, vomiting, diarrhea and constipation, bloating, gas, burning sensation in chest, dry mouth change of taste, fatigue, tiredness, fever, depression. Avoid spicy food, gargle with salt in lukewarm water, avoid sweets food as sugar, honey, it make condition worse. During diarrhea do not eat fried or high fiber foods, instead consume more liquid/soft-blended food.

During the terminal phase IV, nutrition is crucial. Nutrition helps quantity and quality of life.

Are you aware that women are 2.5 times more susceptible to HIV than men? 64% younger people 15-20 years living with HIV/AIDS are women and girls. So concern for women and girls is our responsibility. Focusing on them is important to prevent new infection. High-risk behavior of men makes many women vulnerable to HIV. Women friendly health care, support, education reduce possibilities fit sexual violence against women can accelerate the spread. Do not discriminate any one can get HIV.

Accidental exposure to HIV—needle stick injuries, mucosal surface exposure, skin exposure, occupational exposure, i.e. Nurses, laboratory technicians, physicians, delivery of HIV positive women – the precaution to be taken in the operation theaters are universal precautions. It is not the city barber who is spreading HIV. It is lack of precaution that is spreading the disease. The migrant laborers who went to the city for work, back with HIV to their rural community and gives to the spouses and sexual partners. The village is a silent nursery for HIV, with all the innocence and intimate and relationships that are characteristic of rural life.

What is a source material? Is it blood, body fluid or other potentially infectious material? What kind of exposure has occurred? What is the HIV status of the person?

Do not panic—most exposures do not result in infection. The risk of infection varies with type of exposure, the amount of blood involved in exposure. The amount of virus in patient's blood at the time of exposure. Whether postexposure prophylaxis was taken within recommended time.

Immediately following an exposure, needle sticks and cuts should be washed with soap and water. Splashes to the nose, mouth or skin should be flushed with water, eyes should be irrigated with clean water, Sali pricked fingers should not be put into mouth reflex.

Promptly report the exposure to the appropriate authority and condition must be treated as an emergency. PEP should be started as soon as possible, within few hours. PEP determined of exposure code, i.e. EC 1: Intact skin with few drops, short duration. EC 2: Mucous membrane or skin whose integrity is compromised, major blood splash long duration less severe, superficial scratch only. EC 3: Percutaneous exposure, more severe, visible blood on device or needle used in patient's artery/vein.

Testing: Baseline test at time of exposure is mandatory. Repeat test at six weeks following exposure, 2nd repeat test at 12 weeks following exposure.

Laboratory tests: Severe depletion of CD4 cells count is a vital test for staging the disease depending on the decision to start antiretroviral therapy or not is based in healthy subjects level of CD4 are 850 to 1050 but deviations are observed. CD4 counts of 500/mm are within normal range, 350/mm severe damage.

Syphilis serology: Syphilis is common in HIV initial screening test to be done.

Hepatitis serology: Hepatitis B and C are found as co-infections in-patient with HIV patient with abnormal liver function test BHV and HCV.

PPD skin test and chest X-ray, Mantoux routinely recommended – particularly at low CD4 cell count fine needle aspiration of lymph node also is done to confirm TB.

CBC test done.

Lipid profile testing HDL, LDL, Fasting triglyceride and blood glucose done.

Pap smear done.

When did the AIDS drugs arrive? Zidovudine in March 1987, Ritonavir in March 1996, Efavirenl, in September 1998, Abalavir in February 1999.

Gastrointestinal complications in HIV: Almost all patients with HIV infection develop these complaints during the course of their illness. Candida herpes simplex, dysphasia – difficulty in swallowing according to sign and symptoms treatment given.

Hospitals to build positive attitude to HIV patient, no discrimination at home and society. No denying burial to AIDS victims. Government of India indicates the course of action with respect to AIDS. Nutritional education in early stage. Drugs have become affordable to many but not all.

Disposal of dead body: Wash with water. 2:1 sodium hypochlorite solution. Nose and mouth are plugged with cotton swab, soaked with appropriate dilution. Disposal in electric crematorium.

Factors Having Negative Impact on Adherence

- Lack of education about HIV disease.
- Alcohol or drug use.
- Poor social situation.
- Inadequate health insurance.
- Number of medications/pills.
- Frequency of dosing.
- Stringent dosing requirements.
- Presence of side effects.

Interventions to Educate and Explain Adherence (to stick, to cling, state of clinging)

- Take time to educate and explain goals of therapy and need for adherence.
- Develop concrete plan for specific regimen.
- Minimize dosing frequency and number of pills.
- Simplify food requirements.
- Inform patient about potential side effects, and anticipate and treat them.
- Avoid adverse drug interactions.
- Provide written schedule pictures of medications, pillboxes and mechanical aids.
- Recruit family and friends to support treatment plan.

Aims of Pretest Counseling

- To provide information on HIV test and its variables.
- Ensure that the test is informed and voluntary
- Facilitate HIV and others medical risk assessment.
- Promote PPTCT, new HIV infection prevention and appropriate treatment.
- Facilitate the use of social support system and mechanisms.

Aims of Post-HIV Test Counseling

- Appropriate disclosure of test result.
- To facilitate an appropriate and emotional response.
- To reinforce issues discussed in pretest counseling.
- To facilitate action plans.
- To promote continuity in interactions.

Low risk, medium, high depends on type of exposure.

- Protective barriers—gloves, gowns, and water proof gown, apron, eyewears, mask, e.g. major surgical procedures especially orthopedic and oral surgery, vaginal delivery, vaginal exam, IV cannula insertion, removal, handling lab specimens, injections, minor wound dressing, contact with blood, splashing, uncontrolled bleeding.

Identity card to wear the red ribbon – The red ribbon is the International symbol of AIDS awareness. India is second in the World in HIV infections, and Maharashtra state is first in India. Wear the red ribbon to remember those who have died to show respect for those who have been bereaved, and to demonstrate solidarity with those who are infected or affected by HIV / AIDS.

Nurse can counsel and support individuals in their choice in health care. She has to accurately identify the problem, do clinical observation, and collect relevant date of family and community. All health and human development must ultimately constitute overall socioeconomic development.

Her intervention: Give the client support; always wash hands after handling infected area. Administer antibiotics if advised by doctor. Assess the possible causes by history counsel and educate parents in monitoring implement medical regimen. Make dietary modification. Monitor weight, implement oral care, and give tepid sponge bath.

Refer if necessary to hospital for treatment. Advice plenty of fluids and rest, take warm water gargle with saline, have a warm bath, if there is headache, do cold compression, maintain proper hygiene, avoid dust, smoke; be constantly alert, watch for any signs that may indicate any harm, attempt to establish a relationship with family, and observe family behavior.

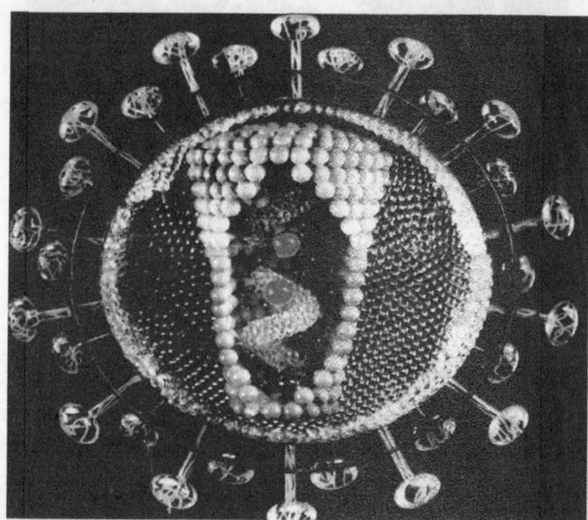

Fig. 19.1: AIDS is caused by a virus known as human immunodeficiency syndrome

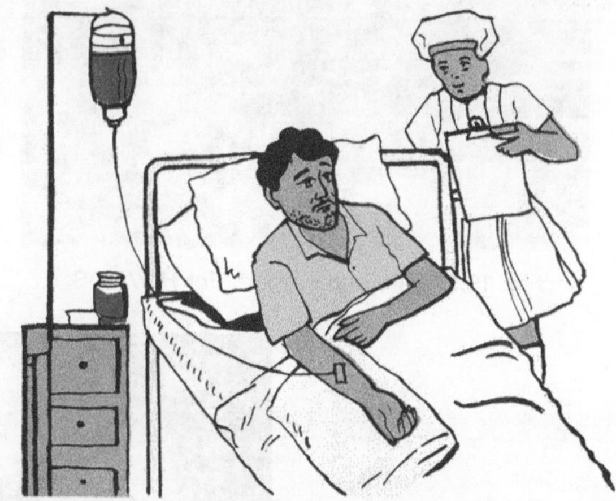

Fig. 19.2: HIV can spread through blood. If an infected person's blood is given to this man, he will be infected

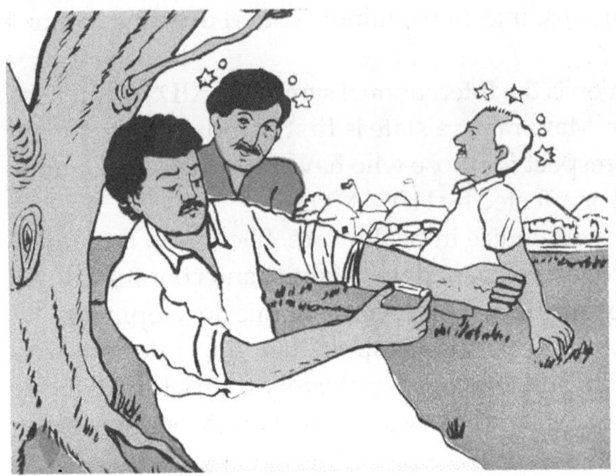

Fig. 19.3: Drug abuse: Using unsterilized needles used from person to person

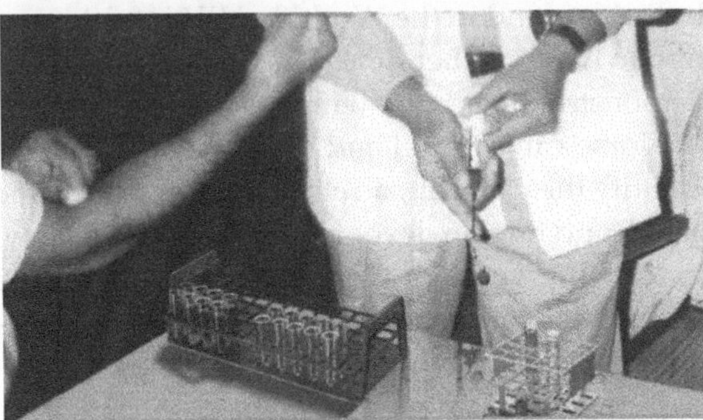

Fig. 19.4: Transmission of HIV infection through occupational exposure, such as needle sticks and pricking and cuts, splashes of needles *(For color version see Plate 4)*

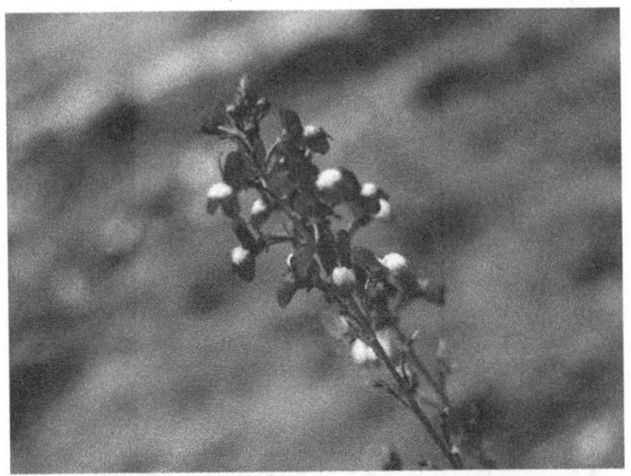

Fig. 19.5: Care and support. For HIV/AIDS

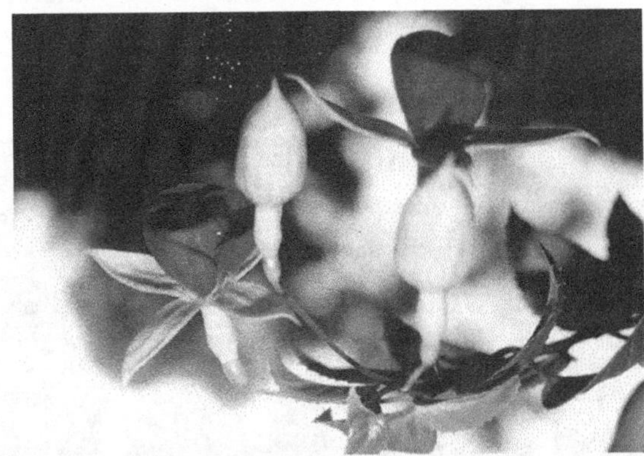

Fig. 19.6: Respect the dignity of person

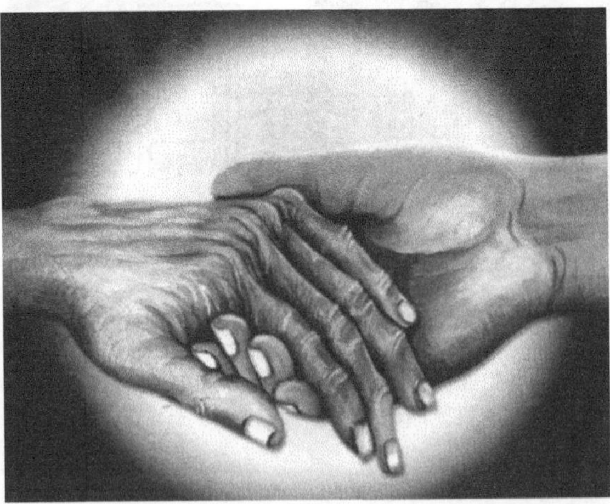

Fig. 19.7: Let us give dignity and respect, the fundamental right to live with self-respect

20 Leprosy: National Health Problem

Leprosy is a chronic infectious disease caused by *M. leprae*, an acid-fast rod-shaped bacillus. The disease mainly affects the skin, the peripheral nerves, mucosa of the upper respiratory tract and also the eyes, apart from some other structures. Leprosy has afflicted humanity since time immemorial. It once affected every continent and it has left behind a terrifying image in history and human memory-of mutilation, rejection and exclusion from society. However, the social picture of leprosy has changed over the last decades.

Leprosy is curable disease. Leprosy is more a social issue than a medical problem. A coordinated approach by the governmental and non-governmental organizations is needed to tackle the problem. The empowerment of people as well as their involvement and support are also crucial. Many times people affected by leprosy become victims of social isolation and rejection. Leprosy is a disease as old as mankind. Due to elimination programs implemented, there has been remarkable improvement in tackling the problem. Complete elimination is no doubt a very ambitious objective, but still a world without leprosy is what every one dreams to see.

Patient has to take multi-drug therapy regularly as per doctor order and follow up with regular treatment. This treatment will also prevent further crippling disability and deformity. Today the global leprosy scene is changing, people are more and more aware that leprosy is caused by germs and it is not caused by punishment from God, or it is not related with the sins of the past, even it is a dreaded disease yet it can be cured and there is no need to fear or run away from person. Today lot of funding agencies ready to help leprosy control projects, where patient affected by leprosy can live with self-esteem and with human dignity.

Maximum number of those affected by leprosy in the world live in to our country. Early detection and uninterrupted medication over a comparatively long period of time are necessary for curing leprosy. However, the stigma attached to the disease compels those affected, and their families, to hide their condition than come forward for treatment. By the time they approach treatment facilities, disfiguring and disabling damages would have set in. Ignorance makes people shun those affected by leprosy and ban them from the mainstream. The irrational fear fed by superstitions that accompany this disease makes it hard for health care workers to involve the general public in bringing about healing. This irrational fear is also transferred even to minor skin disorder like leucoderma making many people lives miserable. Children affected by this condition grow up with a very low sense of self-esteem. These facts should draw the attention of every health worker, especially dermatologists, to the urgent task at hand of restoring health to millions in our country affected by skin disorders.

All skin conditions need care; some, much more than the others. The journey to healing in the case of serious conditions begins when we accept a disorder as just another disease that can be cured. In the absence of such acceptance, the sufferers tend to hide their condition and make it worse. Awareness-building measures should emphasize practice of hygiene to prevent acquiring and communicating irritating skin ailments.

Leprosy is more a social issue than a medical problem. A coordinated approach by the government and non-governmental organizations is needed to tackle the problem. The empowerment of people as well as their involvement and support are also crucial. Many times people affected by leprosy become victims of social isolation and rejection. Addressing socio-economic needs of the people affected by leprosy through community empowerment so as to get awareness is required. All government units and non-governmental organizations should work together to strengthen the existing intervention in leprosy programs like provision of MDT, prevention of disabilities, socioeconomic rehabilitation, training of general health care workers and health education programs to the community and training in leprosy to medical and paramedical personnel.

As all the leprosy cases are not infectious. Precautions to be taken such as avoid congested damp dwelling place, unhygienic living surroundings and ignorance also affects the spread of leprosy. It is also known as Hansen's disease. It is mainly found in warmer climates. It may cause anesthesia or a lack of feeling in the involved limb of the body. All patients need to be isolated during the acute stages. Leprosy is contagious, but the danger of catching it from another person is very slight. Less than 1% of the people exposed to the disease develop leprosy. Unless the person has low resistance and lives in close contact for many years whose body contains large number of bacilli. Leprosy develops in only about 5% of those people married to leprosy patients. Once the disease is under control isolation is not necessary.

It can be diagnosed by looking for skin lesions and test for sensory loss. Any patient showing a positive skin smear, irrespective of the clinical classification, should be treated with the multibacillary regimen. There are numerous other skin diseases, which may mimic leprosy and lead to the wrong diagnosis. Early, correct diagnosis under WHO initiative, and its treatment are available for all patients worldwide, free of cost. Leprosy is not a hereditary disease. Children should be segregated from infectious parents. Give patient your compassion, kindness and free him from prejudice against leprosy that is deep rooted. The whole family lives as a social outcast due to social stigma attached to it.

Early signs are hypopigmentation, thick skin with shiny appearance, loss of sensation to pain and touch, nodules in the skin thickening of earlobes. At least one cardinal sign such as mentioned above present. Later stage deformities develop such as depression of the bridge of nose, wrinkling of the facial skin, loss of eyebrows, stiffness of joints of fingers, shortening and loss of finger and toe due to anesthetic hands and feet. Reconstructive surgeries are available.

Diagnosis is most commonly based on clinical signs and symptoms. A simple test—you will need a clean sharp needle or pin. Tell the person what you are going to do and demonstrate it. The person should be blindfolded or some barrier should be used to prevent him from watching the procedure.

Touch the center of the skin patch with the pin, apply little pressure never pierce or cause bleeding. Ask the client if he feels pain. Test the same area, and also areas of normal skin, with both the sharp and blunt ends of the pin, so that you can compare. The examination should, preferably, be performed in daylight. Any client showing a positive skin smear, irrespective of the clinical classification, should be treated.

The sulphone drugs are most widely used. However, leprosy bacilli resistant to dapsone gradually appeared and period of treatment became longer. Thus treatment with dapsone monotherapy became less and less successful. WHO introduced multi-drug therapy, which is now well-tolerated and accepted by clients and it is highly effective. It rapidly cures clients, interrupts further transmission of the disease and therefore makes elimination of the disease a possibility. Advantages of MDT—it is highly effective in curing the disease. It reduces the period of treatment. Well-accepted by patients, easy to apply in the field prevents development of drug resistance. Interrupts transmission of infection, reduces risk of relapse, prevents disabilities improves community attitude. Conducting leprosy elimination campaigns, promote awareness in the community so that the hidden cases are detected and treated.

Elimination of leprosy will be archived by making MDT accessible to all communities and areas. Treating all registered cases with MDT, diagnosing and promptly treating all new cases, improving quality of patient care, including disability prevention and management, ensuring regularity and completion of treatment, enlisting community support for the program.

In treatment, capsule Refampicin 600 mg is an essential component of the regimens. The drug is given once a month. Clofazimine is most active when administered daily. Ofloxacin 400 mg drug belongs to fluoroquinolone group of antibacterial agents. Dose 400 mg. This drug is not recommended in pregnant women and children below five years of age. Minocycline 100 mg is a member of the tetracycline group of antibiotics is other antibiotic with proven action against the leprosy bacillus. Regular monthly supervised treatment is given for adult and children below 10 years with dose adjusted.

Patient responds to treatment extremely well. Nearly all cases, it can be diagnosed on clinical signs alone. Sing of reaction felt as itching all over the body and pain occurs, do not neglect, but needs to be reported. Also there are certain reactions occur, these reactions are often do damaging to skin, nerves and other tissues, skin lesions become swollen, hot, red and painful. Ulceration may occur damage to the nerve fibers carrying message for sensation and muscle power. It may occur suddenly, during treatment, or after treatment has finished. If late or delay diagnosis takes place, patient will develop disability, deformity.

If it is detected and diagnosed early, it will cure the disease and prevent deformity or else various nerves will be damaged, leading to loss of sensation and muscle power. Deformities are end result of poor treatment, so it is essential to intensified case-detection activities in both family contacts and people in the locality.

Often patient getting burn due to loss of sensation, wrist drop, foot drop, face, nose disfigured can take place. It is important that we learn to differentiate leprosy from other skin disease and not get mistaken with other infections of skin such as psoriasis, skin TB, pellagra, lymphoma, and kaposis sarcoma. Hypo-pigmented patches with loss of sensation, presence of thickened nerves. It is considered an important public health problem as 0.9 million cases detected are found in Asia and Africa.

Infective material of a patient, nose and throat secretions, skin discharges and articles used by the patient acquired in childhood signs of the disease may appear several years later. Also poverty, ignorance, illiteracy, overcrowding, poor hygiene and unhealthy living conditions are important predisposing factors. Genetic factors are suspected, skin-to-skin contacts, direct droplet contacts and some cultural factors promote the acceptable of certain illness and it is not due to bad deeds in life, that a person gets disease like leprosy. Education is the main tool for changing or modifying the health practices. Early case detection, contact survey, group survey, mass survey, examination of household contacts will help us to control this health problem.

In community health, the health nurse should teach the family about the nature of the disease, the need for strict home isolation and family regular treatment, taking care to keeping utensils separate, clothes, towels disinfected, regular taking home visits and follow-up and evaluation is of great importance which will help the patient psychologically as leprosy is curable, preventable disease, helping in controlling the disease is key to success of leprosy free world. Which will enhance in National Leprosy Eradication Program.

Such as there are 5744 centers such as survey education and treatment.

Whereas there are 778 Modified Leprosy Control Unit.

In addition, 40 Sample Survey cum Assessment Unit.

Moreover, 20 Reconstructive Surgery Units.

And 35 Mobile Leprosy Treatment Units. Where on regular basis Modified Leprosy Elimination Campaign takes place from time to time.

Temporary Hospitalization ward facilities too are available.

Religious system too plays active role in the values of attitudes influencing the lifestyles and health activities.

Leprosy caused by bacillus and not by curse or evil spirit or it is not the result of sin. Treatment taken regularly with right dose for long time can brought it under complete control, it is slow disease but leprosy patients are not different from other ordinary people. Early signs of leprosy–light colored patches on skin, specially the face and ears, loss of sensation in fingers/toes, pain in the nerves. Patient should immediately brought to a clinic. People delay in seeking aid because they are afraid. Cause of deformity – burns and cuts are neglected they soon become infected and turn into ulcer. If there is already loss of feeling in the hands/feet is usually permanent. No medicines to bring back the feelings of tingling in the hands.

All skin conditions need care and leprosy much more. The journey to healing begins when we accept a disorder as just another disease that can be cured. In the absence of such acceptance, the sufferers tend to hide their condition and make it worse. Awareness-building and community participation, dispelling misconceptions, therefore, are essential in bringing about a cure. These awareness-building measures should emphasize practice of hygiene to prevent acquiring and communicating irritating skin ailments. We also need to pay attention to the importance of maintaining a glowing, healthy skin. What might initially seem harmless may eventually turn out to be serious. Healthy skin is often an indicator of our holistic wellness, personal hygiene, unpolluted environment, correct eating habits, mental peace and happiness are important contributors for wellness of body, mind and spirit. Skin problem can be prevented through fitting food habits. If you require a glowing skin, drink plenty of water in the morning.

Care of skin by washing and soaking with oil to prevent dry and crack that needs to be inspected, person needs to protect hands and feet from hurting with throne or stone or not protecting foot and wearing badly fitting shoes, shoes that are narrow, nails sticking out badly repaired shoes, inspect your feet, for redness or painful, reset the foot at home, protect it, shoes are as good as medicine. As shoes prevent ulcers, so wear the right kind of shoes, shoes that are made with exact shape of the foot. This we need to take seriously to prevent dangerous deformity and disability.

By taking care and using a cloth, a glove or padded handle, hands, which have no feelings a claw hard, holds the hoe very tightly. Patients think they will not be able to work again, and that their hands are only useful for begging, not true this concept needs to be challenged by rehabilitation and psychological and moral support. Protecting eye and eyelids, which get affected by the germ which settles in the eye causing burning, redness, watering pain, photo-phobia, where some lose vision. Some people not able to close their eyes and cover the eyeballs completely with eyelids, some people do not feel, piece of dust touches the eyeball, so they do not blink – causes wound. Dirt brings sickness, "nursing is not only a service to the sick, and it is service also to the well. They have to teach people how to live."

Leprosy Day is observed on 31st January. There are leprosy homes with a team of staffs such as medical superintendent, medical officer, rehabilitation welfare officer, plastic surgeon, medical social workers, paramedical workers, pharmacist, laboratory technicians, physiotherapist. Clients who do not have homes and forced to live on roads and railway stations can come to such homes and get free of cost treatment. There is physiotherapy, wax bath, exercise, flaccid nerve stimulation, sensory motor testing, moreover, surgical decompression done to prevent further deformity, ulcer-dressing ect. Special department to make soft chappals, gutter splints for stiff finger joints, finger loops sling.

Provision of effective treatment, together with improved case detection methods and prevention of occurrence of disabilities through early treatment and improved management of cases can help to reduce cases. Addressing socioeconomic needs of the people affected through community intervention. A coordinated approach in the true spirit of partnership with all government units dealing with issues surrounding leprosy. Early detection and early domiciliary treatment to control the spread of disease is must. Leprosy is a dreaded disease but it seldom causes death. It may weaken victims, however, can make them weak likely to contact other disease. Training of health workers, family members, giving physical and mental help, rehabilitating person in time of need, guiding expert counseling and with cooperation and collaboration, it can be controlled and world can be leprosy free one day.

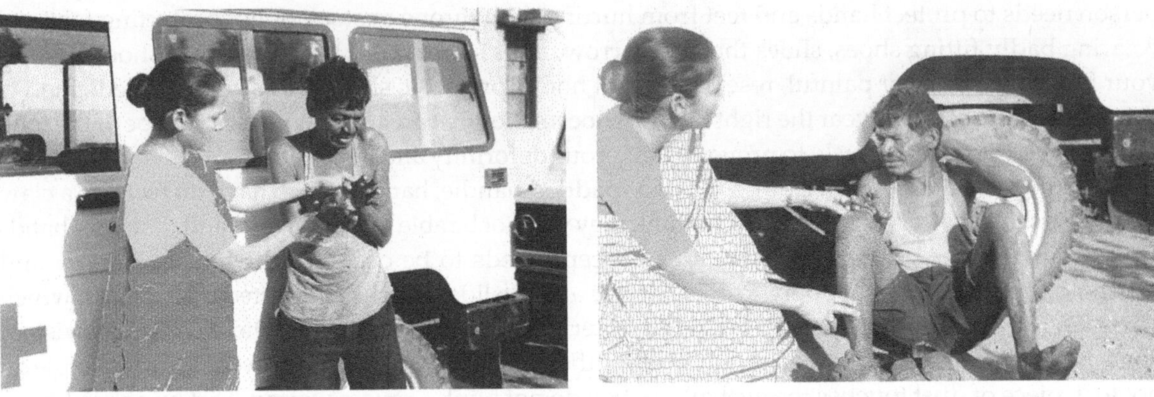

Figs 20.1 and 20.2: Early detection of leprosy and surveillance. Leprosy is curable and can come under control

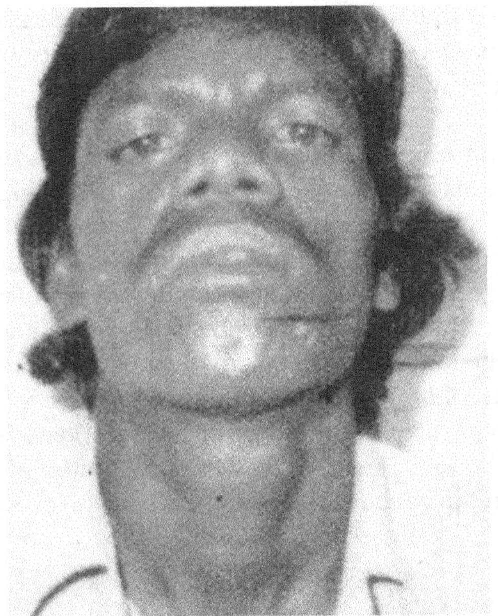

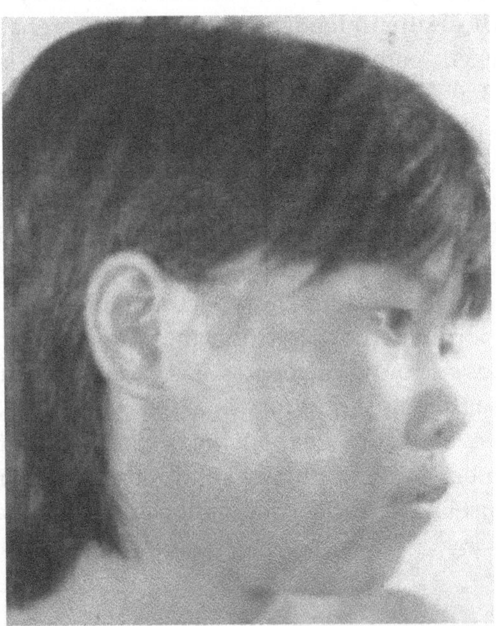

Figs 20.3 and 20.4: Early sings of leprosy–light colored patches on skin, specially the face and ear. Loss of sensation in finger, toes, pain in nerves—do not fear, seek medical aid immediately. Leprosy is caused by bacillus and not by curse or evil spirit or by past sins *(For color version see Plate 4)*

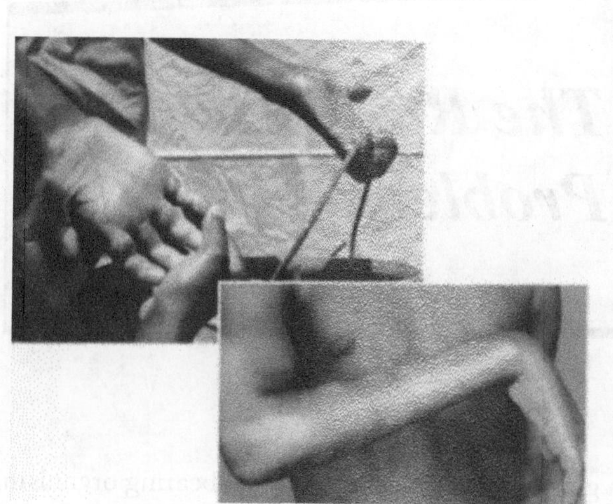

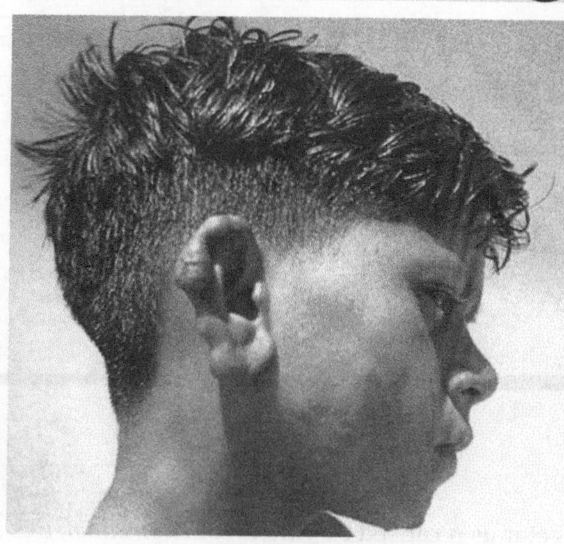

Figs 20.5 and 20.6: Wear soft chappals, gutter splints for stiff finger joints, finger loops sling

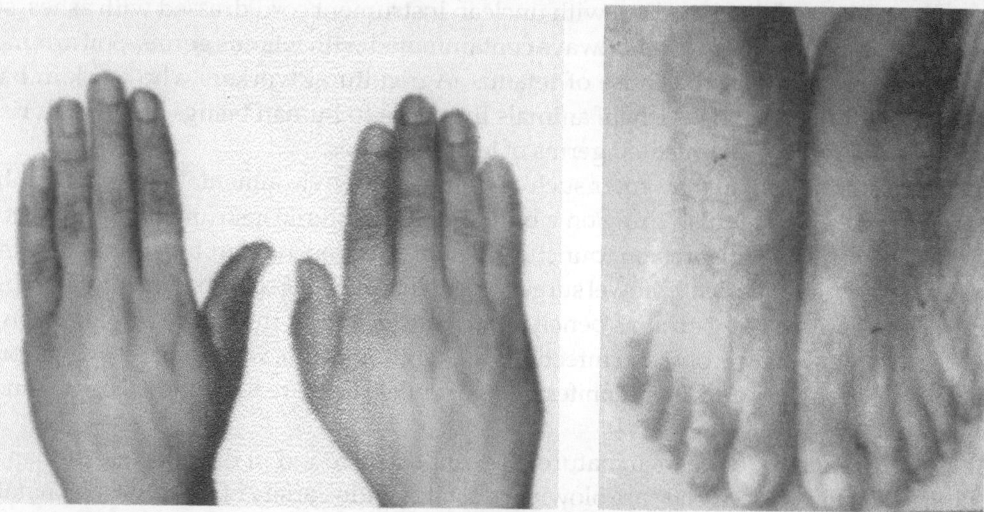

Figs 20.7 and 20.8: Now it is not dreaded disease. It can be controlled by regular medicines, wax bath, sensory motor testing. Flaccid nerve stimulation, decompression to prevent deformity, physiotherapy. Join hands to eradicate leprosy, as it is a national health problem

21 Tetanus: The Rural Health Problem

Tetanus is caused by extoxin of *clostridium,* it is a gram positive, anaerobic spore bearing organism which looks like a drum-stick shape. The spores are highly resistant and difficult to kill them with simple sterilization, this organism lives in soil and dust. The bacilli found in cattle, horses, goats, and sheep where they are excreted in their faeces. All wounds are easily infected, due to trauma, non-aseptic condition like umbilical cord cut with unclean instrument cord dressed with ashes, soil, cow dung and animal manure. Street dirt is always contaminated with tetanus germs. Soil around fields, gardens, in rural area can also be cause of tetanus. Agricultural workers who work in base foot, having houses with floor that is earthen, animals live close to human beings are in high risk when they come in contact with contaminated germs of tetanus spores.

Other factors, this organism may enter such as unhygienic environmental sanitation, unhygienic custom habits, application of dust/dung on wounds, using unsterile instruments, ignorance, lack of PHC services, pin prick, skin abrasion, puncture wounds, burns, human bites, animal bits, stings, unsterile surgery, intrauterine death, bowel surgery, dental extractions compound, traumatic, puerperal (abortion, labor). Foreign body such as pencil, match sticks, put in the ear causes infection such as otitis-media, chronic skin ulcerous, eye infections, gangrenous limb, where spores lying dormant in the wound where they grow and later manifested as disease. These are the different causes and modes of transmission.

As these spores survive for years in nature, the bacilli also found in the intestine of man without causing ill effects to the person. They are blown in dust in a wide variety of situation. Neonatal tetanus is an acute disease caused by this organism and it is clinically characterized by muscular rigidity, painful spasms of the voluntary muscles, lockjaw, and spasm of facial muscles, back, neck, lower limbs and abdomen muscles, which occur at intervals. The mortality tends to be very high, 40–80%.

Today in developed countries it is rare disease. Neonatal tetanus found in newborns is a killer disease and its fatality rate said to be about 80–90%. It tends to occur in areas with poor access to health care. It remains hidden in the community and very often not notified. In early 1980s there were about 1 million newborns were estimated to die annually. Today the decline is due to increase in immunization coverage of pregnant women with a protective dose of TT. Tetanus is important endemic infection in India. Due to lack of hygienic condition together with it daily behavior habits such as lack of handwashing, unclean delivery practices, and conducting traditional birth customs are all important factors affecting disease.

Even today in many of the rural areas there are high rates of deliveries conducted by untrained personnel. Community health nurse has to prevent this by specific action oriented measures in order to note the progress monitoring like regular immunization with booster doses, health education, and clean deliveries by trained personnel needs to be stressed prevention: Active immunization. Preventing neonatal tetanus, all wounds, injury should be properly cleansed as soon as possible after injury, removal of foreign body, soil, dust, necrotic tissue is necessary. Make great effort to provide as much protection as possible in the light of our present scientific knowledge. As it is public health problem and is more found in rural areas, so people should be motivated to follow immunization program. Even today, very few patients ever recover once tetanus has fully developed. Protect yourself now before he is injured.

No human rights without human dignity; no human dignity without human rights. Hence the rights of human persons are essentially the rights of relational beings called to build up the human community. Since society is made up of individual persons, his or her welfare cannot be assured without respect for the dignity and rights of each person. Thus human rights spring from the relational nature of persons. Hence, the rights of the powerless as a class of people in their historical situation have to be defended, others of the kind are landless workers, marginalized farmers and domestic workers. By fighting against the oppression and exploitation of all kinds and helping the oppressed to realize their human dignity; develop their talents and grow into fuller persons as children of God. To experience the strength of solidarity and to fight for their rights, to give them in-depth awareness of their social situation and the true and root causes thereof, to train them to find the solution to their social problems based on their life experience and social realities, to share power and give freedom to make their own decisions Seek a committed and professional approach and is based on professional competence as an answer to the needs of the group of youth it seeks to serve. This is usually done by teamwork.

The face that guides and motivates our work is the one of the poor – helpless, choiceless, a victim of injustices and exploitation, laterally surviving from hand to mouth. The nature of the work, therefore, demands that we be available to the poor and the affected at all times, especially on days of inconvenience or calamity weather natural or man made.

To provide residential accommodation, equipment and material either free of cost or for consideration to the staff and employees of the society and others connected with work to provide for the welfare of the said persons and their dependents and to educate, train, equip and/or assist financially or otherwise in the education, training and equipment of the said persons or other persons for the purpose of the society.

To collaborate, associate with and/or secure participation from other educational institutions and their students, youth movements and their members and other organizations, bodies or individuals in the performing of the society's activities.

To set up, encourage, develop, assist, foster and promote co-operative societies for the economic, and general welfare of people particularly those from socially and economically backward communities and to endeavor for the growth of co-operative movement and inculcation of co-operative principles and values. To organize, conduct research programs and to print, publish and exhibit any journals, periodicals, books and other printed material as well as to produce, purchase and exhibit films, recorded materials, TV programs which promote the objects of the society.

Families in USA—Major changes affecting the families such as alteration in family cycle, divorce, remarriage, breakups, and separation. Adults choose to remain single or choosing to remain unmarried couple sharing same household, divorce increased, birth decreased, increasing proportion of single parent's family. Society changes into structure and functions of the family.

Keeping in mind the well-being of the rural, this forum will collectively strive to maintain and fight against any violation of rural cultural identity enshrined in their world view and in their sacred land. This forum will try to reach to all rural youth, in particular to all those who are the victims of the culture of silence, who neither belong to any organized group nor to any political party, yet are seeking for guidance in their life. Prepare a group of students, who through their intellectual and analytical power will do the research and make their findings available to the maximum number of people. They will also document all valuable works.

It will provide every opportunity for the good and tenacious leadership among the rural people. It will encourage and strengthen the collective community leadership to achieve the political power for the rural. It will fight to lessen the exploitation against rural women to ensure their better participation in the building of just rural society. It will struggle continuously for the better bargaining power of the rural people to bring economic balance in the rural society.

Society is natural to man and it is meant for the promotion of the common good. Law is part of the universal structure of creation, as designed by the creator, the universe is hierarchically ordered. It provides remedy for the social evils. Social obligations have priority over individual desires and wants and hence duty is to be emphasized more than rights.

What are the factors, which help us, evolve vision in our life, in the life of people?

Should we discover new solutions in order to respond to the challenges?

Should we become attuned to the feelings for our people's cause and action?

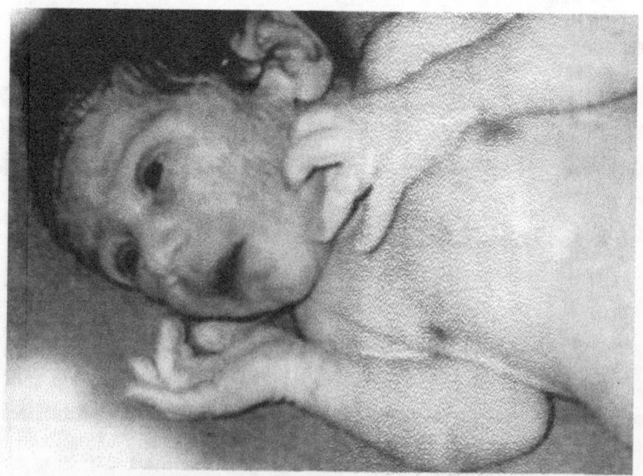

Fig. 21.1: The healthy newborn child

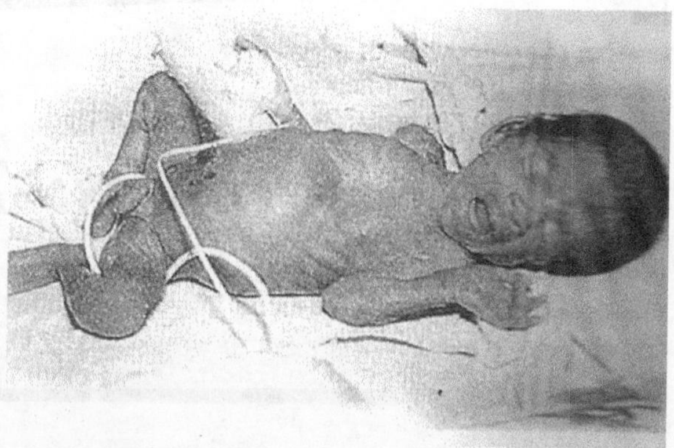

Fig. 21.2: To prevent tetanus, the mother needs to take injection tetanus toxide so that the child is protected from tetanus

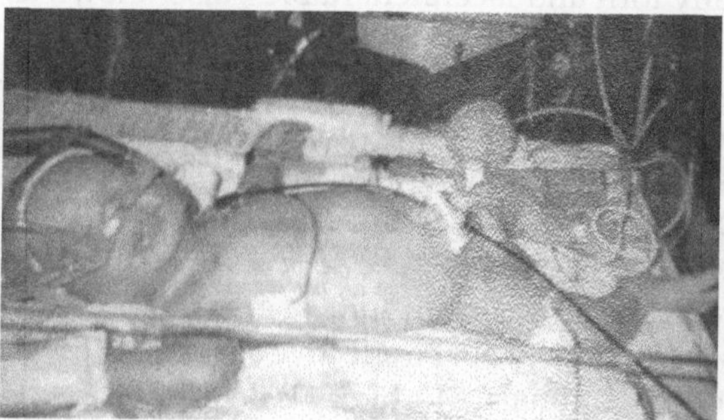

Fig. 21.3: Safe delivery kit in home delivery to be used. Cut the umbilical cord by clean sterile technique. So that tetanus can be prevented in the rural community. To this day, also many children lose life due to this which go unrecorded

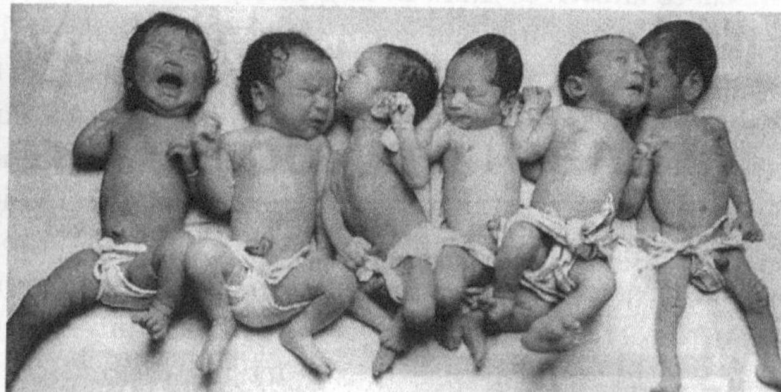

Fig. 21.4: God creates life and mother co-creates. Every child is unique and he/she should be planned and wanted. A healthy child in healthy family is an asset of the community and nation

22 Rabies: The Fatal Disease

Bites of animals are often dangerous. Dog and cat bites are common. Rabies is one of the worst diseases known to man. In dog bites, the flesh is usually torn and lacerated. Rabies, also known as hydrophobia, is an acute, highly fatal viral disease of the CNS. It is primary a disease of warm-blooded animals such as dogs, cats, jackals and wolves. It is transmitted to man usually by bites or licks of rabid animals. There is a change in behavior in rabid dog that becomes ferocious and bites any object. Attacks and bite without provocation. The animal runs away from home and bites all that comes in his way. It is grasping for breath, there is a change of voice that is barks in a hoarse voice.

Despite intensive care, person who developed rabies ends in death. Water appears to be the most effective natural barrier to rabies. In many countries rabies is spreading in spite of great advances in research of field control methods. Available anti-rabies vaccines may not be effective against the rabies related viruses. The virus is excreted in the saliva of affected animals. Morbidity is nearly 100%. The number of deaths are much more than reported. Rabies occurs in all parts of India.

This infection is transferred from wild-life to domestic dogs. A single rabid dog is capable of biting a large number of humans under this infection. Cats can also be source of human infection. Wild life rabies fox, hyena, bat rabies – these bats feed exclusively on the blood of animals and man; the virus may be present in the saliva for 3-4 days, before the onset of clinical symptoms and during the course of illness till death. 80% of bites by proven rabid animals will result in rabies.

Laboratory staff working with rabies virus, veterinarians, dog handlers, hunters and field naturalists face bigger risks of rabies than do public. Licks on abraded skin and mucus can transmit the disease. Dogs have the habit of licking – Aerosols (respiratory) transmission observed in caves in infected bats. Person-to-person it is found rare. The incubation depends on the site of the bite, severity of bite, number of wounds, amount of virus injected, species of the biting animal, exposure of bite face, head, neck, upper extremities and bites by wild animals.

The disease begins with fever, headache and twitching pain, numbness at the site of bite. The patient showing intolerance to noise, bright light and fear of water. Rabies in man is called hydrophobia. Intense spasm at the sight of fluid. Symptoms such as headache, malaise, sore throat and slight fever lasting 3–4 days. 80% patients complain of pain or tingling at the site of bite. Followed by widespread excitation and stimulation of all parts of nervous system; the patient is intolerant to noise, bright light or a cold draught of air, fear of air, spasms, dilatation of pupils of increased perspiration, mental changes include fear of death, anger, irritability and depression.

The symptoms are progressively aggravated and all attempts at swallowing liquid become unsuccessful. At later stage the mere sight or sound of water may provoke spasm of the muscles. The patient may die abruptly during one of the convulsions or may pass onto the stage of paralysis and coma. Death occurs due to paralysis of respiratory tract. Intensive care may allow an occasional patient to survive. Today only 3 persons on record who have been striken with rabies have survived.

Diagnosis made on the basis of history, signs and symptoms of skin biopsy, virus isolated from saliva, serum and CSF taken before 8th day. There is no specific treatment for rabies only case management once rabies developed. The patient should be isolated in quiet room protected as far as possible from external stimuli such as bright light, noise or cold draughts. Relieve anxiety and pain by sedatives. Morphia 30 - 45 may be given repeatedly. Ensure hydration and dieresis. Intensive therapy in form of respiratory and cardiac support given. Patient potentially infectious because the virus may be present in saliva vomits tears, urine or other body fluids. Nurses wear facemasks, gloves, goggles and aprons to protect themselves. Persons having bruises, cuts, open wounds should avoid caring patients.

Those who are bitten by a suspected animal prophylaxis of vaccine are given to neutralize virus before it can enter the nervous system. Every exposure treated as medical emergency. Prompt and adequate local treatment of all bite wounds and scratches utmost important remove virus before it can absorbed on nerve ending. Cleansing, immediately flushing and washing the wound, scratches, and adjoining area with plenty of soap and water running tap at least 5 minutes.

Chemical treatment of wound to inactivate by irrigation with alcohol, tincture, iodine.

Savlon not recommended.

Bite wound should not be immediately sutured; if needs to be suture done with minimum stitches.

Antibiotics and anti-tetanus measure taken.

Observe the animal for 10 days, a dog with rabies soon becomes increasingly restless and excitable. It refuses to eat, and indulge in excessive barking and growling. If animal is not restrained, it may bit many other animals and human beings. Wild animals should be killed immediately and rabies dog should be destroyed when the diagnosis is confirmed. Government health officials should be contacted. If dog remains healthy for 10 days, there is no indication of anti-rabies treatment. Rabies vaccine is unique because it is the only vaccine that is given after exposure to infection.

Technique of Administration of Vaccine: The ideal site is anterior abdominal wall, for this area offers enough space to accommodate the large quantity of vaccines to be injected, injection given deep SC – a fold of skin lifted between the thumb and other fingers patient lying/standing position 37 mm/ 1.5″ long needle.

Dose given according to the class one that is slight risk, only licks on healthy unbroken skin, or consumption of unboiled milk of suspected animal, scratches without oozing dose 2 ml for 7 days.

In class two moderate risk that is licks on fresh cuts, scratches on oozing of blood, minor wounds, then dose of 5 ml given for 10 days, with booster dose for 3 weeks.

In class three sever risk which includes all bites, scratches oozing blood on neck, face, palms and fingers, multiple wounds, bites from wild animals, 5 ml 10 days, two weeks booster dose given.

The patient should be isolated and protected. During the treatment, advise the patient to abstain from alcohol, undo physical, mental strain, steroids drug. Advice the patient about the reactions such as headache, insomnia, giddiness, palpitation, diarrhea, itching, inflammation, pain, edema, anaphylactic shock to report to the doctor.

To prevent virus, wear facemask, gloves, goggles, apron, and avoid direct touching saliva, tears, urine, and body fluids to protect oneself.

Anti-rabies injection should be given to all pets.

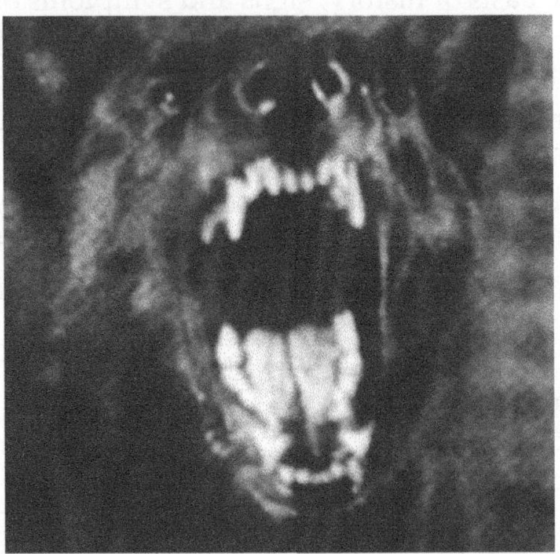

Fig. 22.1: The most fatal disease. 100% fatal once person gets rabies there is no cure. It is the only vaccine given after the exposure

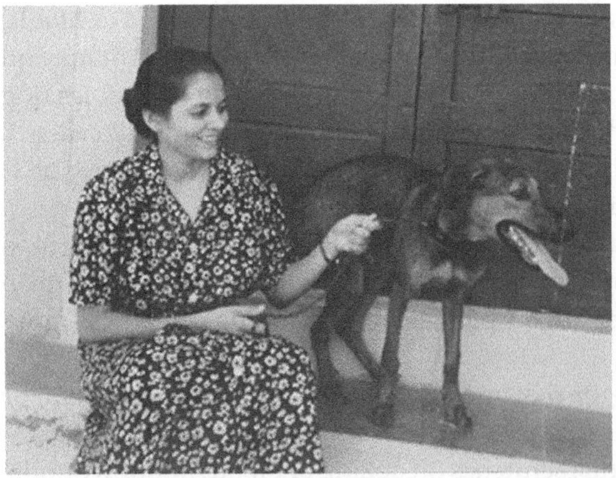

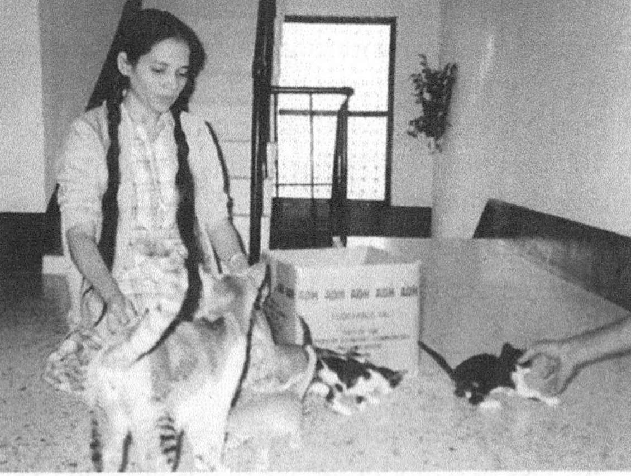

Figs 22.2 and 22.3: Prevent rabies by handling animals with care and giving preventive vaccines to domestic animals

23 Snake Bite: Common Problem in Rural Villages (some amazing facts)

Imagine in the home or outside when you see the snake, people take sticks and run with life behind the snake, isn't it? So much phobia in each of us in case the snake bites us then what I will have gone forever. In addition, because of this fear, poor snake gets killed. In every country, there snakes exist. Total in the world there are 2700 types of snakes found. Water snakes have tail like a fish flat that helps them to swim. Snake has such teeth inward that once he gets prey it cannot escape from his mouth. It attacks by catching with mouth of the prey.

In America, there are certain kinds of snakes who swallow the whole baby chicken, and until the chicken reaches the stomach it does not know what is happening and the snake later vomits away the wings and all that he wants to through later on separately. In monsoon, you find more snake, pythons can swallow a huge goat and deer at a time by suffocating the animal and then after killing break the bones.

Land and water snake both can swim, snakes cannot make hole to live by himself it lives in other animal's house and in cracked places, female snake can lay from 10 to 100 eggs at a time, many enemies of the eggs even snake himself eats its own eggs, twice in a year the snake can lay the eggs. Soon after the birth of babies, they run away from them, every year the snake leaves old skin and gets new skin, baby snakes contain six times more poison than the adult one, if two snakes fight and bite each other they die, it does not drink milk nor keep watch over elders' treasures, it is living as it is created.

Every year in India 3, 15,000 people are bitten by poisonous snakes and among them around 10,000 people die. This is not accurate, as due to lack of notification many people who die are not recorded.

In India, we have 250 types of snake but only 50 types of snake are poisonous. Among the poisonous snakes most of them live in the sea. On land, we have few poisonous snakes. Dangerous to human are cobra, krait, and russel viper and saw scaled viper.

Snakes not have hair, and is cold-blooded animal, heat is not produced in his body, so it is not able to maintain its heat and therefore it likes warm places to hide, and in extreme heat and biting cold, it is not able to survive.

Snake lives up to 12-15 years and python lives about 32 years from known facts. Snakes are non-vegetarians, if possible, regularly drinks water, but if water is not available and easily cannot find water months, it can live without it.

Reptiles that do not possess legs are known as snakes. All snakes can swallow animals thicker than their own bodies because they have amazing jaws. Stretchy ligaments link the upper and the lower half, and the lower jaw is made up of two bones also joined by elastic tissue.

Pythons have the biggest mouths and can even get to grips with a whole goat, pig or antelope. A python will seize its prey in its mouth and then tightly coil itself round the animal's chest, not crushing it but preventing it from breathing.

The king cobra is the longest of all poisonous snakes, reaching lengths of 5-4 m that is 18 feet. It injects so much venom in a single bite that it can kill an elephant in four hours. It is one of the few snakes that make a nest; the female coils on top of their eggs until the young snakes wriggle out.

Snakes do not have eardrums and so cannot hear sounds, but they can sense vibrations such as footsteps. Cobras do not move to the rhythm of the music of the snake charmer's pipe but are probably mesmerized by its movements.

Rattlesnakes can hunt in the dark because they are very sensitive to heat. They have two small pits just beneath their eyes, which are crammed with heat sensitive nerve cells. These can detect a temperature rise of a few hundredths of a degree centigrade. The rattlesnake can very accurately locate a small animal about a meter away. It then shoots its head forward at a speed of 3 meters a second, and its huge fangs inject its victim with a dose of deadly poison. Rattlesnakes are unusual snakes because they do not lay eggs.

Sea snakes come to the surface of the sea to breathe but they can then stay under water for up to eight hours. They are able to do this because most of their body is lung; it even occupies space right into the tip of the tail. Sea snakes are about ten times more poisonous than the most poisonous land snake. They are found only in tropical waters.

The golden tree snake of Malaya can leap from a tree onto its prey. Once launched, it can glide for more than 25 meter that is 80 feet. While in the air it keeps its body rigid and makes it into a hollow shape, which traps air, rather like a parachute.

Saw scale viper roams around in the night, among poisonous snake. It is smallest 30-80 cm long and mouth triangle shape, when angers makes hissing sound, to bite it comes front running and bites, English alphabet 8 makes the bites.

Krait moves around in the night, and found in the bricks and stones also found on the roof of the house, one and a half meter long, color black, stomach white, and stripes on body.

We, in rural areas, of work where so many people work in field and forest are bitten by snakes and due to timely treatment lost their precious life. Through the health education, we can teach the first aid treatment and the recognition of different types of snakes that are poisonous and non-poisonous, the sings and symptoms of its bites.

Most snakes bite only if they are provoked. Not all snakes are poisonous. Even the bite of a poisonous snake is not always dangerous, because the snake bites in its defense; little or no venom is injected. The snakes have to be identified. No anti-venom is necessary if snake is non-poisonous. If it is poisonous, its type must be identified so that specific antivenin can be administered. If the snake cannot be found or identified, it should be treated as poisonous, and general antivenin should be given.

Poisonous snakes are large, have belly scales cover entire breadth of the belly. Vipers large with conspicuous pit between eye and nostrils, head scales present, whereas the non-poisonous are small or moderately large, but not covering the entire breadth of the belly.

Symptoms of snakebites: There will be fang marks, intense pain experienced at the site of the bite of a viper. Areas get swollen and blackened, bleeding might be seen from different places.

Client vomits, collapse and coma follows the bite of cobra or similar snakes, neurological effects are seen, e.g. giddiness, lethargy, muscular weakness spreading paralysis, breathing becomes slow and labored. Respiration ceases it or without convulsions, that is 15 minutes to two hours later.

A bite from a sea snake is felt as a sharp initial prick, which subsequently becomes painless. After 1-2 hours, generalized muscular pain and stiffness develop starting in the neck, shoulders and hips.

Urine becomes brown in color. Respiration failure may occur. No taste in the mouth, excessive salivation, cannot open the eyelid ptosis, drowsy, asthmatic, low blood pressure, fast heart bits, bleeding form nose, mouth sometimes, swelling of lymph nodes, bleeding from the sight of bit.

Lay the client down and reassure him, as it is usually very frightened, though most often its life is not in danger. Apply a broad, form crepe bandage above the bitten area. It should allow entry of a finger. Do not loosen it periodically like a tourniquet. Immobilize the bitten limb with splints to reduce lymphatic flow and spread of the poison. Leave bandage and splint in position till medical care is available; Wash bitten area with plain water or soap. Arrange for immediate transfer to a hospital with killed snake if possible. If unconsciousness, respiratory arrest or cardiac arrest develop, give appropriate first aid.

If the bite is at a place where crepe bandage cannot be applied wash the bitten area and make 3 mm deep cuts through each fang mark with sterile razor blade, so as to cause bleeding and drainage of the venom.

Apply suction to the wound with a pump or mouth through a thin polyethylene sheet to avoid contacts between any cuts on gums and poison. Apply ice pack locally. Keep the client still. If needed, give artificial respiration, for pain tablet aspirin or painkiller can be given. Arrange for transfer to the hospital. Do not suck the blood or go to superstitious doctor where time will pass and client can die, client is kept 24 hours under observation. ASV treatment will be started, if too much blood is lost, then blood transfusion to be given, antibiotics, injection tetanus toxide, special care of a unconscious client.

Blood test: usually blood clots but if blood does not clot then it could be poisonous, urine for albumin test, in naked eyes if you see bloodstain urine, the snake is poisonous, blood uria/creatinin test as the poison spoils kidney, ECG if snake is poisonous it will affect the heart muscles so if needed, ECG can be done.

Prevent that no snake enters in the house, walk on clear clean ground, at night walk with shoes, torch, and keep stick.

There are so many blind beliefs existing about the snakes years hearing from one another and pass onto the next generation. If you kill female cobra, male cobra takes revenge and vice versa. Rat snake if passes in between legs of buffalo, buffalo dies. Snakes head there is a peal diamond. If snake lives 100 years, it gets muschas, poisonous snake while biting turns upside down then poison is emptied. Do not go to the Bhagats to remove the poison.

Save yourself from snake bite, do not keep the heaps of bricks, stones, grass bundles, holes of the rates, firewood keep higher than the floor, cracks of the wall and keep the surrounding clean.

Household water outlet cover it with net, so that snake is not able to enter in the house, if the house is built in the field, then make the wall plaster smooth, and keep the nets to the windows. Do not put hand in the dark where it is not clean. Snake gets frightened of human beings, if you see the snake just stand still, fresh dead snakes do not handle with hand but use stick and try to learn the differences between poisonous and non-poisonous snakes.

Snakes too are God's creation in the nature, so do not simply kill them when you see them in distance places when they do not harm you, take personal precautions as not to get a sting by it and save and prevent yourself by right treatment.

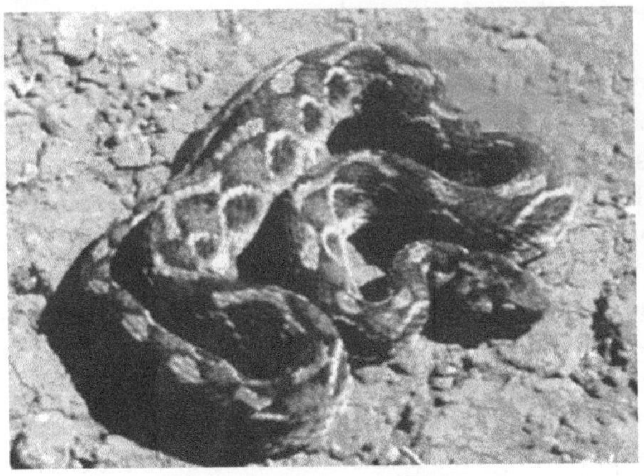

Fig. 23.1: Saw scale viper

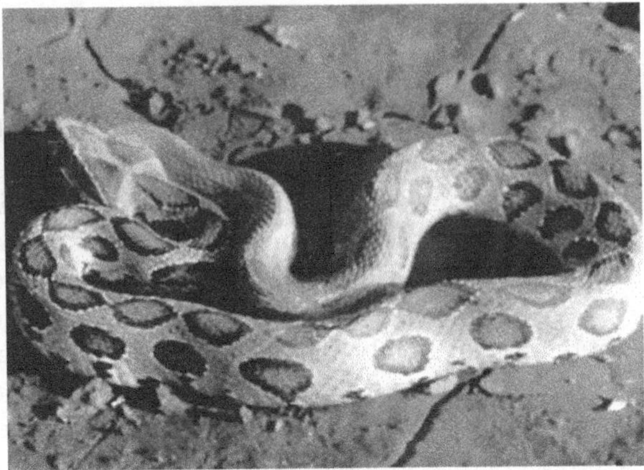

Fig. 23.2: Russel viper

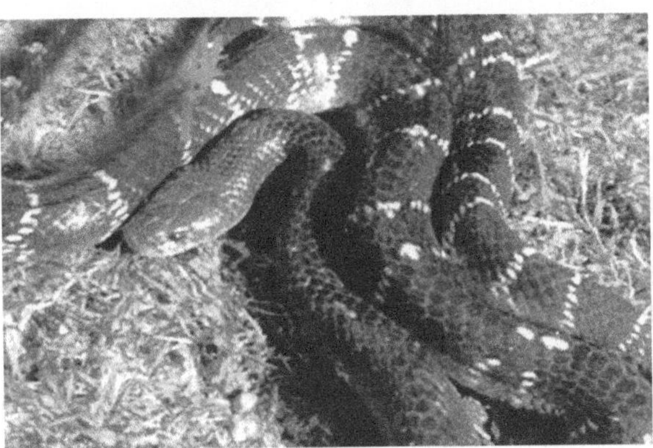

Fig. 23.3: Krait

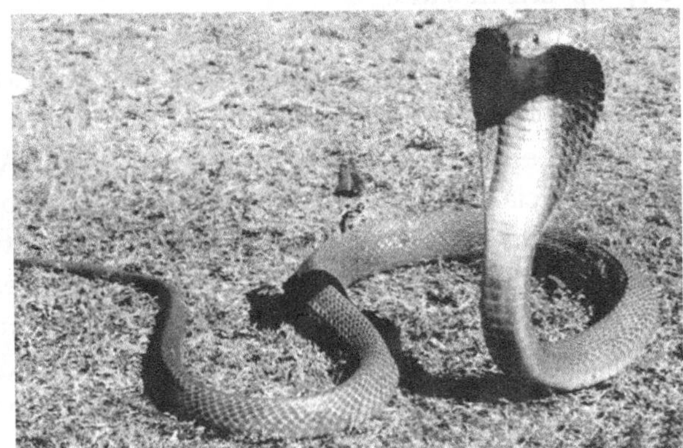

Fig. 23.4: Cobra

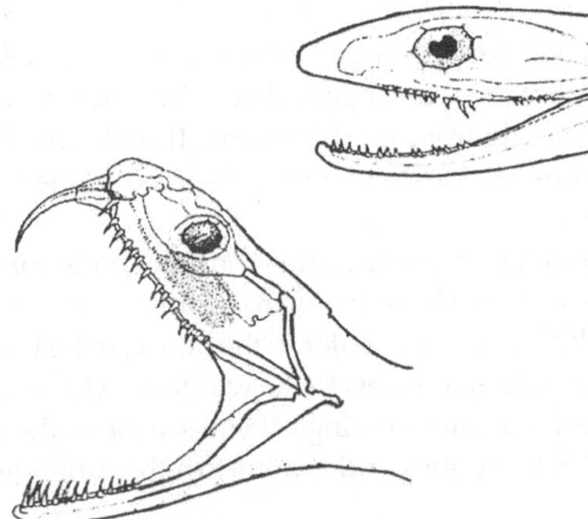

Fig. 23.5: All snakes can swallow animals thicker than their own bodies

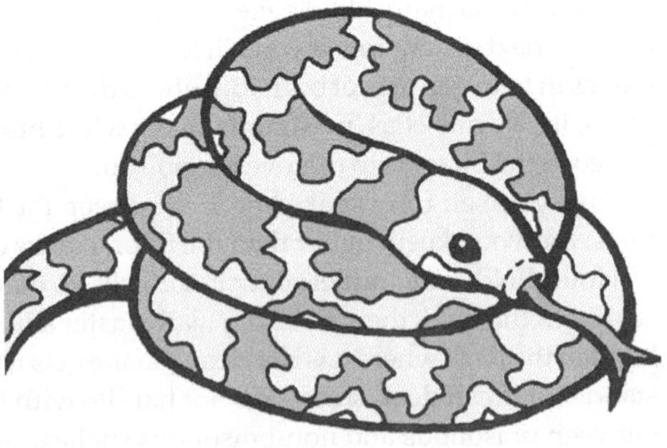

Fig. 23.6: Python has the biggest mouth and can even get to grips with a whole goat, pig or antelope

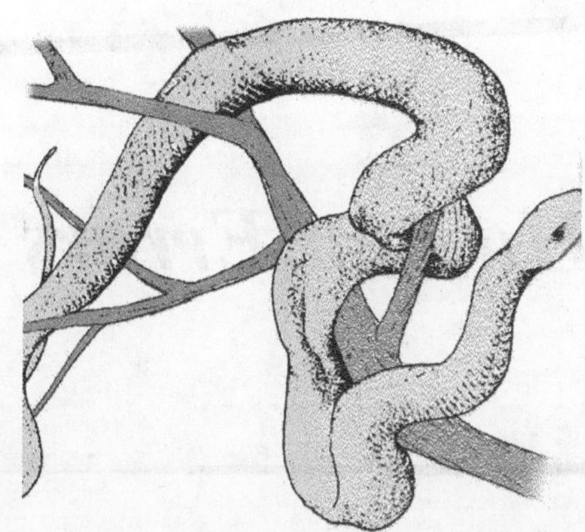

Fig. 23.7: The golden tree snake can leap from a tree onto its prey

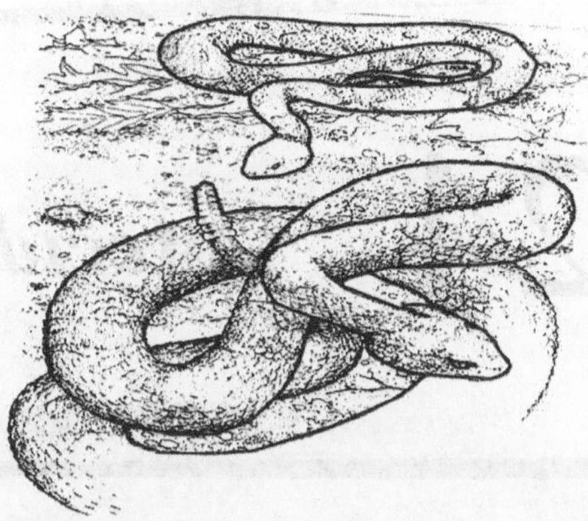

Fig. 23.8: Rattlesnakes can hunt in the dark, because they are very sensitive to heat

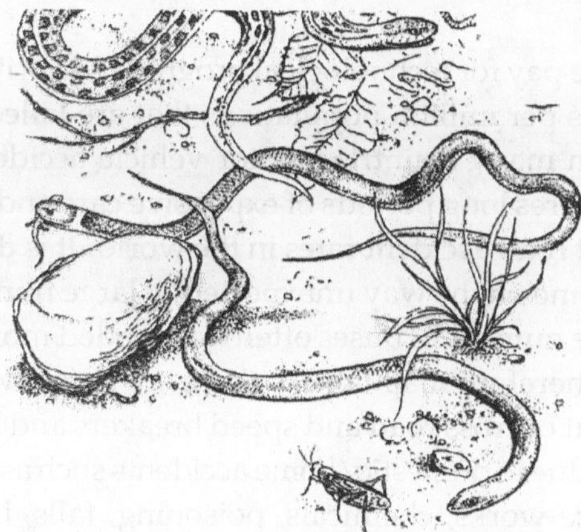

Fig. 23.9: Sea snakes – they are found only in tropical waters. Come to the surface of the sea to breathe but can then stay under water upto 8 hours

24 Accidents: Human Errors

Accident is an unexpected, unplanned occurrence, which usually produces unintended injury, death or property damage.

They are part of the price we pay for technological progress. Majority of accidents are preventable.

There are number of deaths per million populations that are killed in road traffic accidents and disabled and handicapped. In many countries motor vehicle accidents rank first among all fatal accidents. Serious injured requires long periods of expensive care and nursing treatment.

India has one of the highest road accident rates in the world. It is due to large number of animals and roadway bullocks who come on the way unexpectedly; large number of old, poorly maintained vehicles that people use. Large number of buses often overloaded moreover people disregard traffic rules, no traffic discipline is therefore maintained; there are defective roads and its size with poor street lighting, defective layout of cross road and speed breakers and high density of the vehicles.

Another type of accident is due to domestic/home accidents such as drowning, burns of flames, hot liquid, electricity, crackers fire works, chemicals, poisoning, falls, injuries from sharp or pointed instruments, bites and other injuries from animals, epilepsy, and vertigo.

There are other accidents, like gas, kerosene stove, electric shock, keeping drug with reach of children, falls from balconies in high-rise buildings.

Agriculture accidents like handling machines without knowledge.

Industrial accidents remain the tragedy of modern industry and one of its most serious forms of economic waste.

Human factors responsible for accidents such as sudden illness, heart attacks, impaired vision, defective judgment, delay in decisions, poor perception.

Due to lack of body protection not worn such as helmets, safety belts, which increases vulnerability and risk for accidents.

Driving under alcohol and drugs consumption and other social pressures factors are cause of accidents.

Prevention of accidents: Data collection studies bring out risk factors, the circumstances and chain of evens leading up to the accident. Safety education in school is important; drivers should be trained in proper maintenance of vehicles, safe driving, and first aids if accident occurs. The care drivers should use seat belt, compulsory safety helmet, leather boots can protect their lower legs, and children remain seated when they are in vehicle. Alcohol impairs driving ability and increases risk. Drugs like barbiturates impair one's ability to drive safely.

Organization, management of trauma treatment and emergency care services should be fundamental element of health system. Improving roads with proper maintenance, imposition of speed limits, making of danger points signs, reduction of electric voltage, and provision of fireguards.

Strict driving tests and medical fitness, checking regular blood alcohol concentration inspection and seeking ways to make safe environment by new and better methods of altering human behavior.

Medical, social, occupational rehabilitation and compensation to make available so as to prevent and reduce, disability and handicapped that may follow the accident.

Accidents due to rash driving, overspending, jumping signals lane cutting, not wearing helpmates, drunken driving increase 10% accidents. It is a bear negligence, which endangers a person's life, appeal to the youngsters to refrain daredevilry and display their talents in better enterprises. Adhere to the basic traffic and safety norms and do not put self and otters live in danger.

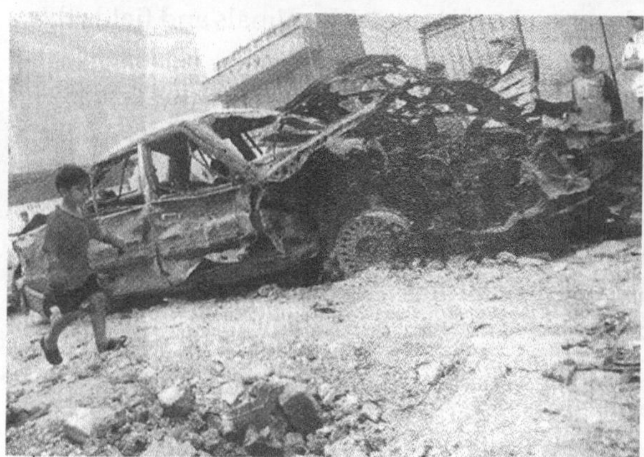

Fig. 24.1: Slow and steady will reach you to destination

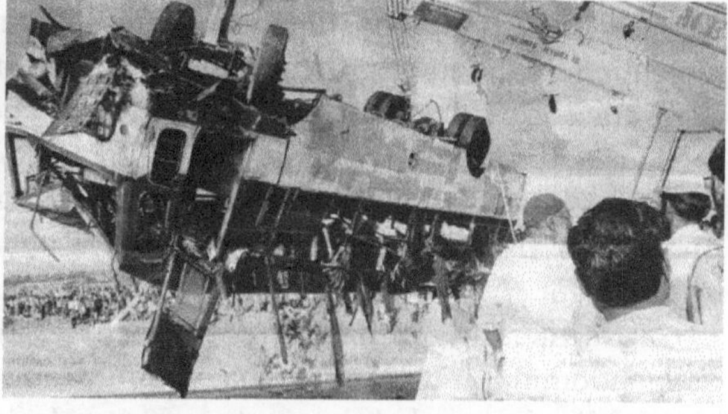

Fig. 24.2: Loss of lives and property: Take care of the precious lives placed in your hand

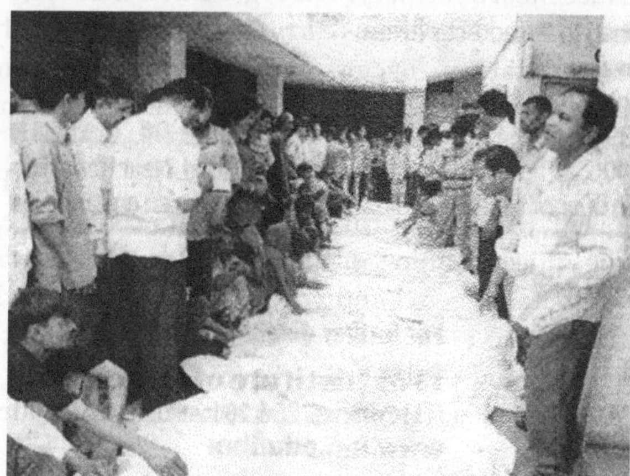

Fig. 24.3: No fault of theirs so many innocent lives lost due to carelessness and human error

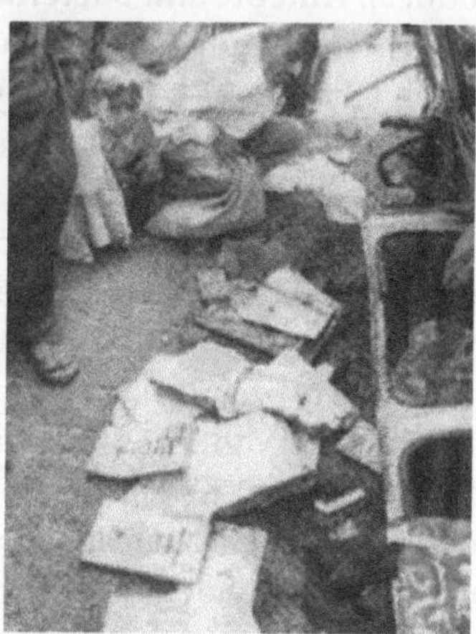

Fig. 24.4: Difficult to accept the sudden loss and pain caused by accident of the beloved ones

25 Gastrointestinal Disorders that Affect Rural Poor

(Food poisoning; diarrhea, dysentery, amebiasis; worm infestation; appendicitis)

Due to lack of personal hygiene, polluted water, unclean food, working with animals and fields there are some health problem that affects the rural community.

Intestinal disorder will usually have a problem with bowel elimination. The manifestation and cause of disturbance/dysfunction could be many one of them is hemorrhage caused by trauma, ulceration, inflation or growth that erodes through a blood vessel. Blood in the stool that is a tray stool/melena can be found out by lab testing of occult blood.

Signs and symptoms of pain and discomfort could be due to obstruction of blood supply to the intestine, which can also cause pain. There is nausea and vomiting results from distention of the duodenum; also due to other reasons such as malabsorption, diarrhea, constipation, abnormalities in fecal content.

Gastroenteritis is an inflation of stomach and intestinal tract that affects small bowel. It is associated with abdominal cramps, diarrhea, vomiting and fever. **Dysentery** is an inflation affecting the colon bloody diarrhea and abdominal cramping. Inflammation occurs more often in children under 10 years of age. Colitis is bacterial dysentery, other dysentery associated with ingestion of contaminated food products. **Amebic and bacterial organisms** cause most dysentery. The organism is transmitted by ingestion of contaminated foods and drinking water. Infected persons carry these organisms in the large bowel. **Cholera** also causes dysentery like manifestations. Bacterial or viral **food poisoning** develops. **Viral gastroenteritis** occurs throughout the world and is common. It often occurs in epidemic outbreaks.

Dysentery is an inflammatory condition affecting the colon. In staphylococcal food poisoning, the bacteria produce a toxin when infected foods are allowed to remain warm for a time before being eaten.

Diarrhea associated with dysentery destroys the mucosal lining of the bowel, leading to fluid leaking into the bowel. Dysentery can be fatal in debilitated, aged and very young persons. Early detection and intervention with fluids and electrolytes are critical to prevent death or disability. Assessment reveals possible vomiting, profuse diarrhea and resultant severe fluid and electrolyte loss. Blood in the stool **Giardiasis** onset is abrupt with nausea, vomiting, excessive foul flatulence, and malabsorption, which causes weight loss.

Best remedy in such occasion is rest, nothing by mouth, replacing fluids. Antidiarrheas and antispasmodics medicines may be given. Community Health Nurse will need to note the number, onset, color, and consistency of stools, eating habits, fairs and festivals, traveling and antibiotic use.

Assess abdominal for bowel sounds, distention, and tenderness. Muscle weakness, fatigue – cessations of diarrhea, decrease in number of stools and solid consistency of stools. Special attention to the diet, rest plan, maintains absolute cleanliness if family shares bathroom.

APPENDICITIS

Appendicitis is another problem during home visits and in emergency takes place in rural areas needs a special attention and treatment. Patient usually comes with severe abdominal pain Community Health Nurse first duty to determine its location; assess rebound tenderness and vitals, fluid and electrolyte status pain medication withheld until diagnosis is confirmed, do not give enema, laxatives or apply heat to the abdomen as this action could lead to perforation. If the rupture of the appendix is suspected, contact physician and shift the client to the hospital.

How does inflammatory bowel disease affect daily life of the rural poor; and what steps need to be taken? How does dietary patterns/habits affect? Clinical manifestation of inflammatory bowel disease and priority of Community Health Nurse intervention. What dietary management is important?

You must ensure safe, standard care and help people to alleviate their problem. Educate them on risk factors and levels of prevention such as chronic constipation, low fiber diet, obesity. Maintain adequate bowel habits (in rural villages women control nature call until it becomes dark to hide themselves as they do not have latrine facilities and that affects health too) avoid gas-producing foods, carbonated beverages, alcohol, smoking, stress alterations in sleep and rest; consume well-balanced diet, exercise daily.

Intestinal disorders are common and it causes problem patients throughout life if they are not treated promptly and completely. Modification in certain behavior to promote health and adaptation to the changes suggested.

Digestive tract/alimentary canal provide the body fluid, nutrients and electrolytes. The raw materials taken in through the mouth and metabolized for energy and tissue building digestion and absorption. Chewing, swallowing food and not eating too fast, person must maintain dental health poorly chewed foods are not readily digested. Even though most organisms are destroyed by the acidic gastric juice. Small intestine complete digestion of food takes place and the residues are then moved on into the large intestine. Where complete absorption of water, formation of feces a expulsion of feces from the body takes place. To provide effective intervention the Community Health Nurse must understand the normal physiology of digestive organs.

Avoid potatoes, breads, jelly, sweetened fruit juice, cakes, pies, cookies, milk shakes, sugar etc.

Take health history: Such as ask when was the problem first noted? Was the onset gradual or sudden? Was it related to food intake? Does the problem occur occasionally or is it persistent? Wheather the pain is continuous or intermittent describe the problem where does he feel pain, does pain spread to the other areas of the body? Is it related to eating, drinking or activity? Does eating, position changes relieve the pain. Therefore, she needs to assess onset, duration, severity, location etc.

Her abilities to encourage and the intake of the right type and quantities of foods. Examine number of meals eaten, away from home regularity of food consumption, assess diverse cultural background, health-related dietary beliefs and practices, dietary practices of religious groups, prohibited foods and beverages she needs to be aware these factors that influences the family nutritional state. Eating is a personal matter. People change outward aspect as clothing and language but culture determines what acceptable and unacceptable foods are. Community Health Nurse must help to categorize nutrition practices as beneficial, neutral or harmful. If it is necessary to change diet for health or medical reasons, suggest few alterations in traditional foods, encourage desirable behavior changes.

Avoid spicy foods, limit caffeine nicotine, hot foods, follow life style change, disorders of mouth, dental carries interfere family nutritional intake.

What lifestyle changes could help the family manage their condition and affect the family?

What teaching is required for medication and dietary management? What disorder manifest in people who consume large quantities of alcohols? What is cirrhosis of liver? The risks faced by the family due to this problem? She has obligation to care for a family with a lifestyle disease. Cirrhosis of the liver can be a very serious and often deadly condition, alcohol abuse accounts for most cases. In the family when person with alcohol lives family goes through emotional experience of anxiety when a person cannot control its consumption; do not judge a person harshly or be unkind to them you have to understand the family and its situation and it is her responsibility to assist the services needs. Look beyond the abusing personality and treat the person and family holistically. She must consider both the physiological and psychological problems associated with many hepatic disorders. Helping family to make appropriate lifestyle changes is an important function of community worker.

Everyday we find something in the news about health maintenance or disease prevention. Research constantly tells us which foods to be taken, unsafe practices, social problems that affect health and well-being.

Food poisoning is also health needs in rural areas:

Watch what you eat, food poisoning is known as acute gastroenteritis, is an acute inflammation of the lining of the stomach and small bowel. Some people are allergic to certain items of food, which, though wholesome to others, may act as poisons to them. Others react poorly to various drugs, chemicals. Food poisoning usually begins suddenly with a feeling of nausea and abdominal craps, followed by vomiting, diarrhea and weakness. Foods used at picnics, in restaurants, and at home are easily contaminated by toxins.

What is food poisoning? What cause food poisoning? What action needs to be taken, what are its sign symptoms and risks? How to prevent it?

It is an **acute gastroenteritis** caused by ingestion of food or drink contaminated with either living bacteria or their toxins or inorganic chemical substances and poisons derived from plants and animals. Caused by chemicals such as arsenic, certain plant and sea foods, e.g. fertilizers, pesticides, and mercury. Bacterial caused by the ingestion of foods and their toxins.

Food brought from street vendors; cooked food that is kept at tepid temperature for long time, such as Wada pav can be rife with a bacteria that causes food poisoning, reheating food; 60% gastroenteritis cases are caused by cooked food that hasn't been reheated properly; cook food to 70 degree celsius and above all it should be piping hot to ensure that it is safe. Pastry biscuits are some of the worst sources so limit them too.

Salmonella food poisoning is common form of food poisoning, wide spread use of household detergents is interfering with sewage treatment, infection from farm animals and poultry through impure meat, milk and milk product, sausages, custards, egg products, rats and mice as they are heavily infected and contaminate foodstuffs by their urine and feces.

Food poisoning on ingestion, multiply in the intestine and give rise to acute enteritis and colitis. The onset is sudden with chills, fever, nausea, and vomiting and profuse watery diarrhea, which last 2–3 days.

Cow suffering from mastitis outbreaks involving milk and milk products. Food like salads, custards, milk and milk products eaten with care. The toxins act directly on Central nervus system. It starts sudden onset of vomiting, abdominal cramps and diarrhea.

The **organism found in feces** of humans and animals, in soil, water and air – outbreaks ingestion of meat, meat dishes and poultry. Food cooked and kept and later eaten spores survive in cooking.

Food poisoning may be mistaken for cholera, acute bacillary dysentery. Lab investigation samples specimen from stool, vomit, and blood for antibodies, environmental study, and data analysis.

Prevention: Meat inspection, personal hygiene, food handles who suffer from infection, wounds, boils, diarrhea, dysentery, throat infection, sanitary improvements sterilization of all work surfaces, utensils – free from rats, mice, flies and dust.

Health education to be given to the food handlers should be educated in matters of clean habits, personal hygiene and through hand washing.

Refrigerator : Proper temperature control, food hot left in warm pantries—a few germs can multiply to millions by the next morning, 'cook and eat on same day' is a golden rule.

Avoid fly born diseases such as diarrhea, dysentery, cholera, typhoid, and gastroenteritis.

Milk born diseases such as cowpox, anthrax, tick-born, bovine tuberculosis, viral hepatitis.

Surveillance: Food samples must be obtained periodically and subjected to lab analysis, if they are unsatisfactory then outbreak of food-born diseases takes place.

It is a common problem in summer – Known as 'stomach flu' meat that is not cooked, mayonnaise based salad, tuna, and chicken salad. Do not cut meat and vegetables on same board.

Follow apt sanitation such as washing hands, food adulteration causes diarrhea. Methods of preservation of food should be scientific. Water, milk born disease adds to food poison.

Food poisoning keep the patient in bed. Encourage vomiting if the food has been eaten within the last one or two hours, for much of it may still be in the stomach. After the stomach is emptied, follow the outline of treatment suggested for acute gastroenteritis, severe cases of mushroom poisoning should be treated in hospital.

Community nurse requires critical thinking, logical judgment. She has a philosophy of life and sets of ideas, principles, goals, standard of values. She is legally and morally accountable person; her actions are drawn from biopsychosocial sciences. Nurse is a socializing agent, she is a advocate and protector. She has to play active role in bringing social change. Nursing is a profession and nursing practice must reflect professionalism, it requires clinical knowledge, judgment, technical competency, and health knowledge, teaching skills, realization of professional responsibilities.

AMEBIASIS

It is the rural health problem where the group needs to be made aware of worm infestation and its prevention methods. Once they understand the causes, its signs and symptoms, its life cycle, its treatment and the complication it can be easy to treat and control in the community. Community health nurse is an important person in this control program.

The problem of helminthes infestation is common in all tropical countries due to prevalent methods of defecation and disposal of excreta. Intestinal infestation adds to the burden of the rapidly growing children whose health status is already compromised by illness, malnutrition and unsanitary living conditions. There are different types of worms.

Pathogenic stains of *E. histolytica* cause it. It occurs at any age. It is a household infection when one individual in a family is infected, others in family get affected. It is closely related to poor sanitation, socioeconomic status, the use of night soil for agricultural purposes favor the spread of disease. It is higher during rains; cysts may survive longer-outbreaks associated with sewage seepage into the water supply.

Transmission by fecal –oral –route. Also by flies, cockroaches, rodents. Avoid eating and handling contamination of water, food, vegetables, and fruits and human feces. Follow sanitation, washing hands after defecation; check the water supply because amebic cysts may survive for several days and weeks in water. Chemical treatment of water, food, hygiene, uncooked food, food handles are major transmitters, they should be periodically examined, treated and educated. Early diagnosis, symptomatic treatment with tablet Metrogyl for 8 to 10 days. (Tinidazole) as per doctor order to be given.

Ascariasis—It is an infection of intestinal tract. Its sign, symptoms are nausea, abdominal pain and cough. Live worms are passed in the stool or vomit. Occasionally they may produce intestinal obstruction, or may migrate into the peritoneal cavity. It is a common helminths infestation; ¼ of world population is infected. It lives in lumen of small intestine, where it moves freely. The eggs are excreted in the feces, they hatch in small intestine, and the larvae penetrate the gut wall and are carried to the liver and than lungs via the bloodstream. Then migrate into the bronchioles – coughed through trachea – and then swallowed by human host in reaching intestine 60–80 days mature. The life span is 1.5 years. Man is the one reservoir.

Hookworm infection: Enter body via feet infection causes chronic blood loss and depletion of body's iron stores leading to iron deficiency anemia; Low birth weight, abortion, stillbirths, impaired lactation, malnutrition. They may occur as single or mixed infections in the same person. The worm measures about 8-10 mm in length, these worms are passed in feces by infected persons. The female parasite lay eggs, which are passed in the feces. A single female may lay 10,000 to 20,000 eggs per day. The eggs hatch into larvae outside the human body in the soil where they grow and develop into infective larvae. These infective larvae enter the human body, the larvae migrate first to the lungs and then into the small intestine. Finally they develop into mature worms in the small intestine and start laying eggs. The time required for this cycle is about 6 weeks. Hookworms are found in the duodenum and upper part of small intestine. Client may suffer from anemia, general debility and loss of body resistance.

Round worms rob man of his food. It is soiled-transmitted helminth eggs remain viable in the soil for months or years under favorable condition. Soil pollution – children play on the ground and contaminate hands and food until all fertile females are destroyed and stools are negative. It is fecal–

oral. It is more common in the children between the ages of 1 to 15 years, with lower socioeconomic status. Abdominal pain, intestinal obstruction, pneumonia due to larva in the lungs, fever and eosinophilia occurs.

The life cycle of round worms is that they live in the upper part of small intestine. It resembles on ordinary earthworm. It measures up to 20 cm–45 cm in length. The female lays eggs in large number, which are passed in the feces. They contaminate the soil or vegetables, given optimal conditions, the eggs take about 10 days to become embryonated when the infective eggs are ingested, they reach the intestine where they hatch into larvae. The larvae penetrate the intestine and migrate to liver, lungs, and the then travel up the trachea to pharynx to be swallowed by the human host.

They reach the small intestine where they become sexually mature in about 6 to 10 weeks. It can be investigated by stool examination for ova or worms.

To prevent roundworm, use boiled water for drinking. Proper disposal of excreta, proper hand washing, and hygienic eating habits to be practiced. Use of sanitary latrines, habit of using foot wears which prevents contacts with contaminated soil in open fields. Cutting the children's nail short. Use of long pajamas to prevent auto infestation, antiprurtic cream can be used to prevent itching, detection and early treatment.

Prevention through good sanitation, safe drinking water, food hygiene, health education, changes in behavioral patterns, mass treatment of deworming, chemotherapy, correction of anemia.

Common risk factors for above mention health problems are overcrowding, improper handling and storage of foods, food handling by infected persons, poor sanitation conditions, and food remaining at a temperature high enough for organism to incubate and colonize easily. To prevent avoid overcrowding, obtain vaccination for viral gastroenteritis, handle food properly, learn storage technique, avoid prolonged use of antibiotics, replacement of fluids and prevention of complications.

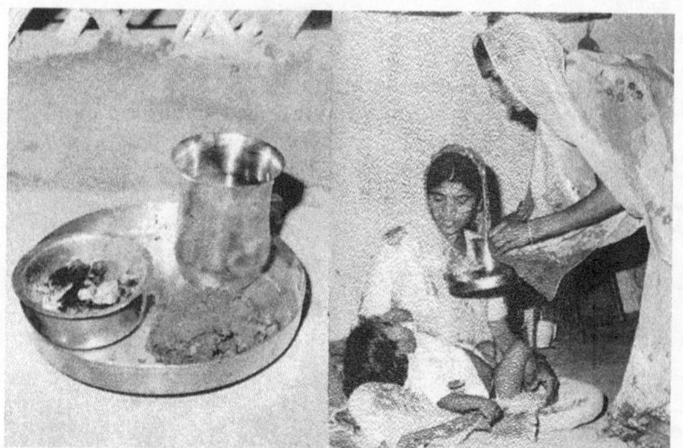

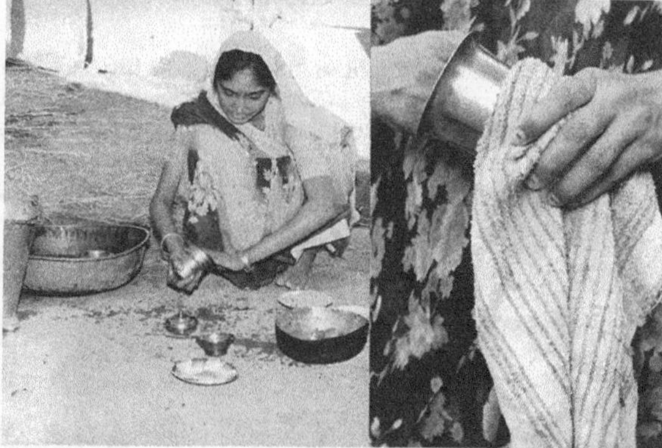

Figs 25.1 and 25.2: Food hygiene and prevention of food adulteration. Food is a potential source of infection and is liable to contamination by micro-organisms, food hygiene in the production, handling, distribution and saving of all types of food. The primary aim of food hygiene is to prevent food poisoning and other food born diseases

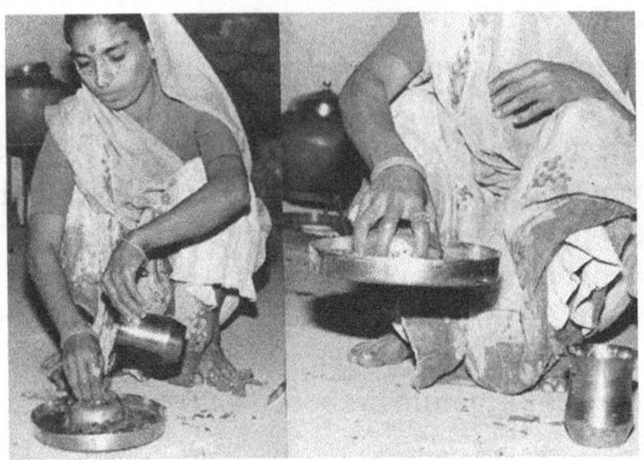

Fig. 25.3: Milk is an efficient vehicle for a great variety of disease. A contaminated vessel, polluted water, flies, dust etc

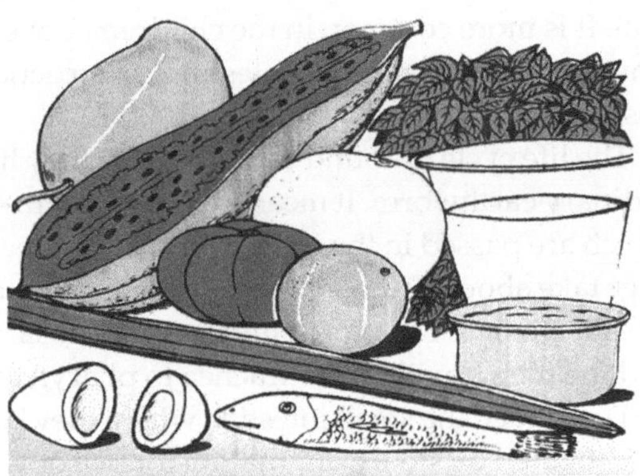

Fig. 25.4: Safe and clean balance diet

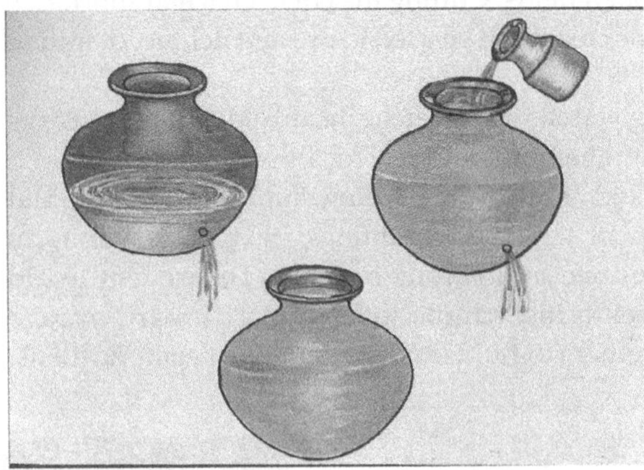

Fig. 25.5: Safe water: Water the liquid of life. It is free from harmful pathogenic organisms. Free from harmful chemical substances. Portable or fit for domestic use. Pleasant to the taste

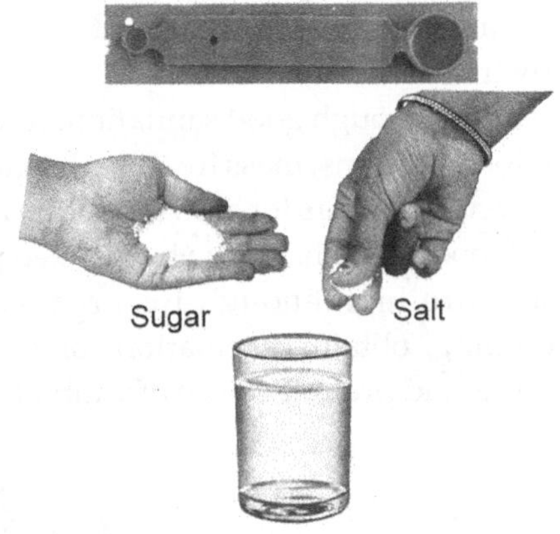

Fig. 25.6: Domestic home made ORS. After food poisoning and diarrhea have oral dehydration therapy

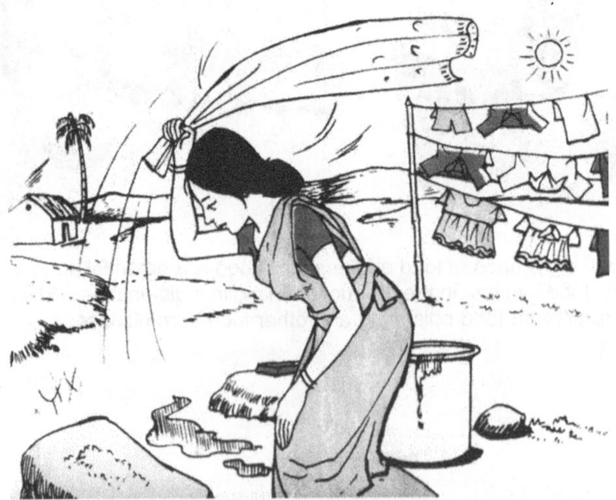

Fig. 25.7: Environmental sanitation and clean surrounding can prevent waterborne diseases and food poisoning and other health problems

26 Living Well with Diabetes

Did you ever wonder how in the world all the various organs of the body know what to do and when to do? With so many different parts all working at the same time it would be easy to produce too much of one thing, too little of another. This is exactly what happens when we are ill, endocrine disorder causes diabetes.

The pancreas is a large digestive organ lying behind the stomach and across the back portion of the abdomen. Most parts of this large gland are busy with the normal processes of digestion through the pancreatic enzymes. But one small portion known as the tail of the pancreas has an entirely different function, for it belongs to the endocrine glandular system. It secretes two hormones, insulin and glycogen. Insulin has much to do with the metabolism of the body. Insulin is the powerful hormone that aids the body in storing nutriment, instead of allowing it to drain away in the urine.

Diabetes mellitus is a metabolic disorder characterized by glucose intolerance. It is a systemic disease caused by an imbalance between insulin supply and insulin demands. Insulin maintains the balance between high and low blood glucose levels. Extra food is eaten but not metabolized, which leads to hunger and the patient loses weight. Elevated blood glucose levels may occur after meals, after stressful events.

Some people are unable to produce enough insulin to meet their own needs. Lacking sufficient insulin, their blood sugar or glucose rises to a high level, while the cells of the body do not receive their normal supply of nutriment. The excess glucose then spills over into the urine. This condition is known as diabetes.

Know your diabetes better to manage it better. Body cells need glucose sugar, which produces energy required for daily life. The food we eat turns in to glucose after digestion. Glucose enters the blood, produced by pancreas, which allows glucose to enter body cells. If it is in the high amounts of glucose in the blood, it results in hyperglycemia. A high blood sugar problem leads to diabetes mellitus.

Diabetes is long-term disease with variable clinical manifestation and progression leads to a number of complications such as cardiovascular, renal, neurological, and ocular disease. Symptoms caused are frequent urination, feeling of always hungry, craving for sweet foods and extra liquids, person always feels tired, has sores that do not heal, gets vaginal infection, sexual dysfunction, and sudden unexplained weight loss. If the family member has diabetes it can run in the family also overweight, numbness and tingling of feet, blurred vision experience by the client.

Clinical classification of diabetes in insulin dependent is most severing form of the disease. Its onset is typically abrupt and seen in individual age less than 30 years old.

Non-insulin dependent is much more common than insulin dependent diabetes. It is often discovered by chance. Its gradual onset and occurs in middle age and elderly if given adequate treatment remains under control.

Malnutrition related diabetes, and other types of pancreatic, hormonal drug induced, genetic and other abnormalities impaired glucose tolerance.

Gestational diabetes—During pregnancy diabetes can be serious. Diabetes babies always weigh more than normal. All pregnant mothers should have a blood sugar test taken and if sugar is high than normal, treatment should be stared.

Obesity—Older people often tend to gain weight and at the same time, many of them will develop a mild form of diabetes because of the strain on the pancreas. It is very important to keep the weight under control.

A family history of diabetes is important when it develops in children. All children of such parents should check the children for diabetes.

Diabetes is one of the leading causes of death in developed countries. It is an iceberg disease affecting about 30 million people worldwide. The major cause of prolonged ill health is coronary heart diseases, retinopathy, and gangrene of a lower extremity, neuropathy, stroke and cataract. It is known as silent hidden killer disease.

Diabetes patients are very susceptible to infections of the skin, such as boils, carbuncles.

Diabetes causes are: Pancreatic disorders defects in the formation of insulin; genetic defects.

Malnutrition affects large number of people, the prognosis is worse in younger person who tends to develop complications. Some people appear to have defective immunological mechanism and under the influence of some environmental 'trigger' attack their own insulin producing cells.

Obesity is a risk factor for non-insulin dependent diabetes, many obese persons are not diabetic also physical inactivity, deficiencies of specific nutrients.

Kidney problems, renal infection may trigger diabetes, marital status, religion, economic status, education, urbanization and change in lifestyle.

The human body is a living engine. It constantly requires food or fuel to keep it going.

People, who lead a sedentary lifestyle, mostly consume flesh foods like fish, chicken, mutton and seafoods in their daily life. Some people prefer fried foods, fast foods, cashew nut, cashew halwa, milk and its products, coconut and its oil.

People who are leading a life of worry, anxiety, emotional stress, and anger.

Lack of exercise, consumption of excess food without adequate work, heavy work without adequate food. Insufficient amount of foods and keeping an empty stomach are not helpful in managing diabetes.

Avoiding starvation and fasting. If there is excess sugar, patient may go into diabetic coma and if it less then normal, can go into insulin comma, maintaining normal level of sugar is an important part of managements of diabetes.

Diabetes is the 5th leading cause of death.

In the first hour or two after meals, insulin concentration rises rapidly in blood and peak at about 1 hour. After meals, insulin concentrations promptly decline even during night insulin concentration are low and constant with a slight increase at dawn; self esteem disturbance related to lifestyle changes imposed by diabetes and its treatment, stigma of having a chronic illness, and frustration at progression of disease despite careful management.

Diet tips which include chapattis, rice small amount, bread, potatoes, porridge and pasta. All vegetables especially green leafy vegetables such as karcha methi, palak, extra helping of salads including cucumbers, carrots, cabbage etc. Fruit one a day or one wati fruit salad, skimmed milk; preferably boiled, grilled foods.

Avoid excess intake of fats and fat products like oil, ghee, butter, fried foods like puris, fatty meat. Avoid sugar, jaggary, honey, jams, cakes and chocolates. Eat less of meat, chicken and cheese and more of vegetables.

Eating a well balanced diet that includes plenty of fresh fruits, vegetables and whole grains/ Choose foods low in saturated fat and sodium.

Avoid meat, eggs, and diary products. Avoid fried foods, rich pastries, cakes, puddings, and sweets. Avoid dry fruits, coconut, papads, pickles, wagers, chips, farsans, and nuts, cheese.

Avoid red meat, organ meats like kidney, brain, liver, and egg yoke. Restrict the intake of fruit juice, restrict the intake of bakery products.

Tests—In fasting, blood sugar test, the client may not eat for four hours but water can be taken. If the patient is a known diabetic, food and insulin are withheld until after the specimen is drawn.

In postprandial blood sugar, these blood glucose levels are tested after meals. Sometimes the patient is given a standard amount of glucose, but most commonly a sample is drawn after a standard meal.

Blood glucose finger sticks- self-testing investigation of self-monitoring devices of blood sugar has revolutionaries' diabetic care.

It can be control with proper interaction of food, insulin or oral medication and exercise.

Regular follow-up and frequent checking of blood sugar and readjusting diabetic medications are very important.

Uncontrolled diabetes may lead to loss of vision, damage of kidneys, recurring infections, gangrene, foot problems, heart arracks, brain damage, and sexual dysfunction.

It is a major cause of disability; blindness, kidney failure, and coronary thrombosis, gangrene of the lower extremities are the severe complications. Hence regular medical check-up and necessary investigations are important. Consult your doctor for the same. Because diabetic patients must realize that they have a disorder, which continues for a lifetime. In the majority of cases there is no cure for this disease. The patient must learn to live with his disability.

Screening of urine examination, Urine tests for glucose, 2 hours after meal, case finding, epidemiological surveys of the population, Blood sugar testing – fasting postprandial or random blood sample need to be done to detect new cases and control in early stage.

Screening 'high risk' people age of 40 and over those with family history of diabetes, the obese woman who show excess weight gain during pregnancy and patient with premature arteriosclerosis.

During pregnancy, diabetes can be serious. Diabetic babies always weigh more than normal. All pregnant mothers should have a blood sugar test taken two hours after a normal meal. If the sugar shows higher than normal, treatment should be started at once.

Prevention: Maintain normal body weight, healthy nutritional habits and physical exercise, adequate protein intake, a high intake of dietary fiber and avoidance of sweet foods, prevention of coronary heart disease.

Genetic counseling: Correction of lifestyle, avoid alcohol, smoking, control of high blood pressure and elevated cholesterol.

When detected it must be adequately treated. To maintain blood glucose level, maintain ideal body weight, small balanced meals more frequently. Diet and insulin and good control of blood glucose will protect against complications. Routine check-up of blood and urine sugar to be done. The diabetic patient must realize that there is no simple solution to his problem. Nor can be cured by having an operation. He must regulate his diet carefully. Omit all free sugar from diet such as candy, cake, ice cream, jam, and pastry. Do not take chances with this disease.

Self care—Responsible for own care, with medical guidance, e.g. drug regimens, self-administration of insulin, abstinence from alcohol, maintenance of optimum weight, attending periodic check-ups, recognition of symptoms associated with glycosuria and hypoglycemia etc. Home blood glucose monitoring is good.

Patient should carry an identification card showing name, address, phone number, details of treatment receiving whenever you go out. All these need education of people.

Retinopathy is a leading cause of blindness in some diabetic patients whose blood vessels of retina get damaged due to which bleeding occurs inside the eyeball causing blurring of vision, black spots. Skin complications are common in them with uncontrolled diabetes. Wounds tend to heal slowly, and boils and carbuncles may appear. If gangrene develops in the feet, amputation may be necessary. Treat all foot infections seriously. Numbness or insensitivity to pain or temperature, extreme sensitivity to touch, loss of balance and co-ordination in toe, feet, legs, hands and arms, symptoms often get worse by night.

Educate the diabetic client not to soak feet in water but use mild soap and clean between toes before that check the water temperature with elbow. Use good lighting, use powder if feet perspire, do not use chemicals, use scissors with rounded edged and cut nails straight, trim nails after bath. Do not go barefoot. Do not use hot water bottles, heating pads or electric blankets. Wear adequate foot protection on cold days. Wear cotton socks to keep feet warm. Do not sit with legs crossed. Bye shoes with thick rubber soles, check insides of shoes before dressing for stones, pins, leather shows are usually best, allow the feet to breath, avoid high heels and shoes with pointed toes. Avoid tight socks and shoes, change daily socks. Be alert for slight of infection, redness, swelling, drainage, pain, foul odors or even slight injuries can become infectious.

Nursing Role in Management of Diabetes

Diabetes is a serious health problem throughout the world. It is estimated one in 20 people that is 12 million people in united state have diabetes. It is fifth leading cause of death, it causes new cases of blindness, and it increases the coronary heart disease. It causes many complications in additional complication of pregnancy.

Abnormal production of hormones present in diabetes. Once the insulin is realest into the bloodstream from the B cells, it is routed through the liver, the fall of insulin level during normal overnight fasting facilitate the release of stored glucose from the liver, protein from muscle and fat from adipose tissues, for this reason insulin is known as the storage hormone.

Normally insulin maintains blood glucose level in normal range, elevated blood glucose levels produces symptoms. Due to osmotic effect shift of fluid balance results frequency of urination, thirst.

Type II diabetes have 50% chance of transmitting the disease to their children. Urine test are not sufficient for diagnosing diabetes mellitus because variables such as age, medications. The result of urine tests for glucose and acetone depend on age, severity of diabetes and renal functions. Factors that can induce falsely elevated values includes resent sharp restricted in carbohydrate , acute illness, restricted activities such as bed rest. Because diabetes is a multisystem, multiproblem disease, it is not a single disease.

In the presence of abnormal insulin utilization, fat metabolism is altered, this results in elevation of lipid, cholesterol and triglyceride levels that are associated with vascular disorders of diabetes.

The management is primarily aimed at achieving balances of diet, many people are well aware that a well-balanced diet is healthy, but most people find it difficult to adhere to a special diet all the time. Maintenance of desirable weight is dietary goal; behavioral modification and fat diet should be avoided. Take into consideration client's occupation, age and activities. Eat according to the prescribed meal planned. Learn to recognize appropriate food portions: Never skip meals; especially clients taking insulin, the body requires food at regular spaced intervals throughout the day. Omission and delay of meals may result in hypoglycemia.

Alcohol is high in calories, has no nutritive value and is areas of concern. Nursing management of insulin administration is proper assessment, education, adjustment to, and side effects of insulin, understand the purpose of insulin, side effects may be manifested. Some clients find it difficult to inject themselves due to fear of the needle. A client with newly diagnosed diabetes needs special explanation. The assessment includes client's mental statues, eating habits, home environment, and attitudes towards diabetes. Also if a client is older, lives alone, or finds it difficult to remember to follow diet schedule, some think that diabetes is not a serious disease if they continue taking medication, client needs to understand the importance of diseases and its ill effect if not followed strict diet. He should also be instructed to contact physician in illness of extreme stress occurs. The client with diabetes may be taking other drugs, which too can affect the blood glucose levels. Medication may have to be changed or dosages adjusted if he is taking glucose lowering agents.

Regular exercise is considered an essential, it contributes to weight loss, reduction of triglycerides and cholesterol, increased muscle tone, and improved circulation. Exercise need not be vigorous, brisk walking is good enough, select exercise and be regulate, client should learn to monitor there own glucose level to see and test after exercise. When the insulin supply is insufficient, glucose cannot be properly used for cellular energy; it responds to cellular starvation, the body releases and breaks down the stored fats and protein to provide to needed energy. More water is lost as ketones are excreted in an attempt to balance the PH value. Vomiting caused by acidosis results in more fluid and electrolyte losses. Monitor blood glucose and urine output, correct electrolytes imbalance and vital signs should be assessed.

In hypoglycemia occurs the client should be able to reverse the situation before medical assistance is required. The client's ability to do this depends on the state of alertness and ability to swallow and the availability of quick acting carbohydrate source. Such as regular soft drink, sugar, candy. Quick acting carbohydrate is convenient for carrying in a purse to be used in such a situation. High fat foods and high protein foods are not to be used initially to correct hypoglycemia. Explore why the situation developed, give additional education to avoid future episodes as repeated episodes can impaired learning and memory. The nurse needs to inform the family about the progress and her calm, competent manner in caring for the client can provide assurance to the acutely ill client and the family.

Chronic complication- angiopathy or blood vessel disease is estimated to account for the majority of deaths in diabetes. Neurotrophic ulceration, muscle atrophy, infection. The client should be instructed to contact the health provider when a blood glucose level more than 250 mg/dl, fever, ketonuria, and nausea and vomiting occurs. Travel for clients with diabetes requires planning. They should have all supplies in carry on luggage and with them all the time. Client should be encouraged in self-management to make major adjustment in special circumstances, such as illness or increased exercise. The treatment plan takes time to learn not all clients are capable of self-management. Home management and improvement of lifestyle is useful strategy. Diabetes once diagnosed, the education and follow-up is life long process. Understand general facts of diabetes and involve family in his care, benefits of exercise, nutrition and medications, proper use of insulin, understand effects of illness and respond appropriately, practice foot care, skin care, dental care, maintain proper hygiene, to prevent complication, understand the benefits and responsibilities of self managements, use effectively available health care system and make use of community resources, rehabilitation of diabetes complications.

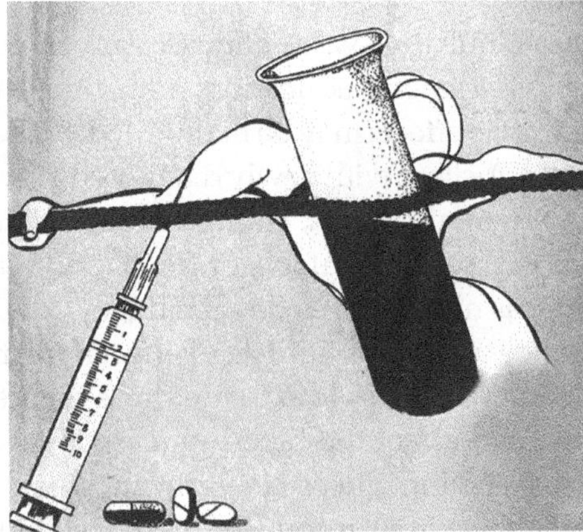

Fig. 26.1: Regular test and doctor order medicines is very important

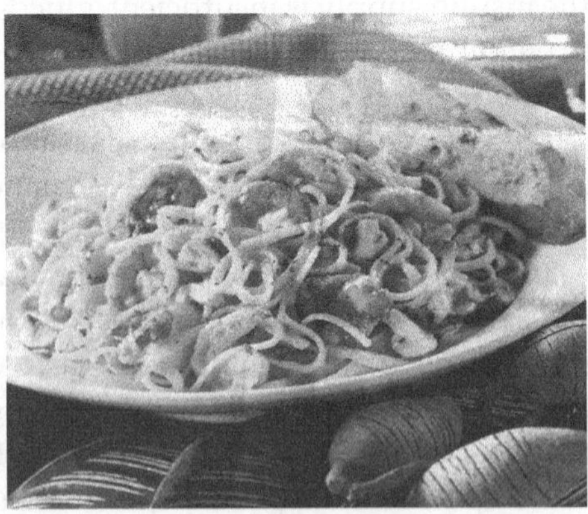

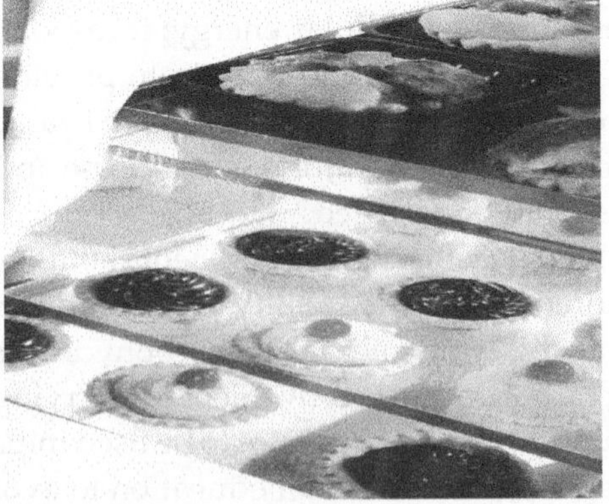

Figs 26.2 and 26.3: Diabetic diet is calculated individually according to the clients ideal body weight, occupation, age and activities. Eat according to the prescribed meal plan. Never skip meals. Diet control and regular treatment can control the diabetics

27 *Healthy Heart*

The human heart is a marvelous organ. It is a strong fist-sized muscle situated in the center of your chest and tilted a little to the left. The function of the heart is to supply blood to all parts of the body. It pumps blood and never stopping even for a moment in its endless activity. Your heart does an enormous amount of work. Naturally, to maintain all this activity, the heart must feed itself. It must also be constantly supplied with oxygen. Coronary arteries the lifelines of the heart provide blood supply to the heart. Like all other tissues in the body, the heart muscle needs oxygen-rich blood to function, and oxygen-depleted blood must be carried away.

Why are the coronary arteries important? Because coronary arteries deliver blood to the heart muscle, any coronary artery disorder or disease can have serious implications by reducing the flow of oxygen and nutrients to the heart, which may lead to a heart attack and possibly death. In many of the large medical centers today, highly trained teams of specialists are now developing newer and more wonderful ways of studying damaged hearts. Cardiology is one of the fastest growing fields. It is mandatory to keep in touch with recent advances.

In the last two decades, there have been revolutionary advances in the management of coronary heart disease. It is of paramount importance to be familiar with the symptoms, preventive measures and methodology of management of this devastating disease. Cardiovascular and cancer are at present leading cause of death in developed countries like Europe, America, which accounts 70 to 75% deaths. It is showing upward trend. Lifestyle and behavior patterns of people are changing rapidly due to ultramodern fast forward lifestyle. Where heart disease puts heavy burden on the lives of people especially if they are poor family with hardships of poverty and economic loss to the family adds to it where there is loss of life and disablement too.

A condition is called congenital cardiovascular disease when it is present at birth. It occurs when the heart or blood vessels near the heart do not develop normally before birth. Heart defects begin in the early part of pregnancy when the heart defects can affect any of the different parts or functions of the heart. In most cases, scientists do not know what makes a baby's heart develop abnormally. Both genetic and environmental factors such as a virus and certain drugs, women who contract rubella during the first three months of pregnancy have high risk of having a baby with a heart defect; genetics appear to play a role in heart defects.

There are many causes, which affect the cardiovascular disease such as **coronary artery disease** that is a narrowing or blockage of the arteries that provide oxygen and nutrients to the heart. It is caused by atherosclerosis that is an accumulation of fatty materials on the inner linings of arteries, which restricts blood flow to the heart, blood flow gets cut off which may result in heart attack, i.e. myocardial ischemia._When heart does not get enough oxygen, patient gets chest pain, i.e. called angina. **Angina** is a sign that patient is at risk of heart attack. Angina is a recurring pain or discomfort in the chest that happens when some part of the heart does not receive enough blood. It is a common symptom of coronary heart disease. Angina feels like a pressing or squeezing pain, usually in the chest under the breast bone, but sometimes in the shoulders, arms, neck, jaws, back or upper abdomen. It is usually relived within a few minutes by resting or by talking prescribed angina medicine. Physical exertion is the most common trigger for angina. Other triggers can be emotional stress, extreme cold or heat, heavy meals, alcohol, and cigarette smoking.

Heart attack results from coronary heart disease. A heart attack occurs when blood supply to part of the heart muscle itself is severely reduced or stopped. This is usually due to atherosclerosis. This can kill or disable someone, depending upon how much heart muscle is damaged. A severe spasm can cause a heart attack. Prolonged pain, unrelieved by rest and accompanied by other symptoms may signal a heart attack.

Warning signs of heart attacks are uncomfortable pressure, fullness squeezing or pain in the center of the chest is accompanied by sweating, light-headedness, nausea or shortness of breath and that lasts more than 30 minutes may be a heart attack. Chest discomfort, fainting, unexplained anxiety, fatigue, palpation, and cold sweat/paleness may occur. When a heart attack occurs, it's critical to recognize the signals and respond immediately. About half of all the heart attack victims wait two hours or longer before deciding to get help. This reduces their chance of survival, because delay in the early phases increases the risk of sudden death. Time is critical. Anyone experiencing the warning signals of heart attack should be taken immediately to the nearest hospital with 24 hour emergency cardiac care.

There are certain risk factors such as related to genetics, gender, age, obesity, stress, anger, smoking, high blood pressure, physical inactivity, diabetics mellitus, high cholesterol LDL from plaque, a thick hard deposit that can clog arteries, clot can block the flow of blood. A high level of LDL increases risk of heart diseases. HDL carries good cholesterol away from arteries, protects against heart attack. The older you become the greater the risk of developing heart disease, partly because arteriosclerosis occurs as a part of the aging process and partly because you have been exposed to other risk factors for longer period of time. Men are more likely to suffer from heart disease than women. If in your family any one parents died with coronary heart disease at young age make sure you go through health check ups with proper health screening which will help you to extend your life. Diabetes run high risk for coronary heart disease, smoking is a single most risk factor, high blood pressure too increase workload of the heart muscles because the heart has to fight to force out blood against a higher resistance, obesity, stress, hereditary factors, consumption of high salt diet leads to risk factor of heat disease.

Chest pain is most common manifestation in heart disease. Ask the client when the pain started. How long the pain episode lasted? What activity the client was doing just before pain? Was he walking rapidly? Was he exposed to cold? Had he eaten spicy foods? What he did to relive the pain? Did he rest, change his position, took the medication? Did the pain radiate to left arm, jaw, back and abdominal region? How many pillows does the client use? How far client can walk, or how many stairs can he climb before becoming breathless? Does he have sudden breathlessness at night? Does he gets awaken with the feeling of suffocation? Does he get shortness of breath when lying down; heart pound experience did he feels any time? Heart bit too fast, or feel the skip of heartbeats. Does he feel dizzy or faint, if he feels such feeling how long this last, or what the client does to relive this sensation? What activity client can perform without getting tired is the fatigue relived by rest.

High blood pressure is very common condition seen in modern life. In most of the cases the true cause is not known. Why does the pressure rise is still a mystery. Hypotension is far less common than hypertension. Heart failure is a serious condition that develops when the heart is no longer able to carry on its normal work. It occurs in most patients with serious heart disease at some time or the other in the course of their disease. Heart's main function is to pump the bloodstream and keep it circulating through all parts of the body. When the heart is tired or weakened by disease, the bloodstream tends to slow down and fluid will gather in certain areas, particularly the ankles and legs. The lungs may begin to fill up with fluid, making breathing difficult. Heart failure may rise from a number of different conditions, such as high blood pressure, coronary thrombosis, kidney disease, rheumatic fever, diphtheria, and low thyroid activity. Anything obstructing the normal flow of blood will eventually produce severe heart failure.

Arteriosclerosis is the process of hardening of the coronary arteries. A healthy coronary artery is normally smooth walled. Angina pectoris is direct consequence of hardening of the coronary arteries in which fatty substances are deposited in the wall of the arteries. Coronary heart disease can be prevented, or at least delayed. An estimated 50 million Indians suffer from coronary artery disease. Modern-day life underlying risks factors ever-growing numbers of heart attacks. The disease is affecting us at a younger age. Risk factors of coronary heart disease play a part in **high blood pressure**, which is the single, most signal to identify individual as high risk for coronary heart disease. Diabetes is two to three times higher risk for coronary heart disease. Genetic factors: Family history, physical activity: Regular physical activity increases concentration of HDL and decreases the body weight. Hormones, arteriosclerosis, type of a personality behavior associated with competitive drive, restlessness, and hostility impatience are more prone to coronary heart disease than calmer, alcohol of high consumption intake 75-gm/day. Oral contraceptive also indirectly affect the disease.

Prevention of coronary heart disease through dietary changes/modification reduce fat intake, consumption of saturated fat, increase vegetables, fruits, whole grains, avoid alcohol, therefore, nutrition, weight reduction, exercise, behavioral changes, health education, self-care, long term follow up, early case detection. Achieve smoke free society by effective information and education. Prudent diet, reduce salt intake, exercise, weight control, change the community as a whole. Identify high risk by simple test by checking blood pressure serum cholesterol, family history with coronary heart disease obesity diabetes, oral contraceptives, smoking etc. It is better to take positive action such as regularly measuring high blood pressure, smoking replaced by chewing gum. Regular drugs, coronary surgery, use of pace makers. During angina pain stop activity, put a tablet of nitroglycerine under your tongue, this reduces the workload of the heart and increases the blood supply to the heart muscle. Avoid activities what provokes angina such as climbing a railway bridge, a large meal, and football play.

Intensive mass education campaign in community promote early diagnosis, treatment, control, preventing sudden attacks death, aspired on anti-coagulant, beta-blockers given as prevention.

Smoking—some people commit suicide by drowning – but many by smoking. It stimulates circulation to raise high blood pressure. It is wide spreading habit. About 25% coronary heart disease causing sudden death occur in men less than 50 years. It depends on the number of cigarettes smoked per day. The filter ones are not protective, which elevates serum cholesterol.

Cues to Cardiovascular Problems

There are certain symptoms found such as fatigue—no energy, more rest than normal necessary, normal activities resulting in tiring. Fluid retention, weight gain, bloated feeling, swelling, tightening of clothing; shoes no longer fitting comfortably. Irregular heartbeats, sensation of heart in throat, dizziness. Dyspnea, air hunger, especially after exertion, pillows necessary for sleep or use of chair. Pain- indigestion, burning, numbness, tightness or pressure in mid-chest, epigastric pain, radiating to shoulder, neck, arms. Tenderness in calf of leg, inability to bear weight, swelling of involved extremity. Aching in calves—distended, discolored, ache in lower extremities after standing for short periods. Alcoholism, anemia, asthma, bleeding disorder, diabetes mellitus, hypertension, kidney disease, pneumonia, rheumatic fever, stroke, influenza, rubella.

Family history should be assessed. Clients sex, race, age are all related to it; certain marital status, role in the household, number of children, coping mechanism, exercise, diet, sleep, support system of the clients life. Use of contraceptives, venereal disease, stress, anxiety, food habits, the number of pack smoking. Hypertension, chest pain, palpitation, wheezing, fainting, leg cramps, shortness of breath, weight gain.

Common assessment abnormalities pulse volume bounding, bruit, distended neck pain, pitting edema of lower extremities or sacral areas, peripheral cyanosis. Age related changes.

Diagnostic studies by radiological chest X-ray, ECG; phonocardiogram, a graphic recording of heart sounds is performed by placing microphone on surface of body; it provides information on murmurs and timing of various sounds.

What Level the Pressure Should be Labeled as Hypertension?

160/95 a systolic pressure greater than 160 mm Hg and a diastolic pressure greater that 95. Accurate measurements are essential for valid comparison of blood pressure. Possibility in source of errors in recording instrumental errors, such as leaking valve, cuffs encircle arm, circumstance that is physical environment, position, fear, anxiety, so on. Sitting position, supine position also some variations are noted. High blood pressure is an iceberg disease. It is major risk factor of stroke heart or kidney failure. The higher the pressure the greater the risk a lower expectation of life. The use of effective drug has controlled blood pressure. Blood pressure rises with age, genetic factor, obesity, salt intake, saturated fat, stress, alcohol, and lack of exercise, hormones.

Why is High Blood Pressure Dangerous?

Hypertension is defined as a sustained elevated blood pressure systolic and diastolic 140/90. Hypertension is a strong familial basis, essential hypertension stars by the age 20 to 30 years. Male have high risk than females of hypertension and cardiovascular disease, 90% of hypertension has no identifiable cause. Risk factor are overweight, smoking, lack of exercise, excess salt in diet, excess alcohol, environmental stress, high cholesterol levels in blood, family history of high pressure.

Complications of high blood pressure—heart attack, stroke, and kidney failure. High blood pressure can be controlled and not cured. Your blood pressure will remain normal just as long as you are taking medicines. Medicines will need to be taken life-long. If you do this, you can feel better and live longer. You deserve to be healthy for as long as you live.

Treatment includes lifestyle measures, maintain normal weight, and decrease salt in diet, stop smoking, decrease alcohol, regular aerobic exercise, and decrease total fats in diet, take fruits and vegetables. Regular follow up for blood pressure monitoring is needed. Blood pressure tends to increase with time. Hence periodic pressure checkup and readjustment of blood pressure medications are needed. Some patients may not tolerate one drug and may need to be changed to another. Yoga/ medications/relaxation techniques have proven benefits in lowering blood pressure. However periodic blood pressure check is needed.

Stroke is acute severe manifestation of cerebrovascular disease. It causes both physical and mental crippling; "Rapidly developed clinical signs of focal disturbance of cerebral function". Lasting more than 24 hrs or leading to death. Due to stroke there are signs of stenosis, rupture of the arteries, dysfunction of the brain, which includes coma, hemiplegia, paraplegia, monoplegia, multiple paralysis, speech disturbances, sensory impairment, etc.

Stroke is a worldwide health problem. It contributes to morbidity, mortality and disabilities, cerebral thrombosis/embolism most frequent form of stroke – followed by hemorrhage. Two-third of patients die within 3 weeks and 48% die within one year due to old age, high blood pressure impaired consciousness. Risk factors such as high blood pressure, Let ventricular hypertrophy, cardiac dilation, diabetes, elevated blood lipids, obesity, smoking, glucose intolerance, blood clotting and viscosity, oral contraceptives etc.

Sign of stroke occurs at any age, in male higher than female. It is slowly progressive disease of who had coronary heart disease, generalized vascular disease. Control arterial high blood pressure, control diabetes, control complications, long-term, follow-up, education and training, tackle by community action. Cholesterol is an extra waxy fat-like substance that occurs naturally in all parts of the body. The liver manufactures it from the fat consumed by us.

Rheumatic fever and rheumatic heart disease cannot be separated. Rheumatic fever is a febrile disease affecting connective tissues of heart and joint. Rheumatic heart disease is a crippling disease. Its consequences include—damage to the heart, increasing disabilities, repeated hospitalization and premature death. It is a preventable disease. It is a problem all over the world. In 33% school age children, 5 – 30 years. It is the most common cause of coronary heart disease and death. The disease may subside or even vanish spontaneously as living standard rise.

Pockets of poverty where socio-economic condition continue to favor rheumatic heart disease. Disease is linked with poverty, overcrowding, poor housing condition, and inadequate health services. Agent is streptococci; rheumatic fever is typically a disease of childhood and adolescence with juvenile mitral stenosis, affects both the sexes equally. In less affluent countries, high-risk group are school age children who are 5 – 15 years and slumdwellers.

Clinical – Fever with profuse sweating, large joints like ankle, knees, elbows and wrists are involved. Brain involvement – manifests abnormal jerky purposeless movements of the arm, legs, and the body. Various types of skin rash appear.

Positive throat culture for group a streptococci. Prevent first attack Rheumatic fever is treating by penicillin. High-risk group children kept under surveillance, e.g. C P 300,000 unit and procaine 600,000 units. Improving living conditions, breaking the poverty cycle, improvement in socioeconomic conditions, evaluation and survey of rheumatic heart disease with random sample of school children.

Cardiovascular disorders are the nation's number one killer. Nurses assess the duration and extent of symptoms, and the clients and family understanding of, perception of and reaction to the illness, patients tolerance to activity, support system, the degree of heart failure. Cardiac transplantation procedure is becoming more and more common. As technology and scientific knowledge progress more hope for patient to cure from cardiac disorders. Nurses who care cardiac patients needs to be more alert, acutely aware of patients prognosis because of the dramatic advances in surgical treatment of children with congenital heart defects many children live into adulthood, and nurses must be skilled in physical, psychological aspect of care when providing. Successful cardiac rehabilitation can be done in the home setting. Bridging hospital care to home. The home nurse must have knowledge of basic arrhythmias, murmurs and extra heart sounds. Teaching medication actions, side effects and method of administration is more successful in the home, where stress levels are usually lower.

Cardiac disorders come in varying degrees of severity. Simple problems such as high blood pressure may be controlled by medication. Nurses see their clients in all stages and health and illness. The dying process is perhaps the most difficult stage to deal with nurses can help make their clients and their families processes less painful. The flow of blood is essential for sustaining human life. High blood pressure prevention in the community is a national problem that individual intervention alone cannot counter. Prevention and early discovery of new cases depends on public health effort. Once a high-risk patients are identified, nurses can teach them how to modify certain risk factors such as diet, sodium intake, exercise. Screening programs provide an opportunity to educate public. Weight reduction, exercise, restriction of alcohol, caffeine restriction, relaxation techniques, smoking cessation, potassium supplements, calcium supplements, and magnesium supplements.

Through research the understanding of cardiovascular disease continues to grow hourly. As a result, the care of people with heart disease is currently one of the most progressive areas in nursing. The human heart beats approximately 72 times per minute, 100,000 times a day and 22.5 billion times in a lifetime. With computer like efficiency it pumps oxygen rich blood into the arterial system. When the heart does not work efficiently, the patients life may be threatened.

What happens to the body when this mechanism begins to weaken and fail? What happens to the tissues and cells when the heart cannot pump oxygenated blood to them in adequate amounts? The normal heart rate is 60 to 100 beats/min. Variations in heart beat are normally caused by exercise, size of the individual, age, gender, hormones, temperature, blood pressure, anxiety and stress and pain. Persons over 65 years of age show changes in their cardiovascular system. These changes include the development of diseases process such as coronary heart disease as well as the physiologic aspects of aging. Heart is remarkable, durable organ. A continuously beating organ that never rests. High incidence of heart disease is a common cause of deaths. Nurses must know to assess the seriousness of its complications. Common symptoms found such as chest pain, shortness of breath, fatigue, palpitation, fainting, and weight gain. Risk factors are stress, types of personality, exercise, diet habits. The heart muscle must have an adequate blood supply to contract properly. When a coronary artery is narrowed or blocked the area of the heart muscle supplied by that artery becomes ischemic and injured and infarction may result.

Avoid food high in sodium—read labels of food carefully as salt is present in large amounts in common commercial preparations such as bakery powder, baking soda, soy sauce. Sodium is often added to some frozen foods, fruits and vegetables. Choose foods that are baked, broiled, boiled, or roasted and without salted gravies and juices, avoid soups, fast foods. Do not add salt at the table, natural spices, herbs and condiments like pepper, chili, lemon and cloves contain negligible amount of salt. Onion and garlic sauce, soy source are all high in sodium. Herb salts onion, garlic contain salt and not recommended.

Low fat, low cholesterol diet, avoid foods high in saturated fats and cholesterol—use vegetable oil instead of butter, avoid gravies, creams, and cheese sauces, avoid fried foods, bake or boil instead, use skim or low fat milk and milk products. Choose lean cuts of meat, remove all poultry skin, and use a wire rack when roasting or baking meats so that the fat can drip off. Fish, poultry have lower fat content. Breast of chicken and turkey are leanest poultry available. Avoid duck and goose. Eat no more than 3 egg yolks per week. Egg whites are low in cholesterol; meat stews, soups and gravies can be prepared in advance and chilled the fat hardens. The fat is the skimmed off. Limit the use of organ meats and shellfish. There are many behavioral activities one can practice to safeguard against high blood pressure, including exercise, eating a low fat, low sodium diet, limiting alcohol consumption and avoiding high stress activities, proper medication use is vital, forget to take medicines, feel there is no need to take regularly as I feel better is not good sign.

Education guide- Daily hygiene of foot care -foot do not soak, use mild soap and wash cloth. Dry well between toes, check water temperature with a bath thermometer or elbow, not toes, to prevent burns, gently rub corns, and avoid cutting, digging or using harsh commercial products. Daily inspect and lubrication- use good lighting put on glasses, report ulcerations, redness, blisters, cracking of skin on the feet, thickening of nails and so on to physician promptly. Rub soothing lotions or lanolin on hands, feet, legs and arms to prevent dryness. Do not use lotion on sores to in between toes. Do not use perfumed lotions.

Dust feet lightly with cornstarch if they sweat. Care of toe nails- use clippers not scissors, cut straight across, no bathroom surgery, and do not use razor blades, if eyesight is poor or you are unable to reach toes, find qualified assistance. Proper shoes and socks- never go barefoot, not even at the beach or in the home. Avoid high heels and shoes with pointed toes. Make sure nothing is in shoes before putting them on feet. Avoid tight socks for absorbency. Change socks daily. Avoid shoes that cause feet to perspire, make sure shoes and slipper fit well and are sturdy enough to prevent from injury. Safety- avoid sunburn. Avoid scratching insect bites on legs to prevent creation of open lesions. Do not use heating pads. Wear adequate foot protection on cold days. Turn lights on in dark hallways and rooms. Do not sit with legs crossed when it doubt, ask for help, have phone number handy. Activity- walking is good but ask physician first. Do not walk if there are open ulcerations elevate feet if they swell. This will help in diabetic related heart disease.

How heart diseases are diagnosed? Diagnostic tests include following tests:

An ECG helps the doctor determine the health of the heart. It assesses heart damage and disease and gives valuable information whether your heart is normal. To do the finding of heart disease first ECG is taken. The ECG records electrical impulses of the heart. ECG records heart's electrical activity as it contracts and resets. It can detect abnormal heartbeats, areas of heart muscles damage inadequate blood flow and enlargement of the heart. If any part of your heart is receiving less blood supply, whether you have suffered a heart attack in the past, if the muscle of your heart is thickened, whether you have holes in your heart, the effect of certain medications on your heart.

Stress test—treadmill is a type of ECG, it is a test performed to measure your heart's health under the stress of physical activity. Which measures how the heart and blood vessels respond to exertion when the patient is exercising on treadmill? A stress test is performed if you are suspected of having heart disease. This test is useful for coronary arterial disease, good screening test, where heart rate, breathing, blood pressure, ECG, tiredness is monitored during this test. The stress test helps determine how fit you are weather a heart problem exists and if it is safe for you to undertake an exercise program. If you experience chest pain, giddiness, shortness of breath or leg cramps; doctor might decide to stop the test. The test is stopped when you achieve your target heart rate; the test takes about half an hour. You can resume your normal activities immediately after the test. The stress test is extremely safe. Rarely have some complications such as chest pain, fall in blood pressure and fainting, irregularity of heart rhythm.

Nuclear scanning can identify regions of the heart where blood flow is limited. A small amount of radioactive material is injected into vein arm. The amount of this material that is taken up by the heart muscle is then recorded using a scanning camera.

Echocardiography—Cardiac ultrasound – an extension of the echo test called the color Doppler by performing an echo; doctor can look into the heart. He can determine the pumping action of the heart, abnormality of valves, any hole in the heart and if the fluid is present around the heart. Echo uses sound waves, which are totally harmless. It uses sound waves to create an image of the hearts chambers and valves. An hand held transducer is pressed against patient's chest – sound waves of the heart are converted into an image that can be displayed on a monitor, which can detect abnormalities in the heart wall motion caused by coronary arterial disease valvular abnormalities can be detected. The pumping ability of the heart, presence and location of holes in the heart, infection of the heart valves, presence of a blood clot within the heart. The echo test is an invaluable minified of information.

2-D echo—Accurate measurements of the heart chambers, cross sectional slice of beating heart – transducer records, patient is asked to move back, side, breathing slowly, holding breath time images are viewed on monitor – recorded on photographic paper and on video tape, 2D echo evaluates the size, thickness, movement, valves, chambers, etc.

Doppler examination: Ultrasound evaluates the direction of blood flow and its velocity. The heart pumping power is normal/reduced, mild/severe, pumping poorly due to cardiomyopathy, abnormal valve thickened, calcified, its tone, blood clot, tumor congenital heart disease, rheumatic heart disease can be detected.

Transesophageal echocardiography is done through throat into the esophagus to evaluate internal heart structure and blood flow congenital heart disease defect detected. This test is used during heart surgery.

Coronary angiography/arteriography/ cardiac catheterization is the procedure performed to find out the state of the heart muscles, valves and the exact location of holes in the heart. It is a testing procedure in which an X-ray opaque dye is injected into the bloodstream, to evaluate blockage, arterial damage. It is done under LA along thin tube inserted into a major leg/arm artery into coronary artery a contrast dye also injected (catheter) to make arteries visible on X-ray, cardiac-catheter also used in infant/children to examine/treat congenital cardiac defect, is known as coronary angiography is a most definitive test for coronary arterial disease. It shows heart chambers, great vessels in X-ray.

Coronary artery bypass graft surgery: There is always a lot of anxiety before any operation. Heart operations probably incite more anxiety than any other surgery. Surgery done to reroute or bypass blood around clogged arteries and to improve blood and oxygen supply to the heart. Borrow a healthy blood vessel a piece from long vein removed and grafted new path. Under general anesthesia given as it is a major surgery where heart – lung – machine used.

Coronary angioplasty — Deposition of cholesterol in the walls of the arteries leads to narrowing or blockage of these arteries. The site and extent of blockage can be determined by the diagnostic procedure of coronary angiography. In which a stent, a wire mesh tube is used to open an artery using angioplasty. They are small spring like metal devices (spring found in ball pen like) a catheter threaded into the heart with a tiny balloon at its tip through an arm/leg vein into the coronary artery. The balloon is inflated to enlarge the blood vessel and open blocked artery. The balloon is deflated and the catheter is removed. A metal coil stent implanted permanently. It re-shapes the blood vessels. During catheter threading X-ray images taken called **Fluoroscopy**. Dye is injected to view the blood vessels, i.e. **Angiogram.**

Pacemaker—The heart's natural pacemaker, located in the upper part of the heart, normally regulates the heart rate. This natural pacemaker, called the sinoatrial node, is a small cluster of specialized cells that produce electric signals at regular intervals. The S-A node automatically increases the heart rate in response to the body's needs for example, during exercise, when a faster blood flow is required. The natural electrical pathway is very important because when the signals reach the lower heart, both ventricles contract, pumping blood throughout the body. This contraction of the heart can be felt as the pulse. Why a heart may need a pacemaker? Sometimes, the S-A node stops working properly and when there is a heart block pacemaker is placed. The pacemaker is an electronic device. It is well shielded from the kinds of electrical interference that are likely to be encountered in daily life, certain sources of electrical interference can slow down or speed up the pacemaker temporarily.

There are numerous blood test studies which reflect the oxygen carrying capacity and coagulation properties. Enzymes are found in blood tissues, they can be elevated because of injury to the muscles, liver, and other organs such as an elevated LDH can mean heart, liver, skeletal muscle, lung or kidney damage.

History and physical examination, serum electrolytes and uric acid, BUN and serum creatinine.

With advanced medicines, healthy lifestyle, new technologies, surgical procedures have declined death and extended lives. Following healthy lifestyle, eating right food choice, doing regular exercise, maintaining a normal weight, avoid smoking, avoiding alcohol, controlling high blood pressure, coping and managing stress, following cardiac rehabilitation programs can prolong life and patient can live happy life. Keep in mind that importance of time is very vital in heart disease to recognize signals and respond immediately. Delay increases risk, time is critical – shift the patient to 24 hours emergency cardiac care, if unconscious before reaching emergency give cardiopulmonary resuscitation. Medication - beta-blockers, nitroglycerine calcium channel blockers and potassium channel openers.

High blood pressure may cause organ damage and the drastic reduction in blood pressure may cause coronary cerebral or renal ischemia. When the blood pressure is more that 210/130 there would be acute vascular damage, acute myocardial infarction, acute LVF, intracranial hemorrhage malignant high blood pressure. Continuous blood pressure monitoring is required.

The walls of the heart consist of powerful muscle fibers that have the power to contract or beat which keeps circulation going. To maintain the right pressure all the vessels have right amount of blood, otherwise tissues of the body waste away and die. Sinoatrial node (SA) transmits electrical impulses and operates like radio station gives signals and regular electric waves. This p waves seen in cardiogram and QRS waves of cardiogram. Though different muscles work as one unit, to maintain its activity heart must feed itself with blood and oxygen.

Heart attacks have a great impact on your family. Your family members get frighten and feel helpless as they watch the doctors treating you, not knowing what would happen. Control your cholesterol, high blood pressure, avoid organ meats, kidney, brain, liver, beef, pork, oyster, lobster, sausages, salami, chicken skin, whole milk, condensed milk, cream, butter, cheese, egg yolk, mayonnaise, ghee, coconut oil, cream filled biscuits, pastries, puddings, chocolates, toffees, ice cream, French fries. Do eat fruits, vegetables, salads, cereals, pulses, egg white, cottage cheese, curd, tea, coffee, fruit juice, potatoes, rice, almonds, and walnuts. Foods are not good or bad. Eating habits are. Quit smoking, do regular exercise, reduce your stress level.

Lead a heart-healthy lifestyle. Restriction of sodium, reduction of weight, restriction of saturated fats, restriction of alcohol, cessation of smoking, reduction of stress, periodic monitoring of BP, regular exercise, modification of lifestyle.

Behaviors that promote health such as sleeping regularly 7 to 8 hours and maintain health; eating breakfast, eating regular meals, maintain weight, positive self-concept and the ability to problem solve, early detection, health promoting behavior and motivation.

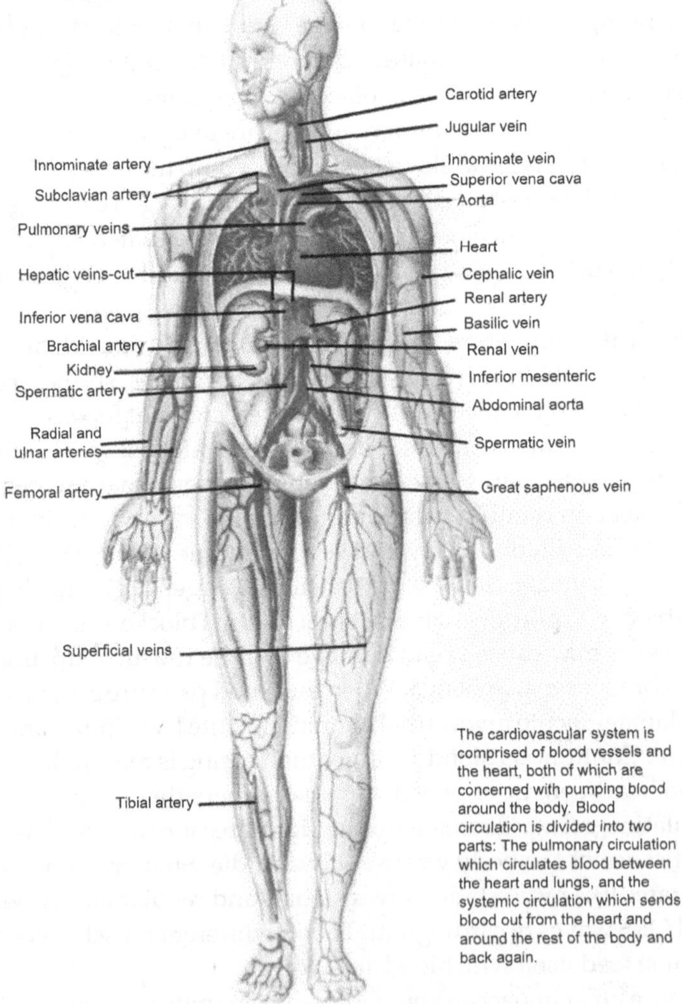

Fig. 27.1: The cardiovascular system *(For color version see Plate 5)*

Coronary Arteries

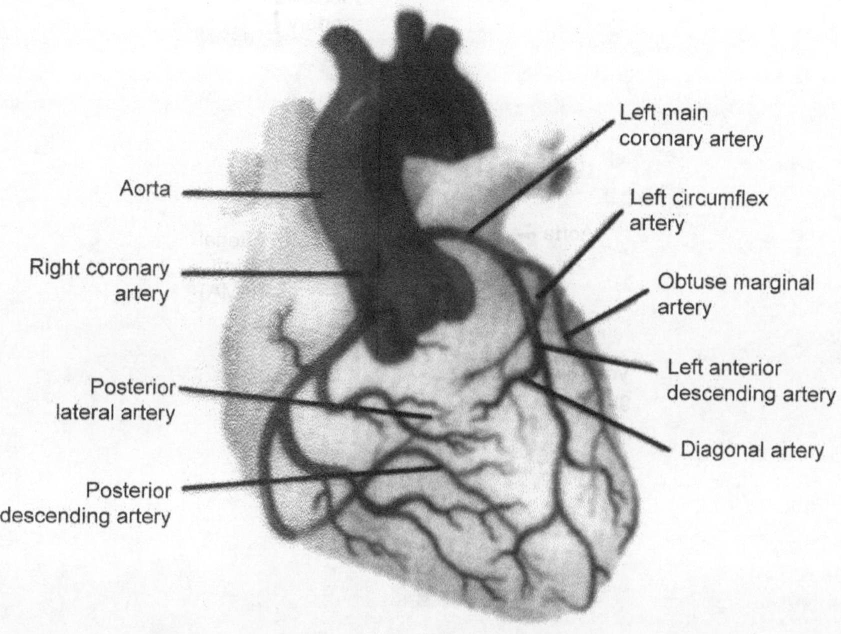

The coronary artery and atherosclerosis

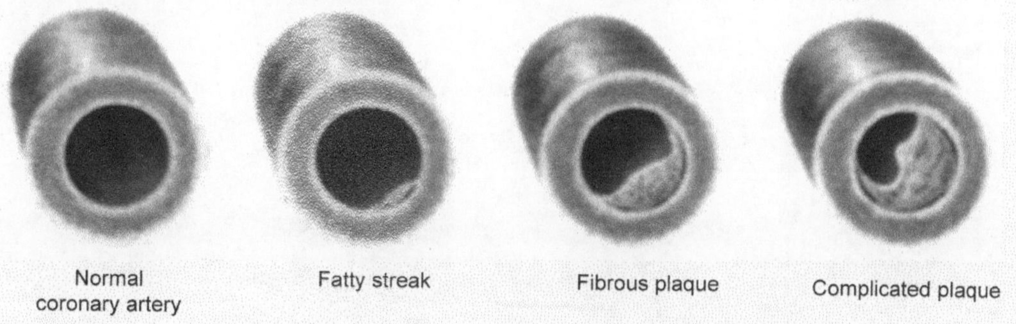

Fig. 27.2: Heart and arteriosclerosis *(For color version see Plate 6)*

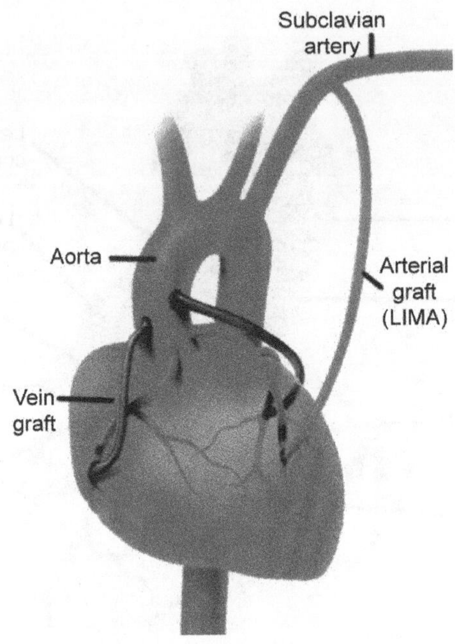

Fig. 27.3: Heart beat: The rhythm of life *(For color version see Plate 7)*

28 Obesity: Increasing Rate of Public Health Problem

Overweight is expressed in terms of body mass index. It is a misconception that obesity is primarily a problem in the affluent countries. It occurs at any age. Infants with excessive weight gain in childhood results in obesity in adults, which is extremely difficult to treat with conventional methods. Men gain weight at the age of 29 to 35 years, while women at the age of 45 to 49 years of age. Genetic factors, physical inactivity, socioeconomic status, eating habits, eating in between meals, preferences to sweet, refined food and saturated fats, food eaten and calories produced equivalent energy needs to be spent or else it deposits in to fat. When people have psychosocial problem, emotional disturbances depression, anxiety, frustration and loneliness they tend to eat more. Excessively obese individuals are withdrawn, self-conscious secret eaters.

Obesity has a family tendency, which runs in certain family. Due to endocrine factor where growth hormone reduces and dries thus, its deficiency causes obesity in certain people. Women do gain a lot of weight after menopause as that has a lot to do with hormones and lifestyle exercise and taking calcium can help. In obese person, fatty mass is increased and content of water is not increased. Obesity can easily be identified at first sight. The longer your waistline, the shorter your lifeline. Extra weight could be due to extra eating. Extra fat puts a strain on your heart, kidneys, and liver and also on the large weight-bearing joints, such as the hips, knees and the ankles. Either we must increase the output of work, or we must reduce the food intake. Putting those large leg muscles to work burn up unwanted calories. Small quantities of food, balance food and regular eating are important. Do not go hungry for long. It takes real will power to lose weight, but it is certainly worthwhile, find value of losing weight.

Watch for those high calories diets such as cashew nut, coconut, cake, chocolate, butter, ghee, ice cream. Your children watch more television, eat more junk food and get more pocket money to spend. Hazards of obesity are coronary heart disease, diabetes, gallbladder disease, and low fertility, lowers life expectancy. Prevention begin in childhood with diet control/changes fiber increase, increase physical activities, one should not expect quick, tangible result. Health education, motivation, helps the patience. 10 years ago, people took the stairs up to their offices. Today they prefer elevator even if they work on first floor. Earlier lunch was brought from home and today power lunch is taken. Ask yourself; is your job hazardous to your health? You do not have to be sumo wrestler to risk your life.

Health is least priority today. Everyone has the feeling that they are healthy, but feeling healthy and being healthy are two different things. Health is only capital that is difficult to regain, better to invest in fitness program today. Fit person has optimal immunity, alertness, a good attention span, flexibility and high energy level. So fit vs fat.

Obesity places an extra burden on the heart, requiring the muscle to work harder to pump enough blood to support added tissue mass. In addition, obesity is often associated with a sedentary life style elevated serum cholesterol and high blood pressure.

Obesity- fitness experts and nutritionists emphasize on the need of a composite holistic plan to reduce weight you want to shed those extra kgs so that you can have a svelte figure and to achieve that results you exercise and compromise with diet. Problems with body image affect both men and women. Most people face it at some stage of their life. Men face pressure to tone their muscle up and look strong. While women face pressure to slim down, tone down and look good. If one wants to achieve a weight loss of few kgs it should be done under tight discipline and authoritative governance.

A composite and holistic plan to be adopted with the help of a professional. Therefore, they may exercise vigorously and not eat properly to achieve the result and hence their body suffers, they become weak and there may arise health problem, so one must consult a proper fitness professional. Fresh fruits to be consumed and workout at any point of time should not exceed. Consume natural foods, no medicines or drugs should be taken to lose weight, over exercise should be avoided, there should not be starvation, slow breathing exercise should be done and fluids like coconut water, fresh fruit juices taken, electrolyte loss also should be monitored.

Obesity—It has been well documented that obese parents often have obese children, parental attitude towards food and eating habits are readily passed on to their children, the nurse must help parents to understand the unique food requirements.

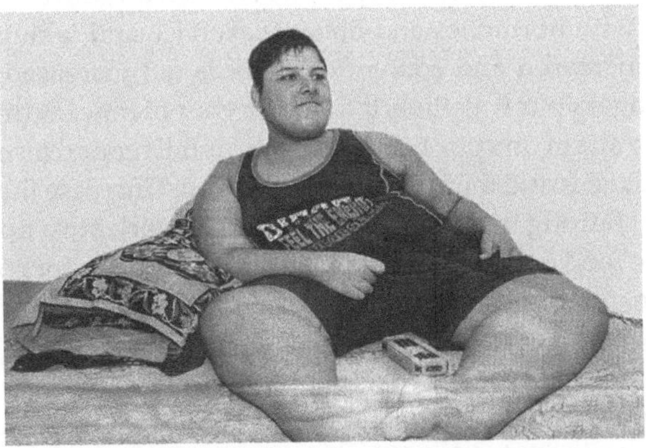

Fig. 28.1: Obesity and overweight

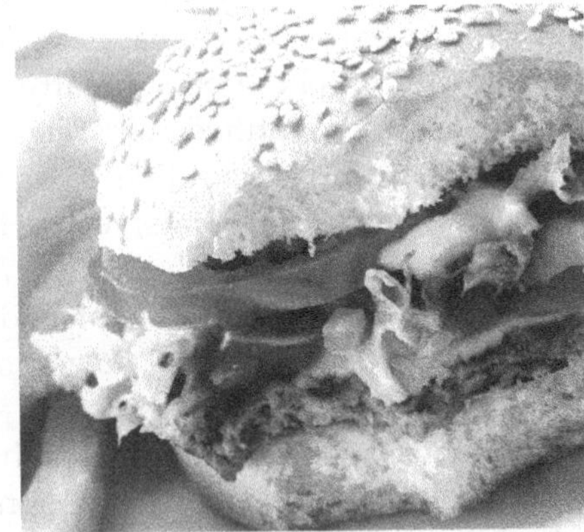

Fig. 28.2: Food that is harmful and has no calories

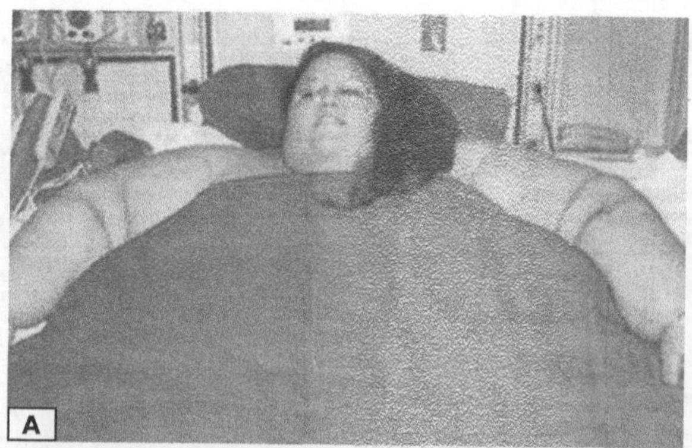

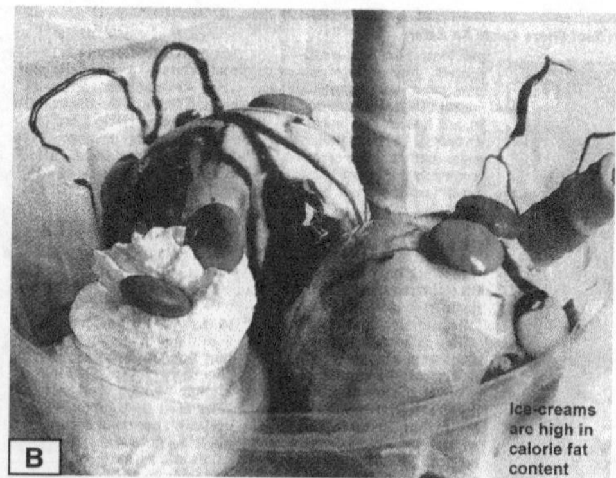

Figs 28.3A and B: Obesity and health problem: Faulty diet is root cause of illness

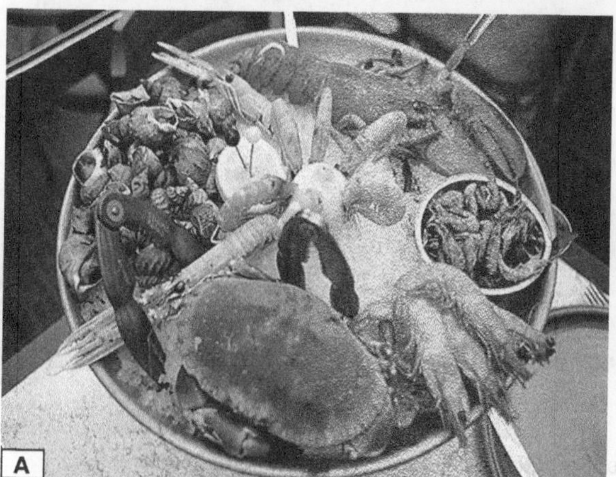

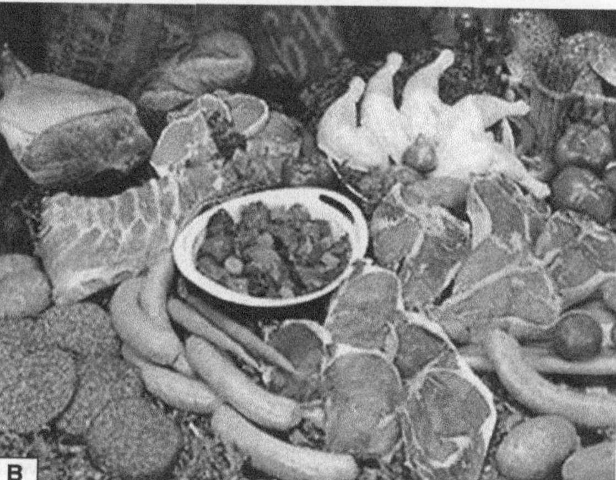

Figs 28.4A and B: Saturated fats. Animal fats are called as saturated fats, and excessive in take of these fats is harmful to body

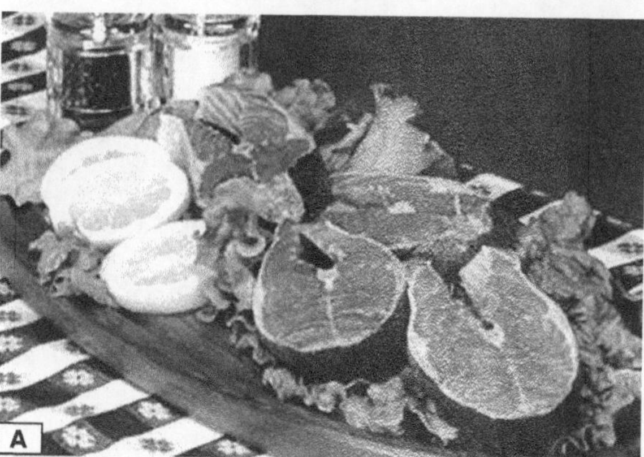

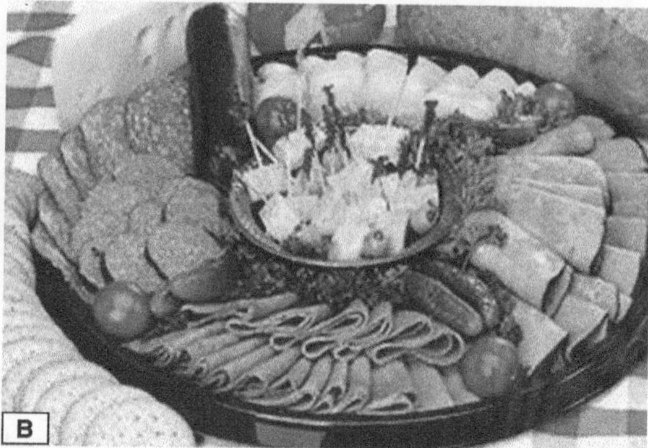

Figs 28.5A and B: Sources of animal fats butter, fat of meat, fish oil, pork, salami. Excessive consumption of saturated fats results in obesity. Consume unsaturated fats as they do not get deposited. Eat right, your lifestyle has a direct impact on your heart. Avoid artery clogging fats, there is no nutritional value in such foods such as chips, ice creams, bread, biscuits, desserts contains bad cholesterol. Your diet can play a very important role in determining the health of your heart. Though all fat diets are not bad use sparingly

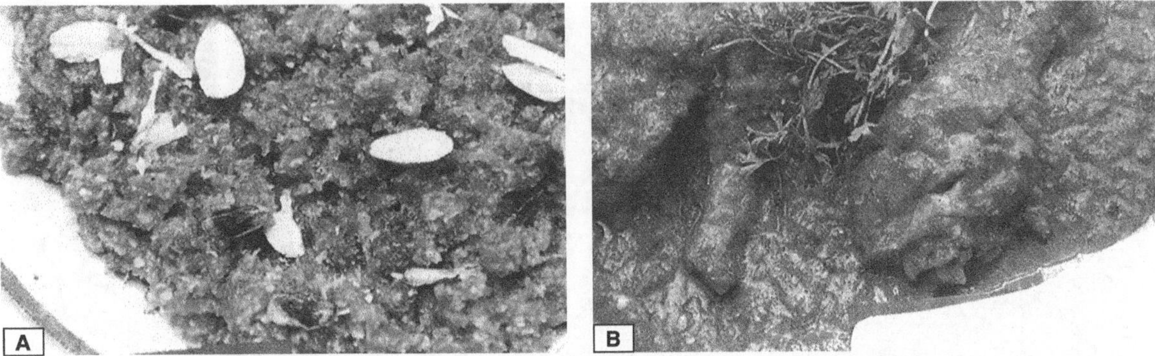

Figs 28.6A and B: Fast food. No time to cook. Routine formed unhealthy habits of ordering foods that gives neither nourishment nor health but can be adding saturated fat make you bulky and unhealthy

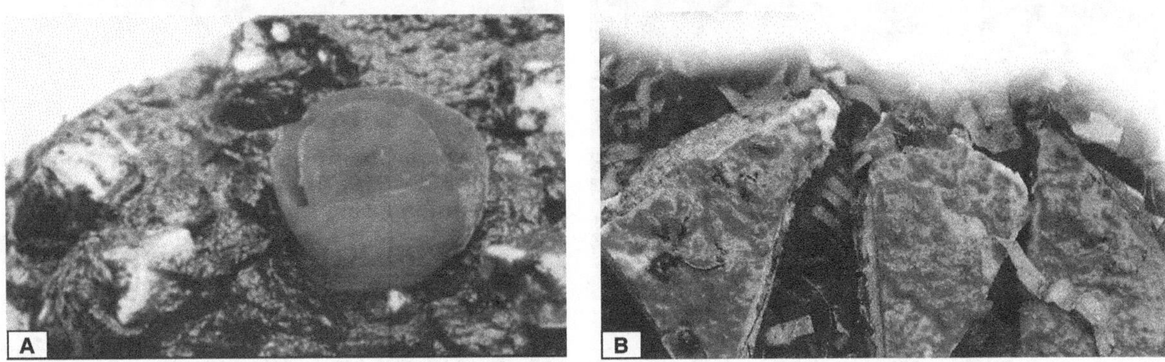

Figs 28.7A and B: Bakery foods and sandwiches fills your stomach and gives you empty calories

29 Prevention and Early Diagnosis of Cancer

Our bodies are made up of cells. Throughout our lives a process of cellular division is continually replacing most of these cells. The process of reduplication is taking place within our bodies all the time. We are unaware of this continual process. This process of cellular renewal, revitalization and reduplication is the very foundation upon which our bodies remain in a healthy state. Certain it is when this happens that the problem is said to be cancerous. Cells in the body begin to reduplicate in an uncontrolled manner. This is how cancer arises.

Therefore, cancer is a group of diseases characterized by an abnormal growth of cells, which has ability to invade tissues and even distant organs, if the tumor progresses beyond the stage eventually leads to death. Cancer can occur at any site, tissue of the body and may involve any type of cells.

So many questions arise in mind such as how does the cancer arise? Can virus cause cancer? Can the AIDS virus cause cancer? Can chemicals cause cancer? Can cancer be inherited? Can hormones cause cancer? Can drugs cause cancer? Can psychological factors cause cancer? What types of cancer are there? What are the most common cancers? Does cancer cause pain? What should I do if I think I have cancer? What tests will my general physician do? What sort of test am I likely to have?

Age is the most outstanding risk factor for cancer. Cancer incidence increases progressively with age; elimination of smoking is key to reduction of risk of many cancers. Consideration should be given to reducing over all fat intakes in the diet. Avoidance of sun exposure helps to prevent actinic skin damage.

There are three rare cancers, which are caused by human T-cell leukemia. The virus tends to set up an inflammatory reaction, and when this becomes chronic and it is possible, that if the cells of the involved tissues become cancerous. Chemicals that cause cancer should be identified and avoided. Like lung cancer, which is linked to smoking of cigarette? Certain foods cause cancer, some chemicals taken in the diet have been shown to promote cancer. Nitrates are used as fertilizers and are ingested on fresh vegetables, which have been shown to be cancer forming. Artificial sweeteners are used in food and drink; preservative which are parts of modern way of living.

Some rare forms of cancer which can be inherited is of eye known as retinoblastoma. Some forms of breast cancer are hormone dependent; in certain cases hormones can beneficially influence the growth of cancerous tissue. In pregnancy, existing cancers of the breast and cervix can be worsened due to certain hormonal levels that accompany pregnancy. Cancer of the vagina was attributable to the estrogen drug that their mothers had received in pregnancy. Some cancers can arise in areas of chronic inflammation such as ulcerative colitis, bowel cancer in certain circumstances, a recognized manifestation of underlying psychological problems.

There are as many types of cancer as there are tissues in the body. The most common sight of cancer is the lung, cervix, breast, uterus, prostate, and bowel. Cancers of the bladder, stomach and the leukemia are also relatively common.

The major categories:

Caremomas: These arise from epithelial cells lining the internal surface of the various organs, e.g. mouth, esophagus, intestine, and uterus, skin.

Sarcomas: These arise from mesodermal cells constituting the various connective tissues, e.g. fibrous tissues, fat and born.

Lymphomas: Myeloma and leukemia arises from the cells of bone marrow and immune system.

Primary tumor: Cancer in the organ of origin.

'Secondary tumor' cancer that has spread to original lymph nodes and distant organs. As diseases advances signs and symptom becomes clinically evident.

Childhood cancer is a stark and heart-wrenching reality. Why do children suffer from cancer? The cause could be chromosomal incompatibility of parents and genetic mutations. Treating childhood cancer emotionally drains out entire team. Doctor's get attach to the child, and feel their suffering. Imagine then how childhood cancer must hurt the client's parents. Often parents need more emotional support. Their whole life turns upside down, what I did to disserve this, why me, I want my child to live, where did I go wrong, guilt, the emotional turmoil is worse then. The lack of control in deciding about the treatment while the baby undergoes biopsies, blood test, umpteen scans, aspirations and operations often gets reflected in the parents themselves reacting psychosomatically. Is there any solution possible? Making the hospital environment friendly to families and making child's family made to feel welcome. Support system is the balm to alleviate such pain. And help them in economic strain.

Childhood cancers are leukemia, brain cancer, spinal cord cancer, retinoblastoma, lyphomas, neuroblastoma, osteosarcoma, Wilm's tumor, etc.

Symptoms are unexplained headaches, persistent nausea, early morning vomiting, diarrhea, persistent fever due to unknown cause, constant tiredness, pallor, general lethargy, constant weight loss, easy bruises, recurrent infections, continued bone and joint pains, unexplained swellings and lumps, enlarge liver and spleen, whitish color behind the pupils, sudden and persistent vision change.

Identifying gynecological malignancies—cancer is the most dreaded disease. The very word cancer spells doom for the patient and disaster for the family. The word cancer sends chills down the spine and uttering it is as though to be similar to announcing a death sentence, most cancers are detected at an advanced stage when cure is difficult. Cancer screening is important by a pap smear of the cervix and pelvic examination yearly for all women who are sexually active. Earlier it is detected and treated, the better the chance for cure or survival. Breast cancer takes a heavy toll every year worldwide. Due to lack of awareness, illiteracy, poverty, and orthodox culture and even after knowledge of the presence of breast lump, the patient comes very late for treatment. Monthly self-breast examination for all women aged 20 and above. Mammography and clinical breast examination yearly for women who are 40 years and older.

Cancer in all forms causing about 12% deaths all over the world. Second leading cause of death [Cardiovascular 21% 1st]. There are various cancer that kills 60% people worldwide. Cancer affects lung, stomach, liver, colon-rectum, esophagus, mouth-pharynx, prostate and lymphoma, breast, cervix, ovary. Ten million new cases are added every year. Cancer is on rising and one of the leading causes of death in India. Cancer is attributed to multiple factors such as environmental factors, food habits, lifestyle, and genetic factors.

Laboratory blood test for cancer condition in which levels may be altered can be detected by doing blood tests such as- CBC-HB% and hematocrit can indicate anemia, nonspecific, may indicate malignancy. Leukocytes-WBC count- leukemia, lymphomas, metastatic disease to bone. Platelets Hodgkin's disease multiple myloma, born marrow suppression. Blood serum test- acid phosphates metastasis prostate cancer, ACTH lung cancer, alkaline phosphates cancer of the bone, liver cancer, lymphoma. Calcium-born metastasis, breast cancer, SGPT, SGOT, metastatic cancer of the liver, testosterone adrenal and ovarian cancer.

Biopsy surgical removal of a piece of tissue from the questionable area. The tissue sample is sent to the pathology laboratory for diagnostic verification.

Reconstructive surgery repair of defects from previous radical surgical resection.

Nurses will ensure that their clients are cared for even in the most adverse circumstances.

Causes of Cancer

The early warning signs of a possible cancer and caution that is change in bowel or bladder habit, a sore that does not heal unusual bleeding or discharge, thickening or lump in the breast or else where, indigestion or difficulty in swallowing, obvious changes in wart or mole, nagging cough or hoarseness. Consult your doctor without delay. Also observe any of the following changes.

Environmental cancer caused by tobacco smoking, chewing. Excessive intake of alcoholic beverages live cancer, beer consumption may be associated with rectal cancer. Due to this there are 3% death recorded. Dietary factors can cause cancer of a stomach, intestinal, bowl cancer, and a breast cancer. Due to certain occupational exposures such as benzene, arsenic, asbestos. Viruses such as hepatitis B and C, complication of AIDS—cancer of lymph nodes and spleen Hodgkin's has viral origin. Others: Sunlight, radiation, air and water pollution, medication (Estrogen) pesticides, costumes, habits, lifestyle – oral cancer. Genetic factors: Leukemia, retinoblastoma.

Many cancers even in their advanced stages do not cause pain. Pain does accompany some cancers, but with modern techniques and therapies such pain can be controlled.

Tests required to detect blood test, sputum or urine, cervical smear, X-ray of the chest, of the skull, various bones and the abdomen, special X-ray of kidney, bone marrow biopsy a sample piece of tissue taken from a particular area of the body. Biopsies of the pleura taken from the chest wall while liver biopsies are taken through the abdominal wall. Fiber-optiscope to observe the lining of the stomach that is gastroscopy, bronchoscope tissue from any suspicious looking areas to confirm diagnosis and it is of crucial importance.

Control: Diet is now considered a major factor in the prevention and treatment of cancer. Many well-known biologists and naturopaths believe that a faulty diet is the root cause of cancer. It is said that of all the natural catastrophes that befall us, the most distressing are those caused by our own behavior. The etiology of most cancers remains vague despite extensive research over the past several decades. Today universal epidemiological consensus exists only regarding certain cancer risk factors.

Cancer is a public health problem. Lifestyle changes can reduce the risk of cancer. Early detection and treatment increase the possibility of a cure. Present medical knowledge in the field of prevention, detection, early diagnosis, treatment after care and rehabilitation is very important in prevention and control of cancer. Control of tobacco and alcohol consumption reduces tobacco alcohol deaths. Cigarette smoking, the number one hazard, who is to blame in this? Keeping personal hygiene, e.g. cancer cervix.

Avoiding or protecting you from radiation, occupational exposures, immunization for hepatitis B, and virus. Avoiding food, drugs and cosmetics, which are containing chemicals. Preventing air pollution, treatment of precancerous lesions as soon as you notice it, paying attention to cervical tears, intestinal polyposis, warts, gastritis, cervicitis, special awareness and motivation through cancer education, especially high-risk groups, motivating people to seek early diagnosis and early treatment. 'Danger signals' are a lump/hard area in the breast, a change in a wart or mole a persistent cough/ hoarseness, excessive loss of blood at the monthly period or loss of blood outside the usual dates, a swelling or sore that does not get better, unexplained loss of weight.

Secondary prevention – cancer registration hospital based client treated by a particular institution, population based registration – surveillance cancer screening is the main weapon – cancer cervix, cancer breast, oral cancer.

Treatment of cancer should be available as surgical removal, radiation, chemotherapy, and today cancer treatment geared to high technology. Relief and freedom from cancer pain is right of patient.

Search for unrecognized malignancy by means of rapidly applied tests, mass screening, selective screening like cancer cervix can detect by the pap smear/test.

Screening for breast cancer – breast self-examination (BSE) – women can find themselves palpation is unreliable for large fatty breast; mammography is specific in detecting small tumors sometimes missed by palpation. Biopsy from a suspicious lesion may end up in a false-position.

Oral cancer is a major health problem in India, linked with tobacco chewing, smoking, alcohol- side of the mouth where tobacco quid kept, cigar, hookah, snuff, betal leaf bidi, nasswar ashes, e.g. smoking with the burning end inside the mouth.

Eliminate tobacco habits from community, needs intensive public education and motivation for changing lifestyle. Through home visits detect oral cancer to control and early treatment. Screening cancer cervix of female age of 25–45 years old. Genital warts, marital status – multiple sexual partners, early marriage, repeated childbirth, oral contraceptive pills and common in lower socio-economic group probably poor genital hygiene this entire situation to be observed and detected if any abnormality found.

Breast cancer is uncommon below the age of 35 years, rises in age 35-50. Family history is high risk.

Those delayed pregnancies late 30s tend to have breast tumors. Early menarche and late menopause are at risk. Hormonal factors – ovaries appears to play a crucial role in developing of breast cancer. Elevated oestrogen and progesterone hormones hold key.

Breast biopsy, diet – high fat diet and obesity, socioeconomic status, radial oral contraceptives – prolonged use of pills, pregnancy before 18 years – younger woman at risk – prevention – reduction of childhood obesity and increasing activities/exercise F/C.

Magnitude of the problem – lung cancer: 'smoking epidemic' it is increasing in industrialized countries – death occurs below 65 age smoking cigarette habit inhalation of puffs nicotine, exposure to passive smoking. The most noxious components of tobacco smoke are tar, carbon monoxide, nicotinic. The carcinogenic or role of tar is well established.

Nicotine and carbon monoxide, contribute to increased risk of cardiovascular disease enhancement of blood coagulation in the vessels, interference with myocardial oxygen delivery.

(Non-filter cigarettes – 'king size' filter cigarettes deliver more tar and nicotine than ordinary).

Other factors include air pollution, radioactivity, occupational exposure to asbestos, arsenic certain dust.

Public information and education, smoking cessation activities, national and international coordination. Awareness about the hazards of smoking national anti-smoking campaign – changes in human behavior or lifestyles associated with smoking. Smoking must be an essential part of the national health policy, (we will loose revenue). Restrictive measures: Control of sales, promotion, health warnings on packets, advertisements, product description showing yield of harmful substances, imposition of limits, taxation, sales restrictions, restrictions of smoking in public places and places of work. 'Cigarettes smoking is injurious to health, government prohibiting laws in closed areas, e.g. cinemas, buses, education institutions and hospitals.

Cessation – has abstinence symptoms sleeplessness, craving for smoking, dizziness, and constipation, to have smoking cessation clinics, nicotine substitutes.

Mass screening as routine public health policy.

Stomach cancer most gastric cancers are adenocarcinomas, linked to improved food preservation practices, better nutrition more rich in vitamins from fresh vegetables and fruits and less consumption of preserved, cared and salted foods.

Patient complains weight loss, fatigue, gastric discomfort – diagnosis – X-ray and biopsy treated by surgical removal of tumor with or without chemotherapy.

Generally have poor survival prognosis 60% survive, 5 years if detected early screening and photofluoroscopy has been used.

Since the ages when cancer diagnosed patient's fear – as it bomb blast – started seeing death in front of eyes.

So many scientific researches – no cure found – no definite cause – reappears, e.g. a fruit apply with stain-narcosis.

ALL: Acute lymphoblastic leukemia; CLL: Chronic lymphoblastic leukemia; AML: Acute mylogenic leukemia; CML: Chronic mylogenic leukemia.

'An impairment of bodily structure or function that necessitates a medication of the client's normal life and has persisted over an extended period of time' chronic illness is long duration in which the patient is permanently incapacitated, are permanent, leave disability.

Non-communicable diseases include cardiovascular, renal, nervous mental diseases, chronic – nonspecific respiratory diseases, blindness, cancer, diabetes, obesity and various other metabolic and degenerative diseases.

Medical care is now enabling client to survive. Consultants should exercise due care and not blindly rely on whatever is prepared by the juniors. The bigger the doctors name the bigger the fees, but what about the quality of service? Very often the well known doctors have no time for the patients and much of the actual work is done by the junior doctors.

Health promoting activities by eating a balance, healthy diet, taking sufficient fluid, exercising regularly, getting adequate regular rest and sleep, eliminating wastes regularly through the bladder and bowels, finding rewarding and satisfying work, exploring new things, communicating well with others expressing love and concerns appropriately, learning how to balance life, wisdom in knowing what to do next and skill in knowing how to do it. Doing good, avoiding harm, obtaining correct and complete information concerning diagnosis. Coping ongoing day-to-day issues and lifestyle changes, strive to have needs met. Have better self-image, have zest for life and feeling well-being.

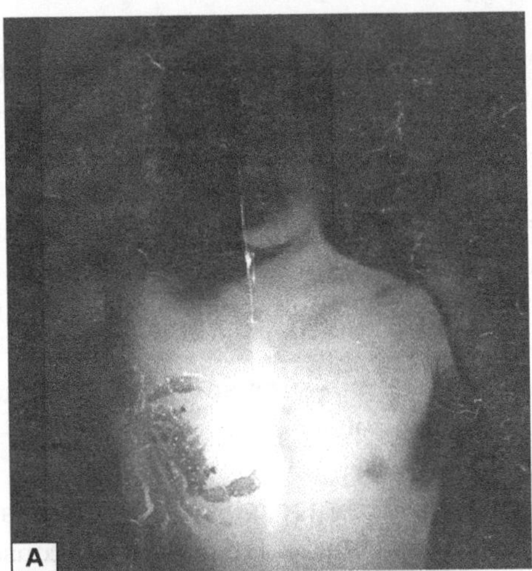

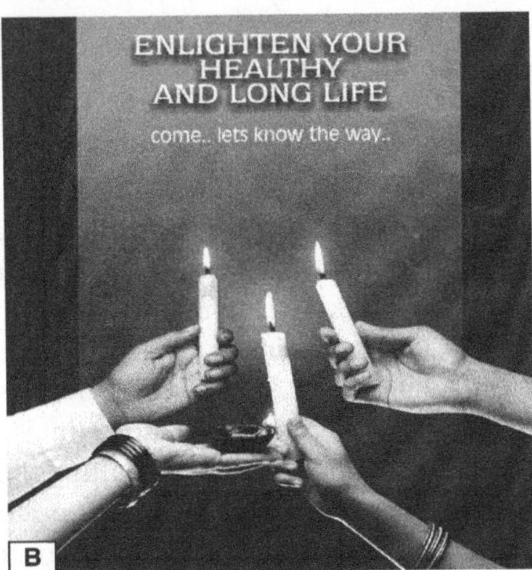

Figs 29.1A and B: Containing cancer. Some chemicals taken in the diet have been shown to promote cancer. Only in exceptional circumstances and with very rare forms of cancer. In the vast majority of cases, there is no real evidence to suggest that cancer can be inherited. Avoid risk factors such as tobacco, exposure to ultraviolet light, chemical exposures at the work place and exposure to ionizing radiation

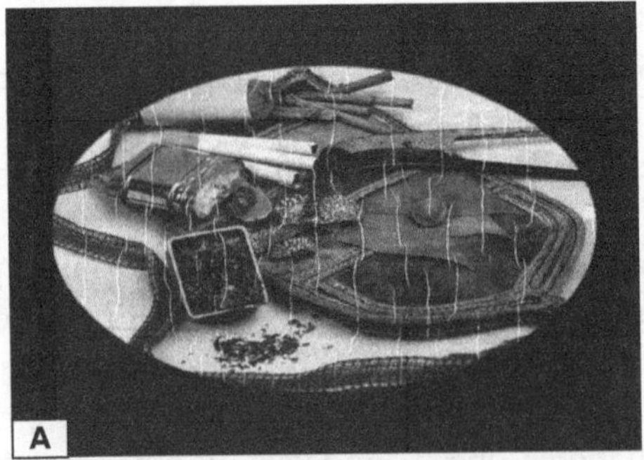

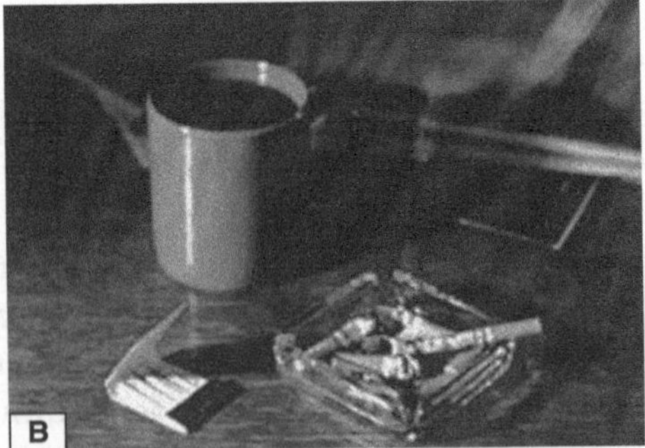

Figs 29.2A and B: Preventing cancer. It is said that of all the natural catastrophes that befall us, the most distressing are those caused by our own behavior

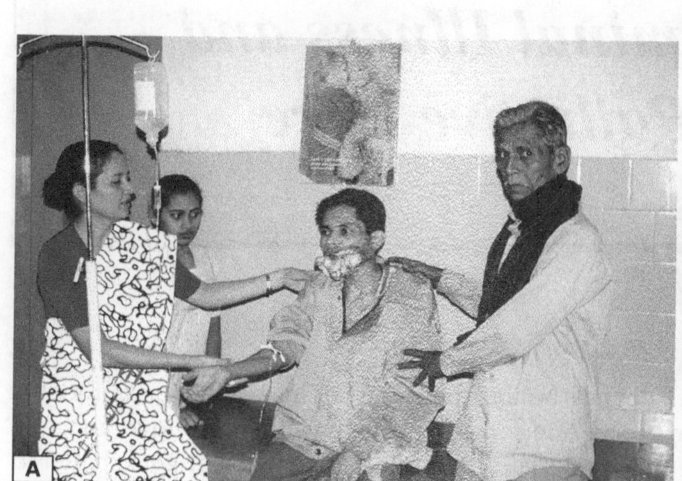

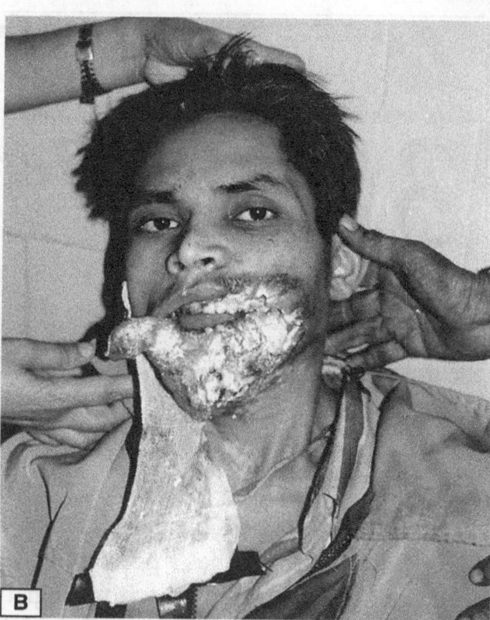

Figs 29.3A and B: Basic care of cancer patient : Cancer as a public health problem. Lifestyle changes can reduce the risk of cancer. Early detection and treatment increase the possibility of a cure. Cigarette smoking, the number one hazard

30 Terminal Illness and Palliative Care

Though cure is not possible, care is possible. Cure fails but care helps. Not dying but living comfortably till one dies. Care enables a person to die in peace. A terminally ill person who needs love, concern, care has also to be treated with integrity and trust. Due to terminal illness, client gets shattered physically, mentally, psychologically, spiritually, socially and financially. Caring for person holistically. Family plays a vital role in caring. Family has various reactions to illness. When family relationships are favorable ones adjustment to illness is better, otherwise other psychosomatic disorders triggers within the family. Terminal illness such as AIDS carries stigma, sense of shame, sense of deep guilt and feels self-responsible for illness. Loss of job, financial constraints, the family into despair, hampers children's education, and drains out energy for caring. Some sudden serious illness such as cancer, HIV, AIDS, impairs the family's equilibrium and coping mechanism breaks down, if the key member of the family bread earner ill, it is worse because it incapacitates and destabilizing the family.

Pain management is an important role of a nurse – pain is a complex concept and experience. Pain is a protective mechanism, some pain has positive value, and pain may serve as a warning signal that the body is experiencing tissue damage, he helps to diagnose cause of the disease and helps in effective treatment. Fear of pain prevents some persons from pursuing potentially harmful activities and may encourage some persons to take care of themselves. Pain varies from individual to individual and even within same individual. Person feels that pain can no longer be tolerated and not able to endure its intensity. Acute pain is unpleasant emotional experience.

Chronic pain is continuous over a period of six months or more, and here we are referring to such pain of terminal patience. Pain that is incapacitating and resistant to usual therapeutic measures, client becomes anxious and frustrated and affects his entire life. Life begins to revolve around the painful condition and the total person and the family is affected.

To relieve pain, accupressure, massage, heat application, cold therapy, externally applied preparation such as ointments, lotions, gel, liniments and balms to achieve some relief. Helping the client relaxation strategies, providing quiet environment and help to relax his leg, back, abdominal muscles, and giving support to the neck with pillow to see that arms and legs are not crossed, rhythmic breathing, soft silent music with the choice of the client, comfortable position and hypnosis to reduce fear and anxiety and ensure optimum sense of well-being. To believe in client, respect his dignity and respond to his pain, collaborate, be with patient and act as a buffer, help to reduce fear and anxiety, consideration of depression and anger and he needs to be assured and assistant, giving support, guidance and counseling.

If the family is counseled and well-informed, family reduces stress in the sick and remain good support with adequate coping skill, self-help and getting to know families who are facing similar problems can give valuable tips. Instill hope and reintegrate them into society. It is difficult when suddenly to lose support assurance and to prepare to live without a person, one has to begin a new and talk out the inner feelings and share deep pain, accept new lifestyle, living on small income, when life is on cross road, psychological trauma and suffering breaks the person. A helping hands and palliative care in such times helps the client gives morally strength to bear.

Every human life is subject to illness. Medical research and treatment in this advanced research still unclear and neither wholly explains not fully overcome suffering. To find value in suffering one has to turn to supernatural power and turn to God for healing. A helping hand needs to give such families' emotional succor. In palliative care, nurses needs an imaginative mind, competence, patience, love, understanding, compassion and ability to listen. The nurse has to develop rapport and trust, confidence in the client then he will open up manifold unexpressed problems and wishes such as fear, anxiety, worry, tension, guilt feeling, hopelessness, and despair and his desire to amend his past life, and to come to terms with his family and with God. The presence of caring loving person will give comfort and ease from anxiety and loneliness.

When pain and distress relieved, client becomes another person. Feels happy and peaceful. When end comes, he has peace and joy. Not the physical pain disturbing but the mental agony and restlessness. Palliative care for life limiting illness prefers to stay at home and die. There magnitude of suffering cannot be ignored. Terminally ill is home bound, room bound, bed bound in prison of his thoughts and fear isolation. They ask not for cure, they need healing and comfort, affirmation, assurance and need our presence. Wants us to listen with our ears with our heart. They want to be belonged and valued. They want peace and hope.

The nurse has to assure him that you matter because you are you. You matter to the last moment of your life and we will help you to live until you die peacefully. Pay him to his call for attention as well as action. Need for evaluation. The joy of life consists in giving what you posses. We may have everything in life, money, power, fortune, fame; still you will not be happy until one learns the art of giving with love. Persons come to us are precious, we would be lost if they are taken from us. Home based counseling deals with fear, grief, and despair and builds us a positive outlook on life. Removes feelings of hopelessness and helplessness in them. Removes stigma associated to sickness, helps them to accept the condition and deal with the issues in confident manner.

Palliative medicine was stress in 1987 and the study and management of client with active, progressive, far advanced diseases for whom the prognosis is limited and the focus of care is the quality of life total care, it requires a broad multidisciplinary approach. No drug relief pain. Life energy is infused with prayer, meditation, music, to reinforce strength and infuse peace, clam of mind. They experience the healing of the spirit. Feels loved and forgiven and coupled with courage person can face any situation even death. When families emotional, economic resources are drained due to medication what is vital at such moment of crisis is momentary help, positive gestures, support from therapist and social worker to reduce the pain and suffering.

Such a terminal sickness chills down the spine. It is when a person has no one to love him that he commits suicide. So long he has friends or dear ones who love him and whom he loves he will live. What is the greatest thing in the world? Love. What does sustain a couple to remain bounded till old age up to death when the physical body and its functions cease? Do you know the love of the old parents? Is life not full of opportunities for learning to love? We want to live tomorrow, and be with, and love back. We love and feel loved. Helping to take control of lives.

Home based care is not the best of care, but it is cheaper, efficient and more appreciated. The most common health needs of people are for care. Care, which provides comfort and support in the time of sickness. To prepare the nurses to shoulder the responsibility of the newer tasks assigned so that they transcend their narrow confinements with wider responsibilities.

They are the sheet anchor of total health care system. To equip oneself with better skill and higher education to accept newer needs of health care, which opens the wide horizon and prospectus to grow. To get better trained conventional roles such as providing health information to the public, evoking individual and community participation, educating people about disease prevention for small family norm etc. To know herself and others better. To study the human behavior and to differentiate between normal and abnormal. Health should mean a lot more than escape from disease/death.

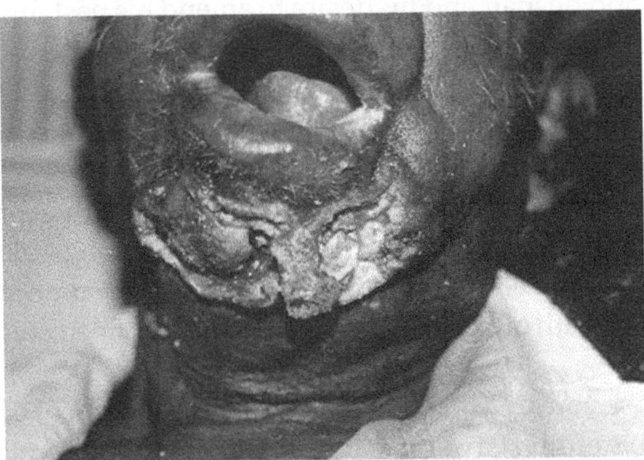

Fig. 30.1: Fundamental right to live with self-respect. Give care and hope *(For color version see Plate 7)*

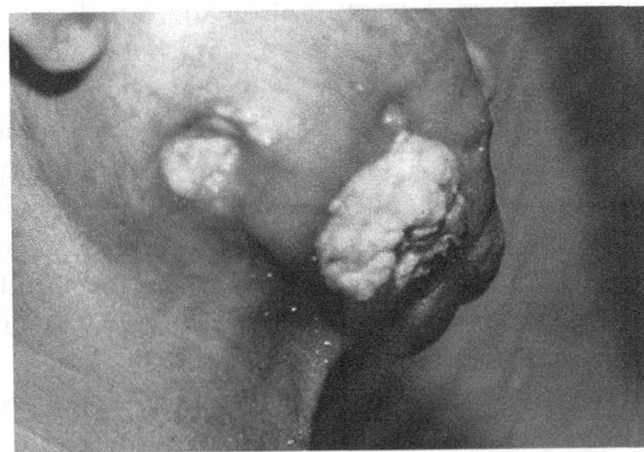

Fig. 30.2: Sharing care and concern for the sick and suffering *(For color version see Plate 7)*

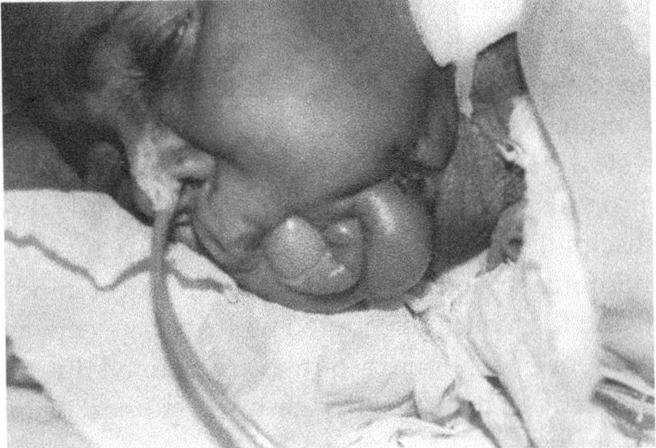

Fig. 30.3: A home from home. Eradicating the crippler. Give support *(For color version see Plate 8)*

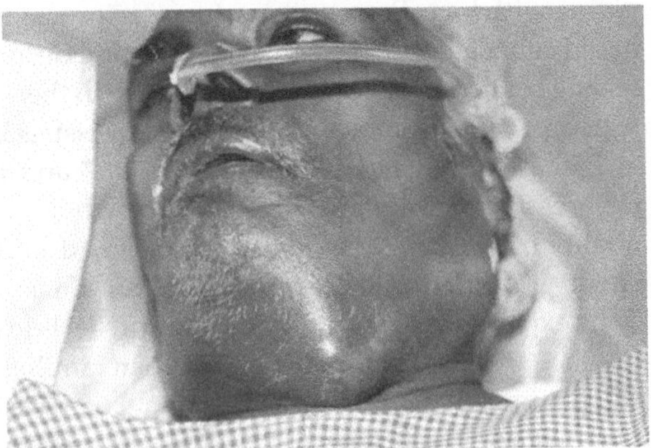

Fig. 30.4: Elevate suffering and pain. Give love and dignity *(For color version see Plate 8)*

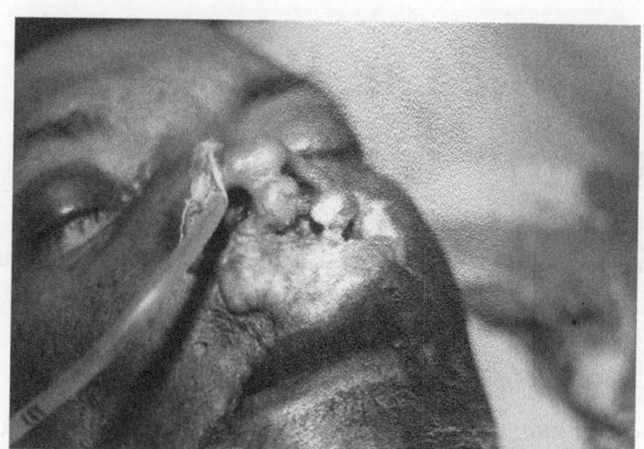

Fig. 30.5: Hold the hands of assurance
(For color version see Plate 8)

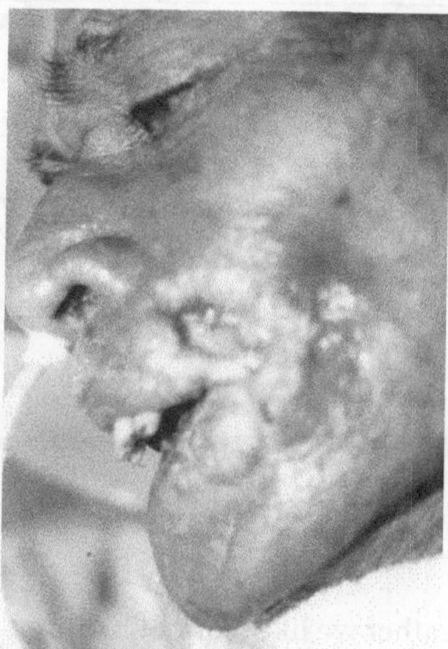

Fig. 30.6: Help to bare pain
(For color version see Plate 8)

31 What Makes a Person Grow Old?

Wheather we like it or not, we are all growing older every day. No one knows when old age begins. Years wrinkle the skin, but worry, doubt, fear, anxiety and self distrust wrinkle the soul. The older population continues to grow. We need proper information to give appropriate care to the older people. Community nurse must understand normal aging changes. Clients may be chronologically old but in functional terms, are active and productive. We wish to stay young and full of energy, but this we cannot do. Aging is both medical and sociological problem.

Younger generation especially of rural poor who live on daily wages from hand to mouth feel great strain to look after the elders due to economic burden. How we can remedy to ensure that the year of retirement of those who have worked hard in its service shall be free from anxiety and help the community to assist the aged to fight poverty, loneliness and ill health by providing them different services. Because old age is not a disease to be cured. It is a stage to be protected.

Life span of man is increasing due to advances in medical sciences and improved conditions. The elders should be made to feel useful, wanted and productive in every endeavor. In time of sickness they need good care and assistance. Therefore, Community Health Nurse needs to guide the family to develop a favorable attitude towards them. We have to use holistic approach, which encompasses understanding the interaction of culture, socioeconomic background, and spirituality as well as the physical, psychological process of the person.

Due to aging, there are losses that are personal as well as social and economic. Among the most devastating experience for them when they lose known people, parents, friends, spouse, children. Also, lose ones home, possessions, pets, employment, social position or financial security.

Aging is a biological process following maturity, with advanced age, the body does not respond as vigorously to illness because of diminished physiologic reserve. Normal changes associated with aging such as decreed contractibility, impaired coronary artery blood flow leads to high blood pressure, heart failure, varicose veins, dehydration, stroke. Decreased speed of neural conduction. Alzheimer's depression, anxiety, sleep disturbance, pneumonia, anorexia, constipation, diarrhea, urinary incontinence, enlarge prostrate, sexual dysfunction, diabetes mellitus, gout, osteoporosis, gait disturbances, falls, fractures, sdpondylitis, accidental injuries, anemia, pressure sores, dermatitis.

These are probably due to the lowering of certain hormones in the bloodstream; this gradual lowering of sex hormones may alter the level of other vital hormones and enzymes, and thus prepare the way for the marked changes of later life. Unfortunately there is no way of turning back the clock of time and preventing these changes from coming on. But we can do much to delay this process by choosing right diet, live sensibly, talking sufficient rest and exercise.

Hereditary influences are very strong in determining the length of person's life. The passing of time always brings subtle changes that cannot be ignored. Sooner or later we must all face up to the profound changes that lie ahead. It depends on the attitude of the mind. To look on the bright side of life inspite of pain and disability is value. Watch out for danger signals. Hardening of the arteries, overweight, arteriosclerosis, high blood pressure, strokes, thrombosis, arthritis, urinary problem, diabetes, digestive disorder, cancer etc.

Healthy aging is not a disease and disease is not aging. Aging is a biological process, which no one can avoid. A little care and caution will avoid many disabilities. Successful aging implies disease prevention; it requires the fulfillment of the physical, social and psychological needs of the older people. It is a process leading to a better quality of life in old age. Self care for healthy aging should start early in life and continue throughout life.

Old life begins at 40, 50, and 60. It is not the year in life that count, it is the life in your years. Growing old is a happier experience than many of us imagine. Young people like to enjoy themselves but this often means behaving in ways that can damage their future health. The harmful effects of alcohol, smoking and poor diet and fitness, fail to exercise because they are convinced that as they grow older they will become miserable. Old age does not mean a decline in happiness. As some young one associate old age with doom and gloom. You can still enjoy life, as you get older with the changed attitude and positive mindset. Look forward for happy and fruitful old age.

Most elders over age 65 are without teeth and those that are present are often diseased or decayed. Dentures may not fit properly, causing pain and discomfort. Weaker jaw muscles and shrinkage of the bony structure of the mouth may increase the work of chewing and lead to increased fatigue when eating. There is decrease of saliva with aging that may cause mucous membrane to become drier. Ear—wax tends to be drier in older people, impacts more easily and taken longer to soften. There is also in some complaints of feeling of fullness, itching or ringing in the ear which blocks having regular assessment. It can be prevented by the care and use of hearing aids and by removing disconnected battery when not in use keeping them clean.

Aging teeth become brittle, drier and darker in color. Teeth become uneven, jagged and fractured after years of crushing and grinding. Gums lose vascular and tissues, elasticity causing dentures not to fit properly. Eating habits often change and malnutrition may be a problem. Diminish taste sensitivity, thinning of mucus and decrease mass and strength and muscles of mastication also occur. Men with genetic tendency develop baldness, axillaries and pubic hair diminish in women, scalp hair becomes thinner and depleted and melanin, causing gray coloring. Older women may develop estrogen production, man may experience balding or receding hairline, oral skin, foot problem arise. Physical limitations create inability to safely insert or remove contact lens.

Constipation, irregular bowl habits and ignoring the urge of defecate, taking low fiber diet and high in animal fats, refined sugar, low fluid intake slows peristalsis, heavy laxative, tranquilizes, iron, diuretics affects the health. If older adults have spinal cord injury or tumor, results in handicap.

Old person feels embarrassed with hearing problem when meet new people, feel frustrated talking with family members when someone speaks in a whispers, difficulty when listening to TV and radio, hampers your personal or social life. To prevent all these eat a variety of foods, maintain a healthy weight, balance your food with physical activity, use sugar and salt in moderation. A good diet is inclusive of protein, minerals, and vitamins.

The future of nursing profession promises dynamic change and continual challenges in the field of senior citizens. Nurses of tomorrow need a broad knowledge base from which to provide care. Nurses of tomorrow therefore need to become critical thinkers, client advocates, clinical decision makers and client educators, counselor and rehabilitator. Through the exercise and tips she helps elders to live longer and healthy life to become stronger, firmer, flexible and energetic, help to fight obesity, high blood pressure, to improve lipid profile, control blood glucose level, improve quality of sleep, reduce stress, improve mood, enhance self-esteem, increase confidence, increase self awareness and control over choices in life.

Helps and guides them to socialize, and adapt to the weather condition, exercise, rest and sleep regularly. It will have net benefit and they will start enjoying activity, feel safe, competent, fit, balance life and will benefit physical as well emotional, unique personal experience, critical thinking, increase cardiac, metabolic output and venous return, improve tolerance and decrease fatigue, feeling better, 30 minutes brisk walk per day. It is never too late to begin an exercise. Nursing interventions are developed to modify the environment for protection from falls, fire, and electrical hazards. Culture that considers personal hygiene to be extremely important is a daily bath is part of their religious duty be encouraged.

Certain precautions need to be taken by elders is drive in familiar areas, do not drive during rush hour, avoid driving at dusk or night, go slow, and keep car in good working condition. Avoid eating, chewing or smoking while speaking. Avoid speaking from another room or while walking.

She can hold their hands, convey assurance and concern, by linking a person with religious organizations, helping them to attend to the social needs and to help to obtain information about mutual help group to remain connected in time of need.

There are other physiological changes occur such as organ and tissue changes associated with aging; cervical spondylitis (impaired balance), loss of lung compliance, dilatation of aorta, reduced stroke volume, reduced maximum cardiac rate, systolic hypotension, osteoporosis, constipation, osteoarthritis, loss of position sense (impaired balance), muscles weakness and wasting, impaired glucose tolerance.

When an elderly client is no longer able to care for him, the younger members of the family have some real decisions to make. Whenever possible, older client should be allowed to remain in their own homes as long as feasible. Be careful not to restrict their activities too much. Fortunate are the old client who have keen interests and active mind. Otherwise caring for an elderly client is not always easy. Nevertheless, whenever possible, it is wiser not to make an issue out of these, but develop forbearance, tolerance and endurance, respecting their dignity and upholding their self-respect as much as possible. Honour thy father and thy mother was the part of the divine law given to the human family long long ago. So much depends on the attitude of the mind. Nothing is more certain than the passage of time and the changes that come with it. Wheather we like it or not, we are growing older every day. There is nothing new about the desire to stay young. However, aging is inevitable that happens to all human who live on this planet.

Old person works whole life very hard for the upliftment and betterment of the family. Nevertheless, suddenly children grow and on their own elders are cornered and they feel without purpose and sudden slow down. You wish you could turn back the clock, and start rushing again. The period of your life that you earned for all your working years, does not seem to hold the same appeal anymore. You begin to feel this is the beginning of old age, and it is downhill from here.

Well, do not despair. You are not the only on who feels this way. Nevertheless, do not dishearten, believe there is life after 60 and you will find it flourishing, begin brisk walk, feel energetic, shed off negatives from mind, do yoga, meditation, you are as old as you mentally think, think still lots can be done constructively. You have right to live for as long as you wish, and enjoy all the amenities and all that life offers. Find a new meaning of life. It can be beginning of an active new lifestyle where you can display your skills to serve society.

Your loved ones may look after you and tend to your physical needs, but can they cope with your pent-up emotional and psychological needs? To lead active life physically and mentally and get social support if the family fails to provide primary care. To find fulfillment in life despite of age and feel worthwhile again, making an active contribution to society where they will be instill a sense of self worth and pride in their dignity.

Search for meaning and purpose of life, peace of mind to handle your feelings, change your mental imagery with wholesome and positive image. After retirement, find alternative ways of enhancing your self-esteem, recognizing your self-worth, as you are free of the pressures of working life, is a time to learn new skills or time to learn and discover hidden talent. Without work, your time, energy may be spent in developing alternative skills. With aging comes increase confidence and ability to cope with changes, able to cope with whatever life throws at them. They have learnt to deal with so many complexes, distressing, pleasurable, exciting, dull and stressful events a wealth of experience, skills, knowledge is accumulated throughout life and is a valuable resource, which should not be lost.

If there were a negative imbalance what would you like to do about it? What ambitions do you have which you have not yet achieved, life after retirement can be a time of fulfillment and or loneliness and boredom when life loses its point. All this depends on your attitude and positive approach. Family life is an important element in your life to enrich relationship together. However, fit and active you may be at 65-70 there is bound to come a time in natural order of things when you will slow down. Your joints will stiffen; death may rob you of someone you love. Death is one thing in life is certain and inevitable, making a will, to ensure that shared property goes to the survivor. Change in body may affect your performance.

Old age is universal problem. As old age advances, degenerative changes take place in the body, many health problems arise. Physical becomes helpless and mentally finds difficult to adjust. Besides they have to adjust to chronic illness, which needs to be integrated.

Preventive strategies to reduce the prevalence of disease and disability to promote physical activity during the day will prevent the common problems of old age, walking 20 minutes each day, stretching and moving all the joints will help to keep fit, it will burn up excess calories, increase calcium deposition in bones, improve muscle function and balance, facilitates regular bowel movements, improves general well-being.

In old age, it becomes easy for the body to adjust if daily routine in fix time for each activity maintained such as sleep, get up, eat, exercise, bath, religious activities, bowl movements, a high residue diet, regular exercise, plenty of water and a fixed time for going to the toilet.

Good dietary habits—Food is a basic human necessity, healthy diet is important from the time of conception to the old age. It remains vital for elderly to maintain activity, resistance to illness, prevent disabilities, over nutrition causes obesity, which can result in problems of weight bearing joints like hip and knee, heart disease and diabetes. Poor dietary habits can result in constipation and also predispose to cancer of the lower bowel.

Age related changes—Sense of taste and smell is reduced, digestion is slowed down, so take small frequent meals, fat intake to be spread over, and loss of teeth, so have soft mashed food, poverty may result in poor diet.

The diet should be prepared according to the needs of older people and easily digestible and presented in attractive way. It should have a variety, avoidance of too much sugar, fat, tea, coffee, and alcohol. Encouraged to eat plenty of fresh fruits, vegetables and high fiber diet and plenty of fluids and water.

Maintenance of good personal hygiene by mouthwash and clean dentures, daily bath, clean clothes, nails are cut and kept clean, hygienic measures should be adopted in preparing meals. Routine medical check up and regular monitoring of the ability to carry out activities of daily living.

Prevention of accidents—Slightest fall may result in fracture, prevented by good lighting in rooms, easy access to the basic needs and items for day-to-day use should be within easy reach.

Promotion of mental health—Happiness, ability to make decisions, ability to take on responsibility, self-esteem, independence, social company, engaging in useful activities, to love and be loved. Keeping mentally alert is just as importance as physical exercise. Therefore health workers can help in arranging social interaction among older people.

Health problems in old age are such as stroke, weakness of one side of the body, speech problem, and balance problem, visual problem. Coronary heart disease, chest pain, difficulty in breathing, palpitations, tiredness and fainting, continuous treatment is necessary. Hypertension, blood pressure tends to increase with age. Routine checking of BP is important. Diabetes mellitus—frequent urination, excessive thirst, loss of weight, requires careful and continuing care to prevent complications. Aging may result in poor eyesight and impairment of vision. Hearing problem, osteoarthritis is common in old age—wear and tear of the joint, pain and reduction of joint movement. The older person becomes confused, restless and apprehensive, depressed, dementiated.

Wheather elders are happy or sad, depend very much their relationship with the family members. Conflict comes with the difference of ages in the community. Younger people find older persons advice outdated and older person openly criticizing young ones and the friction that how the times have changed from his to now. Younger person working finds it difficult to looking after the old. There are hidden and unspoken expectations on the part of the parents from their adult children, which they do not verbalize, and grieve silently, feel the injustice in return for life's investment invested during whole life span for the children.

Due to fast changing world there is such a generation gap felt. Today most of the younger generation is more knowledgeable than their parents. They can access information and travel the world easier and faster than their parent could. In the older days, father was the head of the family, he was the breadwinner and protector, mother homemaker, children learnt from the parents.

We are waking up to a new world economy, and expected to even beat the super powers in the race. This is the one side of the coin, the other side, the fallout, the erosion of the social fabric, especially the institution of family. Values need to be evolved in tandem with the newer socio-economic-psychological demands.

It is difficult to bridge the gap between children, parents and grandparents in the modern world. Technology has widened the gap. We cannot stop urbanization and ultramodern lifestyle. The younger generation moving out for jobs gives them a different attitude, altogether. The exposure makes them more materialistic. The respect the older person enjoyed is vanishing. Roles are all mixed up with the internet, knowledge explosion, and world is their oyster. Salaries their children earn in a week, they perhaps never could in a year, even high qualifications and dedicated years of service. Money as the song goes is the roof of all evil. It is a good servant but a bad master. People who make money the new God, lose their balance. So who has failed modern youth?

The reason of collapse is both parents are employed and have no time to look after children and the children overburden with their academic commitment. Modern gadgets like cell phone, computers have added to their distance. To recreate what is lost, revive afresh, start by creating an environment for facilitating a process of perceiving things differently. Bridging the gap, a mutual responsibility of the young and the old to respect each other. Elders need to provide support that they are there for them and the young few words of love and care. Practice restraint instead of authority by instilling confidence and trust in children; provide the family with a happy and friendly atmosphere. Give the youngsters a patient hearing and respect their views as far as possible, will go long way in creating goodwill among the two generation. Because unhappiness sets in only when the elderly have time to brood; both the sides adjusting with each other and take the sharing experience of elders in right spirit the interaction between young and old. It is just a matter of perception and practicing diverse different values.

There is certain core values irrespective of age all generation should practice. Tolerance and empathy towards elders will never becomes outdated, accepting with grace, the minor omission and commission. Be open to new ideas and suggestions made by the modern generation. Counseling and intergenerational bonding can help to act the bridge between the two groups. Making adjustment and not forgetting the obligation of children towards the parents. Both handle conflict amicably and not rigidly in sticking to their own school of thoughts, while not venturing to see the viewpoints of the young.

Discuss expectations without hesitation. Parents pamper their children when they are young and repent it later. Harmony between both groups is important. As it is the family that needs to deal with its issues, others can only facilitator. The gap arises only when there is lack of respect and understanding; breakdown in quality of relationship of family and community. The younger generation too is facing different challenges and struggles related to modern society and if we can understand their anxieties and problems. What can be done is positive affirmative actions in building on the positive resources where the gap can be bridged.

Helping children to learn positive images through meaningful interaction with older people. It is high time and there is no choice in this modern era of globalization, but to go forward, try to understand and cope with the new patterns that are evolving. Things are changing at a tremendous pace, and we stop even a movement, we will be moving backward.

As today times have changed, elderly abuse, senior citizens not cared for enough, neglecting and abusing is not uncommon, suicide is really a serious risk among older persons specially who live alone, new or worsening health problem, depression and change in support system may indicate suicidal ideation.

Reality orientation, remotivating therapy, loss of autonomy and independence is a real fear among older adults. When to get up, when to sleep, what to eat. It is never too late to change behavior and to improve health status, quality of life. Have low self-esteem, man worries, high levels of alienation, poor self-perception of health and depression. For support, improves quality of life, promotion behavioral change when necessary self cares and self-responsibility emphasis on abilities rather than disabilities, nutrition, stress management is an important function. Risk factors for malnutrition in older adult, population, disease, poor eating, economic hardship, reduced social contact, multiple medications, and weight loss.

The old man tortured over property matters, abandoned in old age homes, yes, times have changed. In traditional old age system, the old aged persons were endowed with power, authority and respect. They were revered because of their wisdom and execution of their duties. Even after retired from active life they were looked after by younger generation. They were considered as wisdom personified.

Today the support system for old aged persons in the form of family support and care is experiencing a change. Today they stand at cross road. Individuals never felt unwanted in past. Today there is opposing value system of the young and the old, therefore the old people find themselves isolated, neglected and even unwanted. Aging is inevitable; it is continuous, universal and irresistible process. Inevitable, physical, biological, emotional, intellectual and personality changes accompany it. We live in society where everything is modernized; they find it difficult to cope up with their various problems concerning physical security, health, finance, loneliness. We all will grow old one day.

The government is offering various benefits like old age pension, higher threshold limit of exemption under income tax, higher rate of interest on saving schemes, exclusive health insurance, travel concessions, railway concessions etc, up to 90% assistance for old age home, day care centers, better health care facilities, protection of life and property.

As abuse of power of attorney is a growing crisis for seniors. Who are at their mercy of their children or relatives? Some cannot wait for them to die and abuse power of attorney. Houses can be sold with the money ending up in the hands of someone other than the senior who owned it, so financial abuse is one of the most common. Where persuading, tricking or threatening the adult out of money, property, or possessions. Cashing pension or other cheques without authorization; using their money not for the purpose, make or change their will, sign legal documents they fully do not understand.

Sometimes loneliness and emotions make situation bad to worse and more traumatizing. Once their savings disappear and no resources left, it becomes difficult to access costly medical aid. They have right to live with dignity, making the health care affordable, the right to good health and safety. There are middle income and lower income senior citizens unable to generate any income out of the home that they live in, majority of elders. Moreover insurance companies refuse to provide you with a mediclaim cover; provided, there is no pre-existing, life-threatening diseases like cancer or kidney failure at the time of taking policy where elders need to pay hefty premium and if they are not capable of paying what? Expensive illness, Government needs to intervene and ensure the policy and not denied to any senior citizens.

In this age of communication, the media has a strong role to play in revolutionizing the social values. They must play a positive role in social/family conflicts. Not as all is lost yet. Maintain good health and make life throbbing. Life is a bonus. Behind the faces of older people are the stories of their lives, their memories, their experiences, their dreams. They have in abundance and yet a resource we rarely remember to tap, wisdom that our elders gift us.

Support services for the older person, schemes for the care of older persons. National policy on older persons to facilitate carrying out of respective areas of operations and action in the direction of human age integrated society. Social security schemes and welfare benefits for the older persons in the organized sector. Retirement benefits, provident fund, pension, and gratuity.

Welfare schemes for the older persons in unorganized sector—Old age pension scheme, old age home, mobile geriatric services, adoption of the elderly, socioeconomic activities for supplementing income, marginal subsidies on purchase of train and flight tickets. The situation of the aged in villages is that they are most helpless because they are neglected by their own families, the families do not pay any attention to the elders. Often they are seen as an economic burden since they are unable to contribute financially to the household. In most families, the elders are kept outside the main structure of the house, which is symbolic of their exclusion from the family.

The elders in this set up are seen as unwanted. They are given very little food, just enough for the survival and existance. This group is vulnerable to sickness and desease. Their dependency on their children is total, since the aged do not have any savings, for every little personal need they have to ask their children for money, which is often demeaning and degrading. The situation is at times pathetic. Most of them feel dejected and depressed. Reasons for the neglect are complex, it is embedded in the sociocultural ethos but most important reason is economical. The vast majority of villagers live below poverty line, so most families find it difficult to support the elders economically. We have to play a significant role in restoring human dignity and improving the quality of life of the elders who are at the periphery of the rural village society. As whole life what they earn is spent on marriages of children and building house and when they are old and children grown up whom they have educated through the sacrificing there dreams, do not care for them.

United Nations principle for older persons on 16 December 1991—The United Nations General Assembly adopted resolution 46/91 containing to add life to the years that have been added to life. Government was encouraged to incorporate the principles into their National programs whenever possible. Independence—Older persons should have access to adequate food, water, shelter, clothing and health care through the provision of income, family and community support and self help.

Have the opportunity to work or to have access to other income-generating opportunities. Be able to participate in determining when and at what pace withdrawal from labor force takes place. Be able to reside at home for as long as possible. Remain integrated in society, participate actively in the formulation and implementation of policies that directly affect their well-being and share their knowledge and skills with younger generation.

Be able to seek and develop opportunities for service to the community and serve as volunteers in position appropriate to their interests and capabilities. Benefit from family and community care and protection in accordance with each society's system of cultural values. Have access to health care to help them to maintain or regain the optimum level of physical, mental and emotional well-being and to prevent or delay the onset of illness.

Have access to social and legal services to enhance their autonomy, protection and care. Be able to enjoy human rights and fundamental freedoms when residing in any shelter, care or treatment facility, including full respect for their dignity, beliefs, needs and privacy and for the right to make decision about their care and the quality of their lives. Be able to pursue opportunities for the full development of their potential. Older people should be able to live in dignity and security and be free of exploitation and physical or mental abuse. Be treated fairly regardless or age, gender, racial or ethnic background, disability or other status, and be valued independently of their economic contribution.

Aging is an inevitable process in every ones life. As we grow old, the health needs also vary. Our concern should be helping the aged to live happily and to their satisfaction. As age grows each system of the body is impaired and gives rise to disorders. The bones become brittle and tend to break more easily, weakening of the supportive tissues lead to hernia, prolapses of the internal organs, and memory of the recent events decline.

Aging is a normal physical and behavioral change that occurs as one mature and advance in age. Provide them bright light for reading; use lamps that do not have glare. Use dim light burning in bedrooms and bathrooms at night. Provide safety rails at the sides of the bed to protect the client from falls. Place the furniture in a convenient place, talk slowly and distinctly; use simple language with short sentences with lowering the pitch of the voice. Relieve anxiety and reassure the client. When body parts function in harmonious way and at the optimum level, life is successful and happy. Change your perception you will change your response.

Elder abuse—Times have changed in traditional social system, the old person were endowed with power, authority and respect. They were considered as wisdom personified. The support system for old in the form of family support and care by kith and kin is experiencing change. Today they stand at the cross road, the traditional family norms and values were a great source of security and care. Today they find themselves neglected, isolated and unwanted. Bodily harmed, sexual abuse, confinement, mental anguish, verbal assaults, name calling, threats, forced isolation, frightening, treating as a child, withholding food, drugs.

Fear related to illness. Fear of pain, loss of body parts or mutilation, fear of abuse or neglect, fear of being punished for past behavior or lifestyle, fear of death. Fear of strange place such as health care or treatment facility, fear of being the subject of experimental treatment, fear of equipment of diagnostic procedures to treatment regimens. Fear of ones feelings hurt, fear of being alone or isolated from significant others, fear of burdening others. For most persons what is known is much less frightening than that which is unknown.

Remember today where you are tomorrow it will be me. The body becomes old but the desires to live remain the same. Our old parents have lost hearing, or diminished sight, due to aging but they have not lost the human dignity. Uphold their dignity and self-esteem till the last breath of there life. When you breathed first, when you came on this earth as newborn baby, your parents were there near you, when your parents breath last be at their side. Even if you do not go to holy places for pilgrimages will not matter but if you do neglect your duty of not looking after your old parents you will have to answer and will not be spared by God who is living in your old parents. What so ever you do to the least of my people you do unto me the Bible says. By this you shall know me.

Old age and death may be considered as a sign of fulfillment of our Dharma/duty in this world and passing to the eternal life, where the reality is seen face to face. There is an eternal life waits with God. No more pain, no more suffering, only heavenly bliss one with Gods spirit.

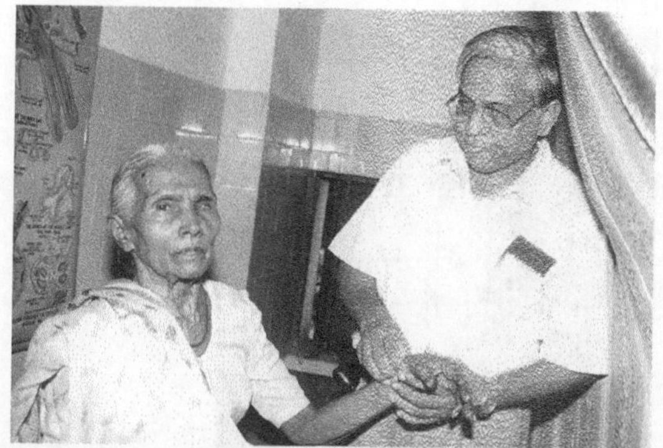

Fig. 31.1: Healthy aging: Aging is a biological process which no one can avoid

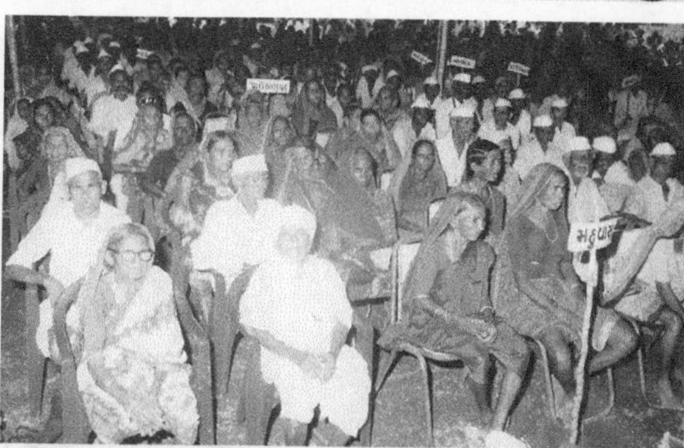

Fig. 31.2: A little care and caution will avoid many disabilities. Give then human dignity and respect they deserve

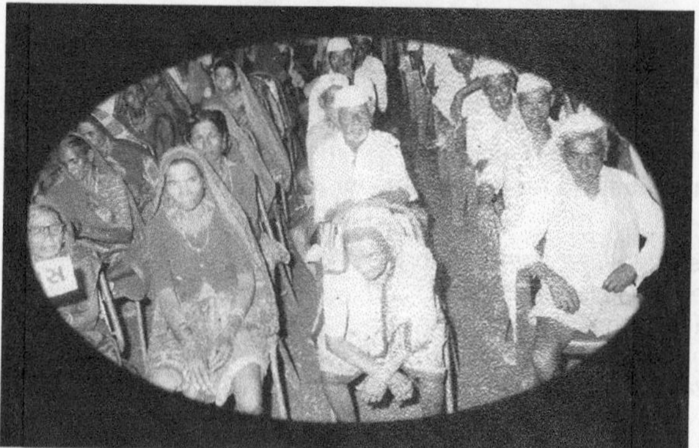

Fig. 31.3: Successful aging implies disease prevention. It is a process leading to better quality of life

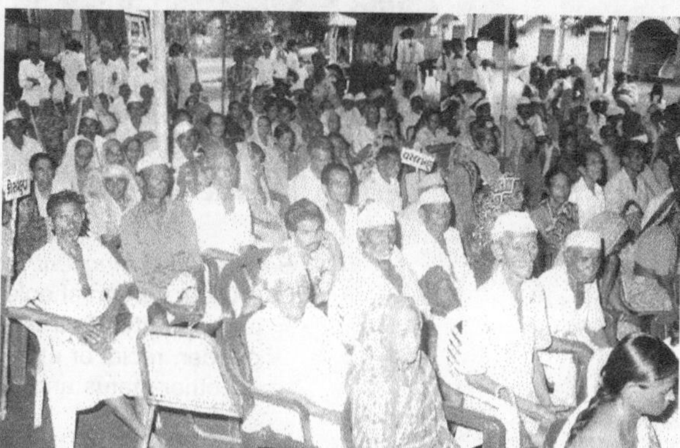

Fig. 31.4: Aging is not a disease and disease is not aging

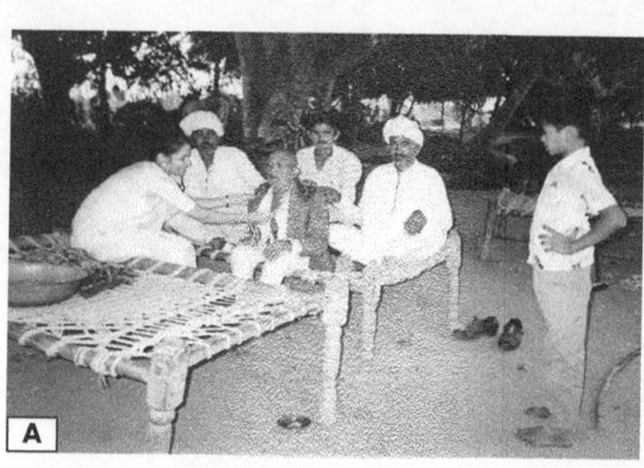

Figs 31.5A and B: Prevention strategies for healthy aging are:

- Promote physical activity
- Maintain daily routine
- Proper dietary practices
- Routine medical check-up
- Promote mental health
- Good personal hygiene

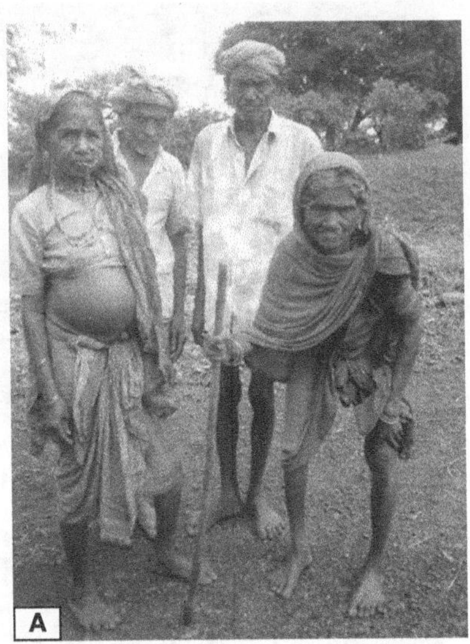

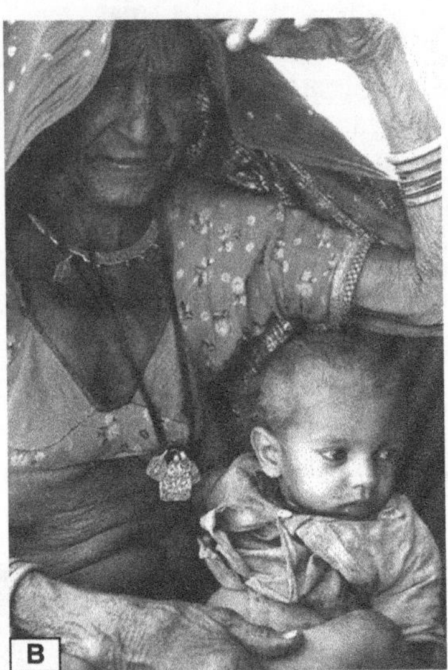

Figs 31.6A and B: Older person should remain integrated in health care, Family and community support. Older person should have access to adequate food, water, shelter, be able to reside at home for as long as possible

Behind these innocent faces, there is a pathetic story.
Older person should be able to live in dignity
and security. Be treated fairly, regardless of age,
gender, racial or ethnic background, disability or
other status and be valued independently

32 Death: The Unknown Path

Life and death are two sides of the same coin and the coin is soul. When the soul assumes a physical body it is life and when it discards the physical body once the purpose as designed by the almighty is completed, it is death. Life and death are transitory phases. Our physical bodies are vehicles for the soul, for its journey towards the ultimate destination, uniting with the supreme soul. That is salvation. Every beginning has an end and every end has a beginning. Then why fear death? However, it is sometimes normal to fear the unknown or unfamiliar. Most people prefer to die at home, having the people they love around them and being in familiar surrounding which lessen their own feeling of fear and uncertainty.

Death is easily understood as the departure of life force from the body. It is a complete physical separation from the body and all earthy belongings and attachments. Death gives meaning to human existence. It sets a limit on our time in life urging us to do something productive with that time as long as it is ours to use. Death is not something destructive. It can be viewed as one of the most constructive, positive and creative elements of culture and life. It is one of life's unchangeable. Denial is a resistance to the prognosis of death, to a feeling of loss.

Why me? It is a refusal to recognize definite physical changes. The client bargains with God that if only I could complete this or that, meet so and so and then I could die, fulfill this last task and would be ready etc. A more suitable approach is to respond honestly. With acceptance comes peace. Acceptance is an active and creative attitude towards the life that remains. One cannot avoid the inevitability of death. When death seems imminent, a family is feeling devastated by a wild range of feelings.

Your role is to share the pain, touch the person, be silent, give love and hope of peace, and accept death as a part of living. The death of a person brings deep feeling of grief to family and friends, for the nearest and dearest it is a personal loose and for some life can be utterly lonely. God is a source and giver of life, which has to return to him back, God is the author of life and hope of the just. We come from him and we have to return to him. Death is a mystery and no one can escape this reality of death. You do not know when, how, where, it will strike you. You will have to trust in the almighty in his mercy for the deliverance and ready to face the inevitable.

After the sun set, there is a promise of sunrise, after the Good Friday there is Easter. Hope in the shadow of death. Not a single family remains untouched by death. The dying person needs purification, cleansing, surrendering, forgiving, which will help him to recover or accept death peacefully. God himself has walked this root.

Death opens the doors of heaven. Body becomes one with the universe where the mother earth embraces us. Whatever we have, the money, power, prestige, belongings all one day we have to leave and go empty handed as we had come to this earth. Death does not see your age or your wealth. Life is short and momentary. Once the breath of life is gone we are zero. All have to face death equally without any exception or partiality. The poor man dies and the rich wealthy man dies. Only God can save us from this.

Each of has seen death of our dear and near ones in our friend circle or in our relation. Every child is born today going to die tomorrow; every living thing in the nature is born and dies. No way can you avoid this fact of life. Every creature fears and shivers with the thought of death. Each one has their dreams and plans for life and they want to fulfill them and live long. Death is like cycle of day and night which goes on. Sometimes one lives life as if they have come to stay permanently upon this earth.

Sometimes it is very painful when people die unprepared. They get up and go out never to return back home. Accidental death, sudden death is very hard for the family to take it in if the person is a bread earner or young it becomes still traumatic. Sometimes death strikes the only son, daughter, and if she is already young widow who has sacrificed life for that child dies leaving the person alone we get anger on God and tend to lose faith.

Yet life needs to go on inspite of it not easy to handle. Persons limit to stretch and tolerance barks down. How do you help or console such families to face these challenges? At what and at whom can they look and live for? The mystery of death cannot be answered. When the call comes from above, person just have to leave everything and follow. Only we can submit to God who gives life and who takes away there we do not have the choice. In history, we have so many incidence of great people dying all of a sudden when they were at the peak of their career and prime of their life in lime light, unavoidable yet true cannot be explained in human terms death and after death what happens to this soul. Only faith, hope and religious beliefs give us consolation and strength to bear.

Death is a final truth and without going through the dark night one cannot see the dawn of the morning. Body is perishable and the soul is imperishable. We are created from the earth and one day we will become one with this earth. Death will come into life like a thief without warning without one knowing, one stork and finished, the World ends for that person. Only his good work and the memories remain alive. Empty handed we come and the same way we will return to God. What we have on earth nothing will come along with us. The rising sun will have to set. Neither your mother nor father or anyone else will accompany you on this journey you will have to go alone. So all will have to face this reality one day, so be courageous and live life to the full while you are still alive.

When we die where will I go? What will happen to me? Dying gracefully, joyfully is important. It is the final thing you get to do. Death is a part of life. One who does not know how to die, or is unwilling to die, cannot live. If you are afraid of death, even if you live a thousand years and do everything that you wish to do, still something better could be done. This is the way of life. But death is perfect; death does not need anybody's assistance. Look at this life right now, inhalation, exhalation, if next inhalation does not happen, that is it…that is how fragile this life is, people always think death is something that happens to somebody else, it is not so, it will happen to you and me. If you remind yourself everyday that you will also die, you will be conscious and you will want to make every moment of your life as beautiful as possible. Those who are constantly aware of this fragile nature of existence they don't want to miss a single moment. They cannot take anything for granted; they will live purposefully enlightened and awaken life.

The reality of death comes in many guises; it can be a cruel shock or a blessed release from pain. It can be lingering and distressing, sudden and violent or quiet and peaceful. All of us wish a gentle death in familiar surrounding with loved ones in attendance. Elderly people can die in road traffic, accidents, intensive care unit or hospital ward, to die at home in bed or in favorite armchair. Changes in life deterioration and suffering are most difficult to bear for human mind. If you have a good friend who will listen, non-judgmentally, allowing you to mirror your thoughts and clarify your feelings you will probably find that you feel better for talking, certain things one want feels comfortable to talk to person whom one trust. If the duration of life of a person is expected to be limited, then the quality of what life remains becomes especially important. Let us live every moment.

As long as there is breath in the body, there is hope. Little things can be very important. The dying person should have his most precious belonging around him, within reach social and emotional needs. It is important to help the dying person not to become bored. He should be able to see as much of his friends and other relatives as he wishes, without getting overtired. There are times when death is positively longed one get upset at hearing an elderly person express his desire to die. To want to hold on to a well-loved parent and to keep him with us is natural, an honest acceptance by each individual of his own limits is the key to inner peace and psychological balance. People who have been ill for a long time or who are very elderly may die so quietly that you hardly notice that last breath. Do not be afraid to hold the dying persons hand and to talk to him even if he cannot reply. Hearing is the last of our senses to go so your voice will comfort and reassure him. After death and funeral, life for the family is not same, you will need to pick up thread, pull yourself together and be gentle with yourself.

Signs of approaching death—Death, as occurring when respiration and circulation are irreversibly stopped and no movements are apparent. Facial appearance changes, sunken glazed eyes, changes in the sight, speech and hearing. The pupils fail to react to light, respiration become irregular, shallow and very slow and strenuous, client may be restless due to lack of oxygen, absence of all reflexes- sign of clinical death. Maintain clients dignity, meeting the special needs according to his religious customs, be sympathetic to the family, the relatives should be given enough time to be with dying person. Cleanliness and appearance are important until the end.

It is physician who declares the death of the client, he is legally dead when only the physician certifies. If death is caused by accident, suicide, homicide, poisoning should be brought to the notice of the legal authorities and body should not be handed over without written permission. Custom varies in relation to the care of the body after death. The eyes are closed immediately and body straightened, mouth closed, head elevated on a pillow, ornaments are removed and body clean and neatly dressed in clean clothes. The body is moved to the mortuary with an identification tag. If the relatives are present, the body may be handed over to them. The client's chart with all details about the cause of death certificate to be sent to the office of registers birth and death.

Death is a part of our life. We are born to die little each day. Every time we pass through from one stage of life to another something in us dies. The innocence and the spontaneity of children die, to the daring of youth, to the reasoning of maturity. All flower fades, a leaf falls, a raindrop evaporates, a breeze that passes away, a caterpillar to butter daily. We test death in moment of loneliness, when we live in bitterness, hatred, and isolation we create our own death by the way I live.

Death is a natural part of nature and human life. Nursing care for critically ill and dying needs alertness, observation, and resourcefulness, sympathy. Nearing death client should not be alone, relatives are present, and nurse gives consolation to the near ones. Sometimes death comes suddenly; sometimes, it comes over several days or weeks. The process of dying is a progressive failure of the vital functions. The central nervous system, circulatory system, and the respiratory system, and shown by various physical signs. Signs of clinical death are absence of temperature. Pupils do not react to light, absence of all reflexes. Person goes various psychological stages like denial, anger, and depression. Understanding and acceptance of the person, sympathetic, warm, considerate, and relatives should be given enough time with the dying.

Care of the dead body—Doctor declares and confirms. Adjust bed in flat position, body placed perfectly straight position, eyes close immediately, one pillow could be under the head. Mouth close and jaw bandage applied, jewelleries removed, body washed, nails cut, plug cotton swab, clean gown wear, hair brushed and arranged neatly, and body taken to the appropriate place. If the death is by accident, suicide, homicide, poisoning, snakebite it should be brought in the notice of the legal authorities, without their written permission body should not be handed over to the relatives.

Death is a mystery to most of us. While we are uncertain as to how and when it will come. We are certain that it will. All things compounded die to change form. The question is: Are we prepared for the event? There are two options before us. Not to think about it or try to understand the prospect and when it does. There is transition and impermanence all around us. In death, is certain of new life as in nature, old leaves fall to give rise to new shoots.

In cosmic happenings stars are collapsing every second to give rise to the new. Our own body sees constant death of cell that gives way to new ones. What we perhaps fear most about death is fear of the unknown. Perhaps no friends, family, known faces, possibly all alone in a foreign land. In addition, what we are afraid of is the ignorance about who we really are, how we eventually die and what form we assume is the result and many factors, and how we live over life and how we eventually die. Catholics who advocate the strict use of life support measures and strictly forbid euthanasia.

Giving the news of a client's death or critical condition over the telephone is difficult. Do not give bad news first and prepare the family for the anticipatory grieving. Disposal of the dead body ceremonies very from community to community, culture to culture and from one religion to other religion.

It is said in West Africa, one particular tribe carry the dead to the forest and leave them to the devoured by beasts. Some throw the dead into sea and river. Some Tibetans leave the dead bodies in the cemeteries near the village to be devoured by the beast. Parsees place the dead in round tower called the tower of silence to be devoured by birds. In Egypt, the practice of mummification, Hindus burn the dead where they carry the body on bamboo or wooden bed and take to ghats for cremation, sometimes the incomplete half burnt bodies remains are thrown into the river. Cremation of bodies in the cities uses furnaces and exhumed. This is easy and sanitary method. Christians and Muslims bury their dead where they use coffin of wood that is used be easily destroyable for fast disintegration of the bodies. Trees to be planted around the cemeteries so as to absorb the carbonic acid gas let out during the disintegration process dissimilated easily.

Conclusion—Perspective in palliative care- nursing care with advanced disease final stage of life-dying, normal dying process, the control of pain and other symptoms, the terms hospice care, palliative care and end of life care. Client centered care- need to address better care at the end of life. It is family center care. Client passes the stages of denial this cannot be true, I will be just fine after this; angry I do not know how my wife will get alone after I am gone. Acceptance- I have no regrets, I' have done everything, I have wanted.

Palliative care does not emphasize cure but rather provide relief of suffering by managing symptoms and maximizing quality of life of clients and their families facing the problems associated with life threatening illness, through prevention and relief of suffering by means of early identification and impeccable assessment and treatment of pain and other problems. Death as normal and natural the dying process is profoundly individualized. Symptoms vary not only in frequency and intensity but also in the distress experienced by clients. Agitation, frequent moving an inability to get comfortable groaning not relaxed, clenched teeth, tightened fits, distressed, frowning, seating, restless, fast heart rate. Indicators of imminent death- family members must be informed about the changes to expect so that they feel as prepared and can recognize death is approaching.

Clients impaired urinary elimination due to renal failure, impaired gas exchange, disturbed sensory perception, acute confusion, death anxiety, or fear due to physical discomfort. May feel unfinished business or special concerns. The dying process can be a time of emotional crisis for many patient and their families. When facing the last days of life should be given the opportunity to express all concerns about issues that matter most of them. Support the family while they accept the finality of their loss. Experiencing the pain and the loss. Finding way to move forward in life. The nurse is the bearer of light along the path of the unknown as the client and family attempt to make sense of life's greatest mystery death. The nurse can promote a healthy and positive dying experience for all involved.

Accept the reality of the loss, experience the pain of the lost, and adjust to the environment in which the decrease in missing remembers the deceased with moving forward with life. They need the manifestations of normal interventions of grief. What the future may look like without person who has died; offer opportunities to repeat the story of the death. The family coping tasks in terminal illness are important.

Today community nurse is different from that of past years. With expansion of health services in the country the nursing practice both in hospital and in the community is facing a great challenge. Hers is not an easy task to perform, as she has to work with sick, old, poor, uneducated and varied types of sickness where she needs to be equipped with abilities to cope these situations. She has to establish relationship and understand the community point of view to become effective instrument and to bring about necessary change in society. She has to march the journey into the community to bring health in all forms.

Essence of Gita – Why are you unnecessarily worrying? Whom do you fear? Who can kill you? Soul is not born, nor does it die. What has happened for the best, what is happening is happening for the best. What will happen will happen for the best? Do not brood for the past. Do not worry about the future. The present is on. What you have lost, that you are weeping? What had you brought that you have lost? What have you made that has been destroyed?

You brought not anything what you have, you got from here, what was given, was given here, what you took from this universe. What you gave, you gave unto this universe have come empty-handed and shall go empty handed. What is your today was somebody else's in the past and will be somebody else's in the future. You think it was yours and are deeply engrossed in it. This attachment is the cause of your sorrow.

Change is the law of life, what you call death is life itself. In a moment you are a millionaire, in the very next you are a poor man. Mine, your, small, big, ours, theirs, remove this from your mind, and then everything is yours and you are everybody's. This body is not your, nor are you of this body. Earth, water, air, fire and ether comprise this body and unto this shall it return. But the soul is eternal, than what are you?

Surrender unto the Lord, He is there for ultimate support. He who experiences this is completely free from fear. Whatever you do offer it unto him. By this, shall you forever experience eternal bliss.

A life giving, living will and testament – (Nani A Palkhivala)—When I die give my sight to the man who has never seen a sunrise. Give my heart to one who has known the agony of the heart. Give my blood to a youth pulled from the wreckage of a car so that he might live to see his grandchildren play. Let my kidneys drain the poison from another's body. Let my bones be used to make a crippled child walk. Burn what is left of me and scatter the ashes to the wind to let the flowers grow. If you bury something, let it be my faults and my prejudices against my fellowmen. Give my sins to the devil. Give my soul to God. If you wish to remember me, do it with a kind deed or word to someone who needs you. If you do all I have asked, I will live forever.

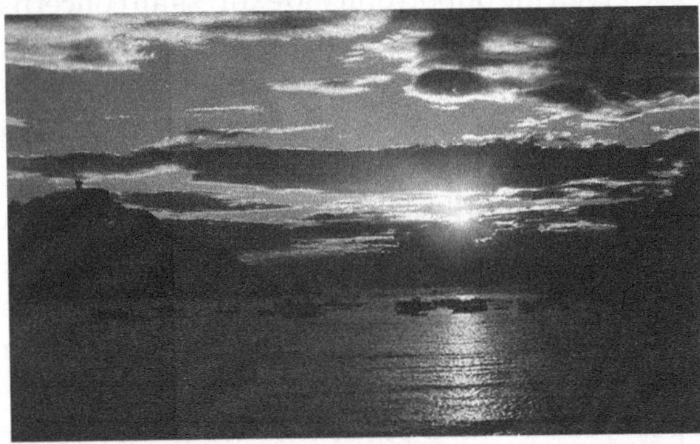

Fig. 32.1: The unknown journey

Fig. 32.2: Giving hope that there is light after death

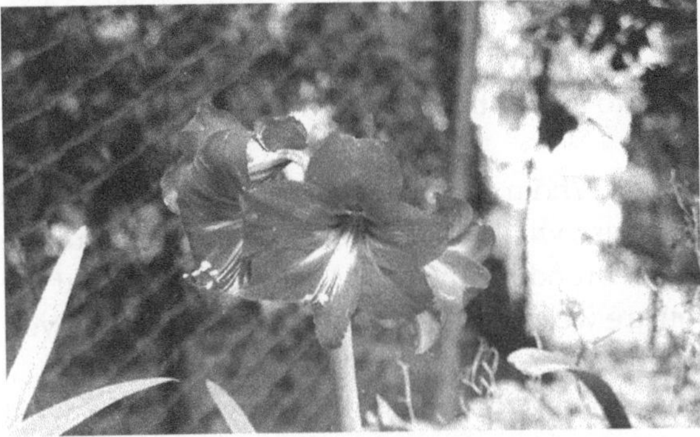

Fig. 32.3: Physical life ends and spiritual life begins

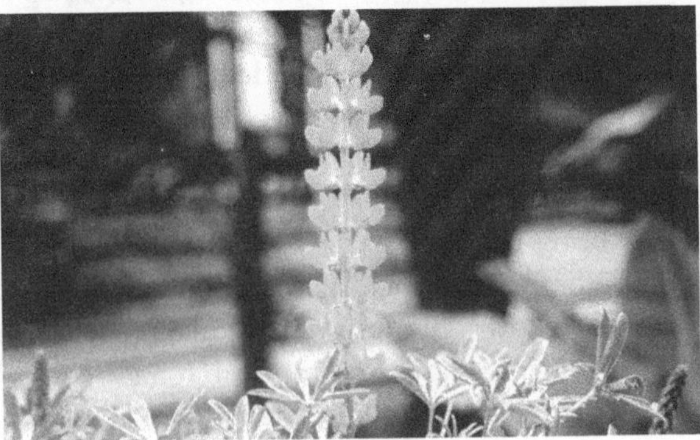

Fig. 32.4: There is life after death

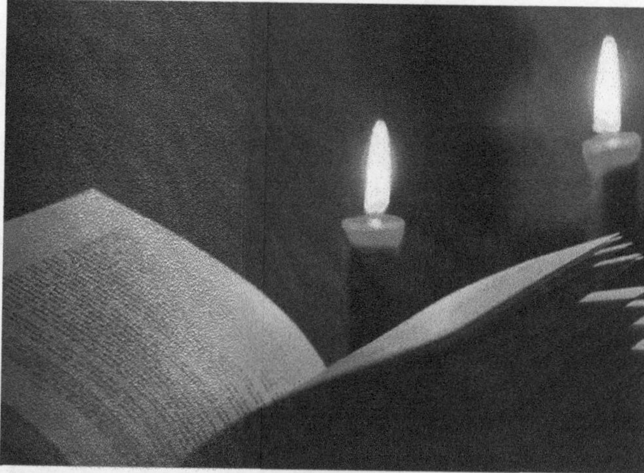

Fig. 32.5: Death a physical separation of body and a soul's journey to the unknown world. With death, life is not ended. New life is born. Make it as a positive experience. Death is an inevitable reality and mysteries of life

Index

I

K

L

M

N

O

P